Manual of STEMI Interventions

Manual of STEMI Interventions

Edited by Sameer Mehta MD FACC MBA

University of Miami Miller School of Medicine,
and Lumen Foundation, Miami, FL, USA

WILEY Blackwell

Registered Office(s)
John Wiley & Sons, Inc., 111 River Street, Hoboken, NJ 07030, USA
John Wiley & Sons Ltd, The Atrium, Southern Gate, Chichester, West Sussex, PO19 8SQ, UK

Editorial Office
9600 Garsington Road, Oxford, OX4 2DQ, UK

For details of our global editorial offices, customer services, and more information about Wiley products visit us at www.wiley.com.

Wiley also publishes its books in a variety of electronic formats and by print-on-demand. Some content that appears in standard print versions of this book may not be available in other formats.

Library of Congress Cataloging-in-Publication Data

Names: Mehta, Sameer, editor.
Title: Manual of STEMI interventions / edited by Sameer Mehta.
Description: Hoboken, NJ : Wiley, 2017. | Includes index. |
Identifiers: LCCN 2017014480 (print) | LCCN 2017015848 (ebook) | ISBN 9781119095439 (pdf) |
    ISBN 9781119095422 (epub) | ISBN 9781119095415 (cloth)
Subjects: | MESH: Myocardial Infarction–therapy | Anticoagulants–therapeutic use | Stents
Classification: LCC RC685.I6 (ebook) | LCC RC685.I6 (print) | NLM WG 310 | DDC 616.1/23706–dc23
LC record available at https://lccn.loc.gov/2017014480

Cover design: Wiley
Cover images: (From left to right) © Feverpitched/Gettyimages; © Ryan McVay/Gettyimages;
© Nils Versemann/Shutterstock; © kupicoo/Gettyimages

Set in 10/12pt Warnock by SPi Global, Pondicherry, India

Printed in Singapore by C.O.S. Printers Pte Ltd

10 9 8 7 6 5 4 3 2 1

Contents

List of Contributors

Thomas Alexander MD
Kovai Medical Center and Hospital,
Coimbatore, India

Laura Álvarez MD
Lumen Foundation, Miami, FL, USA

Juanita Gonzalez Arango MD
Lumen Foundation, Miami, FL, USA

Miguel Vega Arango MD
Lumen Foundation, Miami, FL, USA

Yousef Bader MD
Cardiovascular Center, Tufts Medical Center,
Boston, MA, USA

Andreas Baumbach MD
Bristol Heart Institute, Bristol, UK

Neeraj Bhalla MD
Department at BLK Super Speciality
Hospital, New Delhi

Freddy Bojanini MD
Lumen Foundation, Miami, FL, USA

Roberto Vieira Botelho MD PhD
Eurolatino Medical Research, Lumen
Foundation, Miami, FL, USA

Estefania Calle Botero MD
Lumen Foundation, Miami, FL, USA

Hans Erik Bøtker MD PhD FACC FESC
Department of Cardiology, Aarhus
University Hospital Skejby, Aarhus,
Denmark

Miguel A. Campos-Esteve MD FACC
Cardiac Catheterization Laboratories,
Pavia Hospital Santurce, San Juan, Puerto Rico,
USA

Antonio Colombo MD
Interventional Cardiology Unit,
San Raffaele Scientific Institute, Milan,
Italy; Interventional Cardiology Unit,
EMO-GVM Centro Cuore Columbus,
Milan, Italy

Juan Corral MD
Lumen Foundation, Miami, FL, USA

Suzanne de Waha MD
University Heart Center Luebeck,
University Hospital Schleswig-Holstein,
Luebeck, Germany

Landy Luna Diaz MD
Lumen Foundation, Miami, FL, USA

Daniela Parra Dunoyer MD
Lumen Foundation, Miami, FL, USA

Jose Escabi-Mendoza MD FACC
Cardiac Care Unit and Chest Pain Center,
VA Caribbean Healthcare System, San Juan,
Puerto Rico, USA

Denis Fabiano de Souza RN
Research Nurse, Eurolatino Medical
Research, USA

James J. Ferguson III MD
St Luke's Episcopal Hospital,
Texas, USA

Wladimir Fernandes de Rezende MBA
Dax Tecnologia da Informação, Brasilão

Francisco Fernandéz MBA
CIO ITMS do Brasil

Alexandra Ferré MD
Lumen Foundation, Miami, FL, USA

Francesco Giannini MD
Interventional Cardiology Unit,
San Raffaele Scientific Institute, Milan, Italy

Juliana Giraldo MD
Lumen Foundation, Miami, FL, USA

Cindy L. Grines MD
Detroit Medical Center, Heart Hospital,
Detroit, MI, USA

Timothy D. Henry MD
Cedars-Sinai Heart Institute, Los Angeles,
CA, USA

Gerd Heusch MD FACC FESC FRCP
Institute for Pathophysiology, West German
Heart and Vascular Centre Essen, University
of Essen Medical School, Essen, Germany

David Hildebrandt RN
Cedars-Sinai Heart Institute, Los Angeles,
CA, USA

Yong Huo MD
Peking University First Hospital, Beijing, China

David G. Iosseliani MD FACC FESC
Moscow City Center of Interventional
Cardioangiology, Moscow, Russian
Federation

Thomas W. Johnson BSc MBBS MD FRCP
Bristol Heart Institute, Bristol, UK

Navin K. Kapur MD
Cardiovascular Center, Tufts Medical Center,
Boston, MA, USA

Sasko Kedev MD PhD FESC FACC
Medical Faculty, Ss Cyril and Methodius
University, and Director, University Clinic of
Cardiology, Skopje, Macedonia

Julius Cezar Q. Ladeira DDS MSc
ITMS do Brasil

David C. Lange MD
Cedars-Sinai Heart Institute, Los Angeles,
CA, USA

Fernando Lapetina-Irizarry MD FACC
Cardiology Department, Pavia Hospital
Santurce, San Juan, Puerto Rico, USA

David M. Larson MD
Minneapolis Heart Institute, Minneapolis,
MN, USA

Azeem Latib MD
San Raffaele Scientific Institute, Milan,
Italy; Interventional Cardiology Unit,
EMO-GVM Centro Cuore Columbus,
Milan, Italy

Michel Le May MD
Director of the Coronary Care Unit, and
Director of the University of Ottawa Heart
Institute Regional STEMI Program, Ontario,
Canada

Joshua PY Loh MD
Consultant at the National University
Heart Centre, Singapore, and an Assistant
Professor at the Yong Loo Lin School of
Medicine, Singapore

Cindy Manotas MD
Lumen Foundation, Miami, FL, USA

Sameer Mehta MD FACC MBA
University of Miami Miller School of Medicine, and Lumen Foundation, Miami, FL, USA

Nestor Mercado MD
Detroit Medical Center, Heart Hospital, Detroit, MI, USA

Isaac Yepes Moreno MD
Lumen Foundation, Miami, FL, USA

Sebastián Moreno MD
Lumen Foundation, Miami, FL, USA

Ajit S. Mullasari MD
Madras Medical Mission, Chennai, India

Daniella Nacad MD
Lumen Foundation, Miami, FL, USA

Estefania Oliveros MD
Lumen Foundation, Miami, FL, USA

Samir Pancholy MD FACC FSCAI
Wright Center for Graduate Medical Education, Commonwealth Medical College, Scranton, PA, USA

Tejas Patel MD DM FACC FESC FSCAI
Apex Heart Institute, Ahmedabad, Gujarat, India

Marco Perin MD
Lumen Foundation, Miami, FL, USA

Carlos Otávio Lara Pinheiro BSc
Dax Tecnologia da Informação, Brasilão

Maria Teresa Bedoya Reina MD
Lumen Foundation, Miami, FL, USA

Sergio Reyes MD
Lumen Foundation, Miami, FL, USA

Olga Reynbakh MD
Lumen Foundation, Miami, FL, USA

Daniel Rodriguez MD
Lumen Foundation, Miami, FL, USA

Orlando Rodríguez-Vilá MD MMS FACC FSCAI
Cardiac Catheterization Laboratories, and Associate Chief of Medicine, VA Caribbean Healthcare System, San Juan, Puerto Rico, USA

Ivan Rokos MD
UCLA, California, USA

Neil Ruparelia PhD MRCP
San Raffaele Scientific Institute, Milan, Italy; Imperial College, London, UK; EMO-GVM Centro Cuore Columbus, Milan, Italy

Roopa Salwan MD
Cardiology and Interventional Cardiology, Max Super Speciality Hospital-Saket, Delhi, India

Márcio Sanches MD
ITMS do Brasil

Theodore L. Schreiber MD
Detroit Medical Center, Heart Hospital, Detroit, MI, USA

Michael Schweitzer MD
Lumen Foundation, Miami, FL, USA

Sanjay Shah MD DM
Apex Heart Institute, Ahmedabad, Gujarat, India

Holger Thiele MD
University Heart Center Luebeck, University Hospital Schleswig-Holstein, Luebeck, Germany

Maria Botero Urrea MD
Lumen Foundation, Miami, FL, USA

Alicia Henao Velasquez MD
Lumen Foundation, Miami, FL, USA

Vincenzo Vizzi MD
Bristol Heart Institute, Bristol, United Kingdom

Yan Zhang MD
Peking University First Hospital, Beijing, China

Tracy Zhang BS
Lumen Foundation, Miami, FL, USA

Preface

Fifteen years ago, I performed my first door-to-balloon STEMI intervention. The beauty of that procedure, as well as of more than 2000 since then, has remained pristine. Almost every procedure has either saved a life or preserved left ventricular function. Often, both. In a front page article on June 21st, 2015, the *New York Times* reported that cardiovascular disease is no longer the #1 killer in the Unites States on a count of the strides made with STEMI interventions. This is amazing progress whose implementation has been seismic – in our massive country, from less than 4% of primary PCI being performed in 1999, we now have a STEMI nation. As a result, almost every patient can now receive a quality primary percutaneous coronary intervention (PPCI) anytime and anywhere. I believe that achieving a nationwide capability to perform PPCI is one of the biggest success stories in modern medicine.

Progress in PPCI has also occurred worldwide. At the 2016 Lumen Global STEMI meeting in Kuala Lumpur, Malaysia, 15 developing countries representing 3.8 billion populations, presented their STEMI programs. Universally, they reported improvements in both the STEMI process and procedure and major reduction in cardiovascular mortality. I have been humbled to have contributed to these developments. Until this date, I believe, I am the world's sole STEMI-only performing cardiologist. This was a massive individual undertaking that required enormous personal and financial sacrifices, recalibration of lifestyle and brutal hard work. It was through sleeping in the trenches of STEMI interventions that I mastered the procedural techniques. In particular, this included a kaleidoscopic appreciation of thrombus – its dynamic nature, its varied morphology and its diverse presentation based upon the duration of chest pain. Slowly and methodically, my observations about thrombus in STEMI lesions led to formulation of a Selective Strategy of Thrombus Management, based on thrombus grade. I have adopted this methodology in my last consecutive 1000 procedures and have found it to be universally applicable. These techniques are described in detail in this textbook.

Allow me to dwell a little further in my personal journey. In 2002, when I took an unprecedented decision to devote an entire career to STEMI Interventions, I followed the fantastic dictum of Mahatma Gandhi, "In matters of conscience, the opinion of the majority does not count". I followed this call to conscience and abandoned a thriving interventional cardiology practice. I began a STEMI-only meeting and wrote an entire textbook on STEMI interventions. This fundamental trust in STEMI interventions has now led to my helping to create STEMI networks and educational, research, and training endeavors in 27 countries. I have also begun to use telemedicine to provide access for millions of patients to PPCI, and in creating a public campaign for reducing gender disparities. In pursuing this crusade, I attribute much of this success to the magnificent procedure of PPCI and its fantastic ability to predictably and safely save lives. I was simply fortunate in recognizing these attributes ahead of others!

This textbook, my sixth on the subject of PPCI, is an earnest effort to incorporate the most important lessons that I have learned, and to amalgamate them with current scientific data, guidelines and recommendations from the American College of Cardiology and the European Society of Cardiology. For ease of understanding, the textbook is divided into five parts – Guidelines, Thrombolytic Therapy, Physiology; the STEMI Procedure; the STEMI Process; Global STEMI Initiatives and Future Perspectives. I hope that this structure will comprehensively and seamlessly cover the critical areas. As in previous texts, the chapters on collating the illustrative cases was the hardest and it took months to select cases, to digitize the cineangiographic pictures, obtain pre- and post-procedure electrocardiograms and do so from five different hospitals where these I performed these procedures.

World experts have contributed to several chapters and I am deeply gratefully to these brilliant cardiologists for their work and for their support.

Most of my work in STEMI Interventions, beyond composing this textbook, would not be possible without the supreme sacrifices of my immediate family, to whom this work is dedicated – to my wife Shoba, and to our children Aditya and Kabir.

Part I

Guidelines, Thrombolytic Therapy, Pharmacology

1

Compendium of STEMI Clinical Trials

Juanita Gonzalez Arango MD, Miguel Vega Arango MD, Estefania Calle Botero MD, Isaac Yepes Moreno MD, Maria Botero Urrea MD, Alicia Henao Velasquez MD, Daniel Rodriguez MD, Daniela Parra Dunoyer MD, Maria Teresa Bedoya Reina MD, Sameer Mehta MD

Introduction

As we constructed our fourth textbook of interventions for ST-elevation myocardial infarction (STEMI), the need for including a chapter on clinical trials was paramount. To provide a complete compendium of relevant STEMI guidelines and clinical trials, two distinct chapters have been created. We recognize that this information is easily obtained from searching the internet; however, we deemed it important to present in this book the most up-to-date guidelines and clinical trials. In this chapter, we have divided the trials into stents (Table 1.1), no-reflow (Table 1.2), thrombectomy (Table 1.3), percutaneous coronary interventions for non-culprit lesions (Table 1.4), and the role of left ventricular support devices (Table 1.5). In Chapter 2, we have separated out those guidelines from the American College of Cardiology and the European Society of Cardiology. These topics are discussed further in various chapters of the textbook. However, we firmly believe that a compendium of guidelines and clinical trials will provide a useful summary of these STEMI-related studies.

Manual of STEMI Interventions, First Edition. Edited by Sameer Mehta.
© 2017 John Wiley & Sons Ltd. Published 2017 by John Wiley & Sons Ltd.

Table 1.1 Which stent is most desirable for STEMI interventions?

Study Title	Hypothesis	Cohort	Principal Findings	Conclusion
COBALT: long-term clinical outcome of thin-strut CoCr stents in the DES era [1].	To assess characteristics and outcomes of patients treated with 2 different new-generation CoCr BMS, the MULTI-LINK VISION® and PRO-Kinetic Energy® stents.	1176 patients: MLV ($n = 438$); PRO-Kinetic ($n = 738$).	TLR and TVR were lower in the MLV group. Death, MI, ARC and definite stent thrombosis were similar.	The use of last-generation thin-strut BMS in selected patients is associated with acceptable clinical outcome, with similar clinical results for both the MLV and PRO-Kinetic stents.
Comparison of newer-generation DES with BMS in patients with acute STEMI [2].	Efficacy and safety of newer-generation DES compared with BMS in patients with STEMI.	2665 STEMI patients: 1326 received a newer-generation DES (EES or biolimus A9 eluting stent) and 1329 received BMS.	Newer-generation DES substantially reduced the risk of repeat TVR, target-vessel infarction, definite stent thrombosis compared with BMS at 1 year.	Newer-generation DES improves safety and efficacy compared with BMS throughout 1st year.
Meta-analysis of long-term outcomes for DES compared with BMS in PCI for STEMI [3].	Available literature examining the outcomes of DES and BMS in PPCI after > 3 years of follow-up.	8 RCTs and 5 observational studies. 5797 patients in whom 1st-generation DES (SES or PES) were compared with BMS control arms.	Patients with DES had lower risk of TLR, TVR, and MACE. Incidence of stent thrombosis equal between groups. No difference in mortality or recurrent MI. Those receiving DES had lower mortality.	DES use resulted in decreased repeat revascularization with no increase in stent thrombosis, mortality, or recurrent MI.
Outcomes with various DES or BMS in patients with STEMI [4].	Efficacy (TVR) and safety (death, MI, and stent thrombosis) outcomes at the longest reported follow-up times with DES compared with BMS.	28 randomized clinical trials; 34,068 patients comparing any DES against each other or BMS.	No increase in the risk of death, MI, or stent thrombosis with any DES compared with BMS. EES was associated with a statistically significant reduction in the rate of stent thrombosis when compared with SES, PES, and even BMS.	DES versus BMS was associated with substantial decrease in the risk of TVR. EES had substantial reduction in the risk of stent thrombosis with no increase in very late stent thrombosis.
Benefits of DES compared with BMS in STEMI: 4-year results of PES or SES vs. BMS in primary angioplasty (PASEO) randomized trial [5].	To evaluate the short and long-term benefits of SES and PES vs. BMS in patients undergoing primary angioplasty.	270 patients with STEMI were randomized to BMS ($n = 90$), PES ($n = 90$), or SES ($n = 90$).	PES and SES were associated with significant reduction in TLR at 1year. No difference was observed in terms of death and reinfarction.	SES and PES are safe and associated with significant benefits in terms of TLR up to 4 years of follow-up, compared with BMS.

Study	Objective	Population	Results	Conclusion
PPCI for AMI: long-term outcome after BMS and DES Implantation [6].	To investigate the long-term outcomes of unselected patients undergoing PPCI with BMS and DES.	1738 patients undergoing PPCI for a new lesion. 3 cohorts of BMS (n = 531), SES (n = 185) or PES (n = 1022).	No differences in all-cause mortality or repeat revascularization between DES and BMS. SES was associated with lower rates of all-cause death, nonfatal MI, or TVR compared with PES. Very late stent thrombosis only occurred in the DES groups.	DES are not associated with an increase in adverse events compared with BMS when used for PPCI, neither DES reduced repeat revascularizations.
Safety and efficacy outcomes of first- and second-generation durable polymer DES and biodegradable polymer BES in clinical practice: comprehensive network meta-analysis [7].	To investigate the safety and efficacy of durable polymer DES and biodegradable polymer BES.	60 randomized controlled trials were compared, which involved 63,242 patients treated with DES.	At 1year, there were no differences in mortality. Resolute and EZES, EES and SES were associated with reduced odds of MI compared with PES. Compared with EES, BP-BES were associated with increased odds of MI, while EZES and PES were associated with increased odds of ST. EES and EZES offering the highest safety profiles.	The newer durable polymer EES and EZES and the BP-BES maintain the efficacy of SES. EES and EZES are the safest stents to date.
EXAMINATION trial (EES Versus BMS in STEMI): 2-year results from a multicenter randomized controlled trial [8].	To evaluate the outcomes of the population included in the EXAMINATION trial.	1498 patients were randomized to receive EES (n = 751) or BMS (n = 747).	Rate of TLR, definite or probable stent thrombosis was significantly lower in EES group than in BMS group.	Both rates of TLR and stent thromboses were reduced in recipients of EES.
2-year outcomes after first- or second-generation DES or BMS implantation in patients undergoing PCI. A pre-specified analysis from the PRODIGY study [9].	To assess device-specific outcomes with respect to the occurrence of MACE, after implantation of BMS, ZESS, PES, or EES in patients undergoing PCI.	2013 randomized patients undergoing CA in a 1:1:1:1 fashion to BMS, ZESS, PES, or EES implantation.	MACE rate was lowest in EES, highest in BMS, and intermediate in PES and ZESS. The 2-year incidence of stent thrombosis in the EES group was similar to that in ZESS group, but lower compared with PES and BMS groups.	MACE rate was lowest for EES, highest for BMS, and intermediate for PES and ZESS groups. EES outperformed BMS with safety endpoints and stent thrombosis.
New DES for STEMI: A new paradigm for safety [10].	To compare the long-term safety of new-generation DES with early-generation DES and BMS for STEMI.	3464 STEMI patients were treated with BMS (n = 1187), early-generation DES (n = 1,525), or new-generation DES (n = 752).	At 2 years, new-generation DES had lower mortality, similar reinfarction, and fewer stent thromboses compared with BMS; and similar mortality, similar reinfarction, and trends for fewer stent thromboses compared with early-generation DES.	New-generation DES in STEMI patients have fewer stent thromboses compared with BMS and trends for fewer stent thromboses compared with early-generation DES.

(Continued)

Table 1.1 (Continued)

Study Title	Hypothesis	Cohort	Principal Findings	Conclusion
Safety and effectiveness of DES in patients with STEMI undergoing primary angioplasty [11].	To confirm the safety and effectiveness of DES in patients with STEMI.	370 patients (120 in DES group and 250 in BMS group) with STEMI treated with primary PCI. Patients were retrospectively followed for the occurrence of MACE.	There was no difference in rate of stent thrombosis in the BMS group. Incidence of MACE was lower in the DES group principally due to the lower rate of TVR.	Use of DES in the PPCI for STEMI was safe and improved the 3-year clinical outcome compared with BMS, reducing the need of TVR.
Outcomes with DES vs. BMS in acute STEMI results from the Strategic Transcatheter Evaluation of New Therapies Group [12].	To evaluate the outcomes with DES compared with BMS in patients undergoing PPCI for STEMI.	Patients with STEMI treated with either a DES (1292 patients) or BMS (548 patients). Of those treated with DES, 46% were treated with SES and 54% with PES.	There were no differences between DES and BMS in death, reinfarction, or MACE. DES had lower rates of stent thrombosis and lower rates of TVR. There was a mild increase in stent thrombosis with DES versus BMS from 1–2 years.	DES used with PPCI for STEMI is more effective than BMS in reducing TVR and is safe for up to 2 years.
Clinical outcomes with BP-BES vs. DP-DES and BMS: evidence from a comprehensive network meta-analysis [13].	Safety and efficacy of BP-BES versus DP-DES and BMS.	Data from 89 trials including 85,490 patients. 1-year follow-up.	BP-BES was associated with lower rates of cardiac death/MI and TVR than BMS and lower rates of TVR than fast-release Z-ES. BP-BES had similar rates of cardiac death, MI, and TVR compared with other second-generation DP-DES but higher rates of 1-year stent thrombosis than CoCr EES. BP-BES was associated with improved late outcomes compared with BMS and PES, with different outcomes compared with other DP-DES, although higher rates of definite stent thrombosis compared with CoCr EES.	BP-BES was associated with superior clinical outcomes compared with BMS and first-generation DES and similar rates of cardiac death/MI, MI, and TVR compared with second-generation DP-DES but higher rates of definite stent thrombosis than CoCr EES.
DES vs. BMS in primary angioplasty. A pooled patient-level meta-analysis of randomized trials [14].	Evaluated the risks and benefits of DES compared with BMS in patients undergoing PPCI for STEMI.	6298 patients were randomized; 3980 assigned to DES and 2318 assigned to BMS.	DES implantation reduced the occurrence of TVR with no difference in mortality, reinfarction, and stent thrombosis. DES implantation was associated with an increased risk of very late stent thrombosis and reinfarction.	SES and PES compared with BMS are associated with TVR reduction at long-term follow-up. The incidence of very late reinfarction and stent thrombosis was increased with DES.

Study	Objective	Methods	Results	Conclusions
First results of the DEB-AMI trial. A multicenter randomized comparison of DEB plus BMS vs. BMS vs. DES in PPCI, With 6-month angiographic, intravenous, functional, and clinical outcomes [15].	Test the DIOR® DEB combined with a modern CoCr BMS in PPCI with the goal of obtaining improved angiographic results and comparable vessel healing and preserved endothelial function and fewer malopposed stent struts than PES DES.	150 patients were randomized; BMS implantation (group A), vs. sequential DEB (with paclitaxel) dilatation and BMS implantation (group B), and paclitaxel DES implantation (group C).	In groups A, B, and C, respectively, binary restenosis was 26.2%, 28.6%, and 4.7%, and MACE rates were 23.5%, 20%, and 4.1%, respectively.	In STEMI patients, DEB followed by BMS implantation failed to show angiographic superiority to BMS only. Angiographic results of DES were superior to both BMS and DEB.
DES vs. BMS in STEMI at a follow-up of 3 years or longer: A meta-analysis of randomized trials [16].	To evaluate the safety and efficacy of DES compared with BMS in STEMI patients.	6 studies used SES; 2 studies used PES and the remaining 2 used more than 1 type of DES.	DES use reduced the odds of TLR and TVR. Patients in DES group experienced MACE less frequently than patients in BMS group, which was driven mainly by the decreased revascularization rate. There were no differences in rates of death or MI.	DES continues to be associated with a lower repeat revascularization rate in patients with STEMI, with a small but significantly increased risk of very late stent thrombosis compared with BMS.
Clinical outcomes with DES and BMS in Patients with STEMI: Evidence from a comprehensive network meta-analysis [17].	Safety and efficacy of different DES and BMS in patients with STEMI using a network meta-analysis.	22 randomized controlled trials comparing currently United States approved DES or DES with BMS including 12,453 patients.	At 1-year follow-up, CoCr EES was associated with lower rates stent thrombosis tan PES and BMS, and cardiac death or MI than BMS. SES was also associated with lower rates of 1-year cardiac death/MI than BMS. CoCr EES, PES, and SES had lower rates of 1-year TVR than BMS, with SES also showing lower rates of TVR than PES.	Steady improvements in outcomes have been realized with the evolution from BMS to first- and second-generation DES, with the most favorable safety and efficacy profile thus far demonstrated with CoCr EES.
Long-term outcome after DES vs. BMS implantation in patients with STEMI: 5-year follow-up from the randomized DEDICATION trial [18].	Compared the long-term effects of DES with BMS implantation in patients with STEMI undergoing PPCI.	Patients with a high-grade coronary stenosis with symptoms < 12 hours and ST-segment elevation were randomly assigned to receive a DES ($n = 313$) or a BMS ($n = 313$) in the infarct-related lesion.	Combined MACE rate was lower in DES group. Whereas number of deaths from all causes tended to be higher in DES group, cardiac mortality was higher. The 5-year stent thrombosis rates were generally low and similar between DES and BMS groups.	MACE rate was insignificantly different, but cardiac mortality was higher after DES. Stent thrombosis was the main cause of late cardiac deaths.

(Continued)

Table 1.1 (Continued)

Study Title	Hypothesis	Cohort	Principal Findings	Conclusion
5-year follow-up after PPCI with a PES vs. a BMS in acute STEMI: a follow-up study of the PASSION trial [19].	Evaluate the long-term outcomes of the PASSION trial.	619 patients presenting with STEMI were randomized to a PES group or the similar BMS group.	Occurrence of composite of cardiac death, recurrent MI, or TLR was comparable. Incidence of definite or probable stent thrombosis had no differences in the PES group and in the BMS group.	No significant difference in MACE was observed. stent thrombosis was almost exclusively seen after the use of PES.
Effect of BES with biodegradable polymer vs. BMS on cardiovascular events among patients with AMI [20].	To compare BES from a biodegradable polymer with BMS in PPCI.	1161 patients presenting with STEMI were randomized 1:1 to receive BES ($n = 575$) or BMS ($n = 582$).	MACE at 1 year occurred in 4.3% of patients receiving BES with biodegradable polymer and 8.7% in those receiving BMS. Difference was driven by a lower risk of TVR and ischemia-driven TLR. Rates of cardiac death and definite stent thrombosis were not different.	Compared with a BMS, use of BES with a biodegradable polymer resulted in a lower rate of MACE at 1 year.

AMI, acute myocardial infarction; BES, biolimus-eluting stent; BMS, bare-metal stent; BP-BES, bioabsorbable polymer-based biolimus-eluting stent; CoCr, cobalt chromium; DEB, drug-eluting balloon; DES, drug-eluting stent; DP-DES, durable polymer drug-eluting stent; EES, everolimus-eluting stent; EZES, endeavor zotarolimus-eluting stent; MACE, major adverse cardiac events (death from any cause, nonfatal myocardial infarction, or target vessel revascularization); MI, myocardial infarction; MLV, MULTI-LINK VISION®; PCI, percutaneous coronary intervention; PES, paclitaxel-eluting stent; PPCI, primary percutaneous coronary intervention; SES, sirolimus-eluting stent; STEMI, ST-elevation myocardial infarction; TLR, target-lesion revascularization; TVR, target-vessel revascularization; ZESS, zotarolimus-eluting endeavor sprint stent.

Table 1.2 Management of no-reflow.

Title	Hypothesis	Cohort	Principal Findings	Conclusion
Safety and efficacy of IC adenosine administration in patients with AMI undergoing PPCI: a meta-analysis of randomized controlled trials [21].	Safety and efficacy of IC adenosine in patients with AMI undergoing PPCI.	1030 patients, IC adenosine treatment group (n = 460), placebo group (n = 570).	IC adenosine therapy led to more post-PCI STRes and reduction in residual ST-segment elevation but did not improve TIMI 3 flow, MBG 3, peak CK-MB concentration and post-PCI ejection fraction. Slight trend toward improvement of MACE, incidence of heart failure and cardiovascular mortality but no difference in all-cause mortality.	IC adenosine may be a useful therapy as indicated by improvement in EKG findings. A trend toward improvement was noted in MACE and heart failure events but data are lacking to reach strong conclusions.
IC versus intravascular bolus abciximab during PPCI in patients with acute STEMI: a randomized trial [22].	Safety and efficacy of IC vs. standard intravascular bolus of abciximab in patients with STEMI undergoing PPCI.	2065 patients, IC abciximab (n = 1032) or intravascular abciximab (n = 1033).	IC, compared with intravascular abciximab, resulted in a similar rate of all-cause mortality, reinfarction or CHF at 90 days. Incidence of all-cause mortality and reinfarction did not differ between the treatment groups. Fewer patients in the IC group had new CHF.	IC compared with intravascular abciximab did not result in a difference in death, reinfarction, or CHF. Since IC abciximab bolus administration is safe and might be related to reduced rates of CHF, the IC route might be preferred.
IC versus intravascular administration of abciximab in patients with STEMI undergoing PPCI intervention with thrombus aspiration [23].	Discover beneficial effects of IC over intravascular abciximab in patients with STEMI undergoing PPCI and TA.	534 patients, intravascular (n = 263) vs. IC (n = 271) administration of abciximab.	Incidence of complete STRes was similar. Incidence of MBG 2/3 was higher in the IC group. Enzymatic infarct size was smaller in the IC group. Incidence of MACE was similar in both groups.	IC abciximab does not improve myocardial reperfusion as assessed by STRes, but is associated with improved MBG and a smaller enzymatic infarct size.
Adenosine and verapamil for no-reflow during PPCI in people with AMI [24].	Evaluate the evidence related to the use of verapamil or adenosine for no-reflow phenomenon during PPCI.	939 patients; adenosine group (n = 899) verapamil group (n = 40).	No evidence that adenosine reduced short- and long-term all-cause mortality, short-term nonfatal MI or incidence of angiographic no-reflow (TIMI flow grade < 3 after PPCI, and MBG 0 to 1). Incidence of adverse events with adenosine was increased.	No evidence that adenosine and verapamil can reduce all-cause mortality, nonfatal MI or the incidence of angiographic no-reflow, there was evidence of increased adverse events.
Pexelizumab for acute STEMI in patients undergoing PPCI [25].	Effectiveness of pexelizumab as an adjunct to PCI in improving 30-day mortality from STEMI.	5745 patients. Placebo (n = 2885), pexelizumab group (n = 2860).	No difference in mortality was observed between the pexelizumab and placebo. End points of death, shock, or heart failure were similar.	Mortality was low and unaffected by pexelizumab.

(Continued)

Table 1.2 (Continued)

Title	Hypothesis	Cohort	Principal Findings	Conclusion
Evaluation of IC adenosine or NTP after thrombus aspiration during PPCI for the prevention of MVO in AMI. REOPEN-AMI study [26].	To assess whether IC adenosine or NTP following thrombus aspiration is superior to thrombus aspiration alone for the prevention of MVO in STEMI PCI.	240 patients; adenosine group ($n = 80$), NTP group ($n = 80$), saline group ($n = 80$).	STRes > 70% occurred more in adenosine-treated patients. Angiographic MVO and MACE occurred less often in adenosine-treated patients.	In STEMI patients treated by PCI and thrombus aspiration, the additional IC adenosine results in a significant improvement of MVO, as assessed by STRes.
Short-term effect of verapamil on coronary no-reflow associated with PCI in patients with ACS: A systematic review and meta-analysis [27].	IC verapamil injection may be beneficial in preventing no-reflow/slow flow after PCI.	539 patients; IC verapamil ($n = 266$), control group ($n = 273$).	Verapamil treatment was more effective in decreasing the incidence of no-reflow, CTFC, improving the TMPG and reducing the 30-day WMI. Decreased the incidence of MACE during hospitalization and 2 months after PCI. Verapamil did not provide an additional improvement of LVEF.	IC verapamil injection is beneficial in preventing no-reflow/slow flow, reducing CTFC, improving TMPG, and lowering WMSI. It is also likely to reduce 2-month MACE in ACS patients post-PCI.
Relationship between myocardial reperfusion, infarct size, and mortality. INFUSE-AMI Trial [28].	To compare infarct size measured by MRI in patients with successful (MBG 2/3) vs. unsuccessful (MBG 0/1) microcirculatory reperfusion.	452 patients with anterior STEMI to IC bolus abciximab delivered locally at the infarct lesion vs. no abciximab, and to manual thrombus aspiration vs. no aspiration.	Infarct size was significantly lower in patients with MBG 2/3 ($n = 367$) than in those with MBG 0/1. IC abciximab further reduced infarct size in patients with MBG 2/3 and was associated with a 30% reduction in infarct mass and 90% reduction in MVO. Ejection fraction was higher with MBG 2/3 at 30 days and rate of death was significantly lower.	MBG 2/3 occurs in 80% of STEMI patients treated with PPCI and is associated with smaller infarct size, less MVO, improved ejection fraction, and significantly lower 30-day mortality.
Evaluation of IC adenosine to prevent periprocedural myonecrosis in elective PCI (PREVENT ICARUS) [29].	To investigate the benefits of pre-procedural IC administration of high-dose adenosine during elective PCI.	260 patients; IC adenosine ($n = 130$), IC placebo ($n = 130$).	Greater prevalence of calcified lesions was observed in the adenosine group. Greater prevalence of type C lesions, chronic occlusions, worse pre-procedural TIMI flow, and more severely stenotic lesions were observed in the placebo group.	Pre-procedural IC single high-dose bolus of adenosine does not provide any benefit in terms of periprocedural myonecrosis in patients undergoing elective PCI.

IC fixed dose of NTP via thrombus aspiration catheter for the prevention of the no-reflow phenomenon following PPCI in AMI [30].	IC administration of NTP + tirofiban is a safe and superior compared to tirofiban alone for the prevention of no-reflow.	162 patients; NTP + tirofiban (n = 80), tirofiban alone (n = 82).	NTP group had a lower CTFC, higher proportion of complete STRes, enhanced TMPG 2–3 ratio and lower peak CK-MB value. There were no differences in the final TIMI. LVEF at 6 months was higher in NTP group; incidence of MACE was not different.	NTP + tirofiban via a thrombus aspiration catheter is a safe and superior compared with tirofiban alone in patients with STEMI undergoing PPCI.
New method of IC adenosine injection to prevent MVR injury in patients with AMI undergoing PCI [31].	To examine the role of IC adenosine performed during PCI on the immediate angiographic results and clinical course.	70 patients; group 1 (n = 35) IC adenosine, group 2 (n = 35) placebo.	PCI resulted in TIMI 3 flow after PCI in 91.4% in group 1 and 77.1% in group 2. MBG 3 was observed at the end of PCI in 65.7% and 37.1% respectively. STRes elevation was more frequently observed in group 1.	IC adenosine administration improved the angiographic and EGK results. Seemed to be associated with a more favorable clinical course.
High-dose IC adenosine for myocardial salvage in patients with acute STEMI [32].	Previous studies have suggested that intravascular adenosine improves myocardial reperfusion and reduces IS in STEMI patients.	110 patients; high-dose bolus injection of IC adenosine (n = 56), placebo (n = 54).	No significant difference in MSI was found between groups. Extent of MVO was comparable in both groups, TIMI flow grade, TIMI frame count, MBG, and STRes after PPCI were similar. After 4 months, infarct size was similar in both treatment groups.	There is no evidence that selective high-dose IC administration of adenosine distal to the occlusion site of the culprit lesion in STEMI patients results in incremental myocardial salvage index or a decrease in MVO.
Evaluation of IRA patency and microcirculatory function after facilitated PPCI [33].	To evaluate the effects on clinical outcomes of PPCI facilitated with pre-catheter abciximab with half-dose reteplase, abciximab alone or with abciximab administered immediately before the procedure.	637 patients; half-dose reteplase + abciximab (n = 213), abciximab alone (n = 222), placebo (n = 202).	Patients in combination-facilitated group exhibited higher rates of baseline IRA patency compared with abciximab-facilitated and primary PCI group. There were no differences in the post-PCI corrected TIMI frame count or the rates of post-PCI TIMI flow grade 3 MBG 2/3.	Pre-catheter administration of abciximab alone and in combination resulted in higher rates of IRA patency at baseline. Post-procedural angiographic and microcirculatory variables were unaffected.

(Continued)

Table 1.2 (Continued)

Title	Hypothesis	Cohort	Principal Findings	Conclusion
The impact of pre-PPCI βB use on the no-reflow phenomenon in patients with AMI [34].	To investigate the impact of PPCIβB use on the development of non-reflow in STEMI patients post PCI.	618 patients; βB group (n = 257), no βB (n = 1,358).	Incidence of the no-reflow was significantly lower in the βB group than in non-βB group.	Previous long-term beta blocker use before STEMI is associated with lower incidence of non-reflow in patients with STEMI treated with PPCI.
Clinical and procedural predictors of no-reflow in patients with AMI after PPCI [35].	To identify possible clinical predictors for no-reflow in patients with AMI after PPCI.	Total: 312 patients. Divided into 2 subgroups.	Age > 65 years, time from onset to reperfusion > 6 hours, SBP on admission < 100 mmHg, IABP use before PCI, low (≤1) TIMI flow grade before PPCI, high thrombus burden and long target lesion on angiography were independent predictors of no-reflow.	Occurrence of no-reflow after PPCI for AMI can predict clinical, angiographic and procedural features.
Effect of high-dose IC adenosine during PPCI in AMI: a randomized controlled trial [36].	To assess the improvement of myocardial perfusion and reduction in infarct size with intravascular adenosine.	448 patients; IC adenosine (n = 226), placebo (n = 222).	Incidence of residual ST-segment deviation < 0.2 mV did not differ between patients. No significant difference in secondary outcomes measures.	Administration of IC adenosine after thrombus aspiration and after stenting of the IRA did not improved myocardial perfusion.
Coronary artery calcification score is an independent predictor of the no-reflow phenomenon after reperfusion therapy in AMI [37].	To investigate whether the CAC score is associated with impaired reperfusion during the acute phase of STEMI.	60 patients. Optimal reperfusion (n = 27), No-reflow (n = 33)	CAC score > 100 was associated with the presence of no-reflow. CAC score of non-culprit coronary arteries was higher in no-reflow individuals. CAC score of the IRA correlated negatively with the TIMI flow rate and with the MBG.	CAC score is associated with the presence of the no-reflow phenomenon in STEMI patients.

IC NTP for the prevention of the no-reflow phenomenon after PPCI in AMI. A randomized, double-blind, placebo-controlled clinical trial [38].	To assess whether NTP injected IC immediately before primary angioplasty for acute STEMI prevents no-reflow and improves vessel flow and myocardial perfusion.	98 patients with STEMI, randomized to receive either NTP (60 μg) or placebo.	Compare ST-segment resolution was achieved in 61.7% and 61.2% of NTP and placebo subjects. At 6 months, the rate of TVR, MI, or death occurred in 6.3% of the NTP group and 20% of the placebo group.	In patients with STEMI, selective IC administration of a fixed dose of NTP failed to improve coronary flow and myocardial tissue reperfusion but improved clinical outcomes at 6 months.
Impact of PercuSurge device conjugative with IC administration of NTP on no-reflow phenomenon following PPCI [39].	When administered in conjunction with a PercuSurge device for treatment of AMI, IC NTP is safe and superior to IC administration of NTP for reversing slow flow or no-reflow.	62 patients; intervention ($n = 33$), control ($n = 29$).	Subgroup analysis demonstrated that final MBG and corrected TIMI frame count time were significantly higher in patients with than in patients without the PercuSurge. No significant NTP related adverse events occurred, apart from insignificant transient hypotension.	IC administration of NTP is safe and superior to NTG for improving final epicardial blood flow and microvascular circulation in patients with AMI undergoing PPCI. Combination therapy of PercuSurge device and NTP improved microvascular circulation.

AD, adenosine; AMI, acute myocardial infarction; CAC, coronary artery calcium; CTFC, corrected thrombolysis in myocardial infarction (TIMI) frame count; CHE, congestive heart failure; EKG, electrocardiogram; IABP, intra-aortic balloon pump; IC, intracoronary; IRA, infarct-related artery; LVEF, left ventricular ejection fraction; MACE, major cardiac adverse events; MBG, myocardial blush grade; MI, myocardial infarction; MRI, magnetic resonance imaging (type C lesion from the American College of Cardiology/American Heart Association classification); MSI, myocardial salvation; MVO, microvascular obstruction; MVR, microvascular reperfusion; NTG, nitroglycerin; NTP, sodium nitroprusside; PCI, percutaneous coronary intervention; PPCI, primary percutaneous coronary intervention; SBP, systolic blood pressure; STRes, ST-segment resolution; TA, thrombus aspiration; TIMI, thrombolysis in myocardial infarction; TMPG, TIMI myocardial perfusion grade; WMSI, wall motion score index.

Table 1.3 Is thrombectomy an available tool in STEMI?

Title	Hypothesis	Cohort	Principal Findings	Conclusion
Impact of MT on myocardial reperfusion as assessed by STRes in STEMI patients treated by primary PCI [40].	To evaluate the impact of MT on STRes as a surrogate of reperfusion.	239 patients; MT before primary PCI ($n = 102$) group 1, conventional PCI ($n = 137$) group 2.	A complete resolution of ST-segment elevation occurred in 51.4% of patients in group 1 and in 35.6% of patients in group 2. MT was associated with lower use of stents. Estimate of MACE was not significantly different between 2 groups at 1-year and 3-year follow-up.	In STEMI patients, MT improves myocardial reperfusion, assessed by the percentage of STRes and a lower use of stents. This strategy did not improve cardiovascular outcomes at 1-year follow-up.
Cardiac death and reinfarction after 1 year in the thrombus aspiration during PCI in AMI study (TAPAS) [41].	The TA during PCI in MI improves myocardial reperfusion compared with conventional PCI, but benefit improving clinical outcome is unknown.	1071 patients with STEMI were randomly assigned in a 1:1 ratio either TA (group 1) or conventional treatment (group 2).	Cardiac death at 1 year was 19 of 535 patients in group 1 and 36 of 536 in group 2. 1-year cardiac death or nonfatal reinfarction occurred in 30 of 535 patients in group 1 and 53 of 536 patients in group 2.	Compared with conventional PCI, TA before stenting of the IRA seems to improve 1-year clinical outcome after PCI for STEMI.
Lone aspiration thrombectomy without stenting in young patients with STEMI [42].	TA alone may be a viable option in patients presenting with STEMI or rescue angioplasty.	202 young patients underwent PPCI for acute STEMI; 10 patients had LAT as definitive therapy.	At 1 month, all remaining patients were free of MACE. At 6 weeks, 1 patient had recurrent STEMI after abruptly discontinuing all medication. Follow-up revealed no adverse consequences.	LAT without balloon angioplasty or stenting is feasible and is associated with favorable short- and long-term outcomes.
Effect of coronary TA during PPCI on 1-year survival (from the FAST-MI 2010 Registry) [43].	To assess 1-year outcome in patients participating in the FAST-MI 2010 treated with primary PCI for STEMI.	4169 patients; 2087 patients had STEMI, 1538 had primary PCI, with TA used in 671.	To assess 1y outcome in 30-day mortality and the rate of 1-year survival were similar with both strategies.	In a real-world setting of patients admitted with STEMI, use of TA during PPCI was not associated with improved 1-year survival.

Study	Objective	Study population	Results	Conclusion
TA in PPCI in high-risk patients with STEMI: a real-world registry [44].	Evaluate the effect of TA in real-world, all-comer patient population with STEMI undergoing PPCI.	313 patients; TA (n = 194), Conventional PCI (n = 119).	TA was associated with lower post-PCI TIMI frame count values and higher TIMI 3. Post-procedural myocardial perfusion assessed by MBG was increased in TA group. No difference in clinical outcome at 30 days. Patients treated with TA showed significantly higher survival and MACE-free at 1 year.	STEMI patients with occluded IRA, TA prior to PCI improves coronary flow, myocardial perfusion, and clinical outcomes compared with PCI in the absence of TA.
Rheolytic thrombectomy with PCI, for infarct size reduction In AMI: 30-day results from a multicenter randomized study [45].	RT as an adjunct to PCI reduces infarction size and improves myocardial perfusion during treatment of STEMI.	480 patients; RT as an adjunct to PCI (n = 240), PCI alone (n = 240).	Final infarct size was higher in the RT group compared with PCI alone. Final TIMI 3 was lower in the RT group. There were no differences in TMP blush scores or STRes. 30-day MACE was higher in the RT group.	Despite effective thrombus removal, RT with primary PCI did not reduce infarct size or improve TIMI, TMP blush, STRes or 30-day MACE.
TA during PPCI [46].	Evaluate whether manual aspiration is superior to conventional treatment during PPCI.	1071 patients randomly assigned to the TA group 1 or the conventional PCI group 2 before undergoing coronary angiography.	MBG of 0–1 occurred in 17.1% of the patients in group 1 and in 26.3% of those in group 2. Complete STRes occurred in 56.6% and 44.2% of patients, respectively. At 30 days, rate of death in patients with MBG of 0–1, 2, and 3 was 5.2%, 2.9%, and 1.0%, respectively; rate of adverse events was 14.1%, 8.8%, and 4.2%, respectively.	TA is applicable in a large majority of patients with STEMI, and it results in better reperfusion and clinical outcomes than conventional PCI, irrespective of clinical and angiographic characteristics at baseline.
TA reduces MVO after PCI: A myocardial contrast echocardiography substudy of the REMEDIA trial [47].	To clarify the role of micro-embolization in the genesis of MVO after PCI.	25 patients randomized to be pretreated with TA before PCI of the culprit lesion and 25 received standard PCI.	In patients treated with a TA filter device, WMSI, CSI, WML, and CDL were significantly lower and EF higher; LV volumes were slightly smaller compared with control. The extent of MVO significantly correlated with temporal changes in LV volumes.	TA significantly reduces the extent of MVO and myocardial dysfunction, although it does not have a favorable effect in preventing LV remodeling.
IC thrombectomy improves myocardial reperfusion in patients undergoing direct angioplasty for AMI [48].	Evaluate the effects of MT on myocardial reperfusion during direct angioplasty for AMI.	92 patients with AMI and angiographic evidence of intraluminal thrombus were randomized to either IC thrombectomy followed by stenting or to a conventional strategy of stenting.	Post-procedure thrombolysis in MI TIMI 3 was not different between groups. Myocardial blush 3 was observed in 71.7% of patients undergoing MT and in 36.9% of patients undergoing conventional strategy. STRes ≥ 50% occurred more often in patients undergoing MT. Adjunctive thrombectomy was an independent predictor of blush 3.	IC thrombectomy as adjunct to stenting during direct angioplasty for AMI improves myocardial reperfusion.

(Continued)

Table 1.3 (Continued)

Title	Hypothesis	Cohort	Principal Findings	Conclusion
Impact of TA on angiographic and clinical outcomes in patients with STEMI [49].	Assess the impact of EAC on angiographic and clinical outcomes in patients with STEMI.	535 patients; EAC was used in 165 patients before angioplasty (group 1), 370 patients underwent PCI without TA (group 2).	More patients in group 1 had initial TIMI 0–1 compared with group 2. Final TIMI 3 was the same in both groups. An analysis restricted to patients with initial TIMI flow 0–1 yielded similar results. No difference in clinical outcomes was observed.	Selective use of the EAC results in excellent angiographic and clinical results. Further clinical investigation needed.
Results of MT in STEMI: real-world experience [50].	Evaluate the outcomes of STEMI patients undergoing TA in a real-world setting.	359 patients; 270 thrombectomy (group 1), 89 standard PCI (group 2).	Group 1 had a lower baseline LV systolic function and were more likely to receive IABP support. After adjusting for demographics, initial CK, GFR and IRA, thrombectomy was associated with lower peak CK, but was neither associated with improved LV repair nor with reduced no-reflow.	Thrombectomy in STEMI resulted in lower enzymatic infarct size, but did not reduce no-reflow phenomenon or improve early LV function recovery.
Aspiration thrombectomy for treatment of STEMI: meta-analysis [51].	Evaluate clinical and procedural outcomes of TA-assisted PPCI compared with conventional PPCI in patients with STEMI.	26 randomized controlled trials with a total of 11,943 patients.	No difference in the risk of all-cause death, reinfarction, TVR, or definite stent thrombosis between the 2 groups at 10.4 months. There were significant reductions in failure to reach thrombolysis in MI 3 flow or myocardial blush grade 3, incomplete ST-segment elevations, and evidence of distal embolization with TA.	Among unselected patients with STEMI, TA-assisted PPCI does not improve clinical outcomes, despite improved epicardial and myocardial parameters of reperfusion.
MAT does not impact in short- or long-term survival in PPCI: Insights from the Blue Cross Blue Shield of Michigan Cardiovascular Collaborative [52].	MAT does not impact in short- or long-term survival in PPCI.	12,961 patients; MAT ($n = 4,972$), conventional PCI ($n = 7,989$).	No difference in hospital mortality. MAT was associated with increases in stroke and need for dialysis, and a decrease in post-PCI CABG. No difference in long-term survival observed.	Use of MAT does not appear to be associated with a reduction in mortality in patients undergoing PPCI and routine use of this approach cannot be recommended.

Role of aspiration and MT in patients with acute MI undergoing primary angioplasty [53].	The clinical efficacy of thrombectomy in acute MI remains uncertain.	18 clinical trials randomized MI patients to aspiration ($n = 3936$) and 7 trials to mechanical thrombectomy ($n = 1,598$) before PCI compared with conventional PCI alone.	TA vs. conventional PPCI: MACE significantly reduced with TA. Beneficial trends noted for recurrent MI and TVR. Final infarction size and EF at 1 month were similar. STREs and thrombolysis In MI blush grade (TBG) 3 post-procedure were both improved with TA. MT vs. conventional PPCI: no difference in the incidence of MACE, mortality, recurrent MI, TVR, or final infarction size. Benefit in ST-segment resolution, but not TBG 3, was noted.	Thrombectomy during MI by manual catheter aspiration, but not mechanically, is beneficial in reducing MACE, including mortality, at 6–12 months compared with conventional PPCI alone.
Manual TA is not associated with reduced mortality in patients treated with PPCI [54].	Impact of TA on mortality in patients with STEMI treated with PPCI.	Observational cohort study of 10,929 STEMI patients; 3572 patients (32.7%) underwent TA during PPCI.	Procedural success rates were higher and in-hospital MACE rates were lower in patients undergoing TA. No difference in mortality rates between patients with and without TA during follow-up period. Thrombus aspiration was still not associated with decreased mortality.	Routine TA was not associated with a reduction in long-term mortality in patients undergoing PPCI, although procedural success and in-hospital MACE rates improved.
Clinical outcomes of manual TA in patients with AMI: An updated meta-analysis [55].	Systematically evaluate prospective randomized trials and assess the effects of TA on all-cause mortality, MACE, TVR and MI.	10,756 patients; 5404 controls underwent conventional PCI, and 5352 patients underwent PCI with TA.	A significant reduction in MACE with TA was noted. However TA did not significantly reduce all-cause mortality, TVR, or MI.	Results suggest that adjunctive TA to PCI may be associated with modest benefits related to MACE reduction.
TA during STEMI [56].	Evaluate whether TA reduces mortality.	7244 patients randomized to TA followed by PCI or PCI only.	Death from any cause occurred in 2.8% and 3.0% in TA and PCI only. Rates of hospitalization for recurrent MI at 30 days were 0.5% and 0.9%, respectively, and rates of stent thrombosis were 0.2% and 0.5%, respectively. No significant differences in rate of stroke or neurologic complications.	Routine TA before PCI compared with PCI alone did not reduce 30-day mortality among patients with STEMI.

(Continued)

Table 1.3 (Continued)

Title	Hypothesis	Cohort	Principal Findings	Conclusion
Impact of TA during PPCI on mortality in STEMI [57].	To assess the impact of TA during PPCI on the mortality of patients with STEMI patients.	2567 patients, thrombectomy ($n = 1095$).	Post-PPCI thrombolysis in MI 3 flow was more frequently achieved in TA group. TA was associated with a significant reduction in in-hospital and long-term mortality.	TA during PPCI is associated with a significant reduction in mortality, especially in those with a short total ischemic time.
The impact of IC TA on STEMI outcomes [58].	Evaluate the outcome of aspiration in a "real-world" setting of PPCI.	1035 patients; TA (aspiration group; $n = 189$), standard PCI (standard group; $n = 846$).	No significant differences were noted in the outcome of aspiration vs. standard treatment at 30 days and at 1 year. A significant advantage in favor of aspiration was evident in patients with proximal culprit lesions, anterior infarcts, and right ventricular involvement.	When STEMI involved a large jeopardized myocardium, aspiration was associated with sustained improved clinical outcomes.

AMI, acute myocardial infarction; CABG, coronary artery bypass graft; CDL, contrast defect; CK, creatine kinase; CSI, contrast score index; DAPT, dual antiplatelet therapy; EAC, Export aspiration catheter; EF, ejection fraction; GFR, glomerular filtration rate; IABP, intra-aortic balloon pump; IRA, infarct-related artery; LAT, lone aspiration thrombectomy; LV, left ventricular; MAT, manual aspiration thrombectomy; MCE, myocardial contrast echocardiography; MI, myocardial infarction; MT, manual thrombectomy; MVO, microvascular obstruction; PCI, percutaneous coronary intervention; PPCI, primary percutaneous coronary intervention; RT, rheolytic thrombectomy; STRes, ST segment resolution; STEMI, ST-segment elevation myocardial infarction; TA, thrombus aspiration; TVR, target vessel revascularization; WML, endocardial length of wall motion abnormality; WMSI, regional wall motion score index.

Table 1.4 Percutaneous coronary intervention in non-culprit vessel.

Title	Hypothesis	Cohort	Principal Findings	Conclusion
Culprit-only vs. complete CR during PPCI [59].	Complete CR during PPCI can be achieved safely with an improved clinical outcome during the indexed hospitalization.	120 patients with STEMI and MCS; 95 CR, 25 COR.	CR associated with reduced incidence of MACE, lower rate of recurrent ischemic episodes, MI, reintervention, acute heart failure and shorter hospitalization. Transient renal dysfunction was more common in CR patients. In-hospital and 1-year mortality were similar.	Complete revascularization resulted in an improved acute clinical course.
Complete vs. culprit vessel PCI in MVD: A randomized comparison [60].	Compare safety, efficacy, and costs of CR versus COR in MVD disease treated with PCI.	219 patients with MVD were randomly assigned; CR of vessels ≥50% stenosis ($n = 108$), COR ($n = 111$).	Despite equal MACE at 24-hour strategy, success was higher in COR. MACE rates were similar. Repeat PCI was performed more often in COR group.	CR in MVD was associated with a lower strategy success rate, similar MACE rates.
PRAMI: randomized trial of preventive angioplasty in MI [61].	Whether performing preventive PCI would reduce the combined incidence of death from cardiac causes, nonfatal MI, or refractory angina.	465 patients with STEMI randomly assigned to: preventive PCI ($n = 234$), no preventive PCI ($n = 231$).	Primary outcome occurred in 21 patients assigned to preventive PCI and in 53 patients assigned to no preventive PCI.	In patients with STEMI and MVD undergoing IRA-PCI, preventive PCI in non-infarct CA with major stenosis reduced the risk of MACE.
A randomized trial of TVR versus MVR in STEMI: MACE during long-term follow-up [62].	Primary endpoint was incidence of MACE.	263 patients were randomly assigned to COR group, staged revascularization (SR group) and simultaneous treatment of non-IRA (CR group).	In 2.5 years, 50% of COR group experienced at least one MACE, 20% in the SR group and 23.1% in the CR group. In-hospital death, repeat revascularization and rehospitalization occurred more frequently in the COR group, there was no difference in reinfarction among the 3 groups. Survival free of MACE was reduced in the COR group but was similar in the CR and SR groups.	COR was associated with the highest rate of long-term MACE. Patients scheduled for SR experienced a similar rate of MACE to patients undergoing CR treatment of non-IRA.
Management of MVD in STEMI patients: A systematic review and meta-analysis [63].	RCTs or observational studies reporting about STEMI patients with MVD treated with either a culprit-only or CR strategy.	9 studies with 4686 patients compared culprit-only vs. complete PCI performed during PPCI.	No difference was found for the components of the primary outcome, apart from a reduction in repeated revascularization for complete PCI during the STEMI procedure.	CR performed during PPCI appears safe and offers a reduction in repeated revascularization.

(Continued)

Table 1.4 (Continued)

Title	Hypothesis	Cohort	Principal Findings	Conclusion
Multivessel PCI in patients with MVD and AMI [64].	Optimal percutaneous interventional strategy for dealing with significant non-culprit lesions in patients with MVD with AMI at presentation remains controversial.	820 patients with MVD were subdivided in 3 groups: (1) PCI of the IRA only; (2) PCI of both the IRA and non-IRA during the initial procedure; (3) PCI of the IRA followed by staged, in-hospital PCI of the non-IRA.	In patients with MVD, compared with PCI restricted to the IRA only, MV-PCI was associated with higher rates of reinfarction, revascularization and MACE. MV-PCI was an independent predictor of MACE at 1 year.	In patients with MVD, PCI should be directed at the IRA only, with decisions about PCI of non-culprit lesions guided by objective evidence of residual ischemia at late follow-up.
Early angio-guided CR vs. COR followed by ischemia-guided staged PCI in STEMI patients with MVD [65].	To compare short- and long-term clinical outcomes of early-staged, angio-guided approach and delayed, ischemia-guided treatment of non-IRA.	800 PPCIs were performed; 417 addressed to early-staged, angio-guided PCI of non-IRAs (CR group), 383 incomplete revascularizations (IncR group).	No difference in terms of death and MI was found between the CR and IncR group. MACE-free survival was significantly higher in IncR group, mainly driven by lower incidence of re-PCI.	Early CR based only on angiographic findings in patients with STEMI and MVD is associated with an excess of re-MI and with a higher incidence of MACE.
Non-culprit CA PCI during acute STEMI: insights from the APEX-AMI trial [66].	To examine the incidence of and propensity for non-culprit interventions performed at the time of the PPCI and its association with 90-day outcomes.	5373 patients underwent primary PCI in the APEX-AMI trial; 2201 had MVD; 9.9% underwent non-IRA PCI, 90.1% underwent PCI of the IRA alone.	Death/congestive heart failure/shock were higher in non-IRA group compared with IRA-only PCI group. Non-IRA PCI remained independently associated with an increased hazard of 90-day mortality.	Non-culprit coronary interventions were significantly associated with increased mortality.
In-hospital and long-term outcomes of multivessel PCI after AMI [67].	Outcomes of MV-PCI early after AMI were evaluated.	Patients with multivessel PCI (n = 239), patients with treatment of the IRA alone (n = 1145).	Multivessel PCI group had a higher prevalence of adverse prognostic indicators. 1-year survival free of recurrent infarction and TVR rates were similar between 2 groups.	MV-PCI in patients with MVD after AMI compared with 1-vessel PCI was not associated with an excess risk death, MI, coronary artery bypass graft, or TVR.
Single vs. multivessel treatment during primary angioplasty: results of the HELP AMI Study [68].	With modern non-thrombogenic stents CR with MVD treatment can be safely achieved during the PPCI with a lower need of subsequent revascularization and at a lower cost.	69 patients; culprit lesion treatment only (n = 17), complete MV treatment (n = 52).	Similar incidence of in-hospital MACE. Increase in incidence of new revascularization in culprit treatment group at 12-month follow-up was sufficient to compensate initial higher in-hospital cost, with a similar 12-month hospital cost.	A staged approach to MV treatment during primary angioplasty avoids treating unnecessarily non-clinically relevant lesions.

Importance of CR in patients with AMI treated with PCI [69].	Impact of ICR on short- and long-term outcome in patients with AMI and MVD. Any-cause mortality rate and MACE during hospitalization, within a follow-up period.	798 patients with MVD selected from 1486 consecutive patients with AMI treated with PCI. At discharge, 605 still had at least 1 diseased artery (ICR group); in 193, CR has been achieved (CR group).	Mortality and MACE rates were higher in ICR group than among CR subjects during short- and long-term observation.	ICR is a strong and independent risk factor of death and MACE in patients with AMI treated with PCI.
Randomized trial of CR versus COR in patients undergoing PPCI for STEMI and MVD: The CvLPRIT trial [70].	Feasibility, safety, and potential benefit of CR non-IRA lesions in patients presenting with PPCI for STEMI compared with PCI of IRA alone.	From 850 patients with STEMI, 296 were randomized to receive complete (150) or culprit lesion-only (146) revascularization.	All-cause death within 12 months occurred in 10% of the complete revascularization group vs. 21.2% in the IRA-only revascularization group. There was no reduction in death or MI; a reduction in all primary endpoint components was seen.	CR significantly lowered the rate of the composite primary endpoint at 12 months compared with treating only the IRA.
What is optimal revascularization strategy in patients with MVD in non-STEMI? MV or COR revascularization [71].	To compare MV revascularization with COR in patients with non-STEMI who had MVD.	1919 patients with MVD diagnosed as non-STEMI. Two groups; MV-PCI ($n = 1011$) and COR ($n = 908$).	In-hospital mortality was higher in COR group. Primary endpoints occurred in 241 patients during 1-year follow-up. MVR reduced MACE and non-TVR. No differences in TVR.	Proved the efficacy of MV-PCI (including total revascularization of significant stenotic vessels) in these settings.
Prognostic impact of staged vs. "one-time" MV-PCI in AMI. Analysis from the HORIZONS-AMI Trial [72].	Explore the impact of a single intervention (PCI of culprit and non-culprit lesions together) vs. COR with staged non-culprit PCI at a later date in patients with STEMI.	3602 STEMI patients, PCI for MVD group ($n = 668$); 275 patients (41%) underwent a one-time MV procedure; staging performed in 393 (58.8%).	MV-PCI that included non-culprit vessels during the acute STEMI reperfusion procedure was strongly associated with a greater hazard for 1-year all-cause mortality, MACE, and stent thrombosis.	Suggests that a deferred angioplasty strategy for non-culprit lesions should remain the standard approach for patients with STEMI and MVD undergoing PPCI.
MVR vs. infarct-IRA only revascularization during the index PPCI in STEMI patients with MVD: a meta-analysis [73].	Compare outcome in same stage MV-PCI vs. IRA-PCI in STEMI patients with MVD undergoing PPCI.	15 studies were identified with a total number of 35,975 patients.	Mortality rate was higher in the MV-PCI group compared with the IRA-PCI group. Both incidence of reinfarction and re-PCI were lower in the MV-PCI group. Bleeding complications occurred more often in MV-PCI group. Rates of MACE were comparable between the two groups.	MV-PCI during the index of PPCI in STEMI is associated with a higher mortality and more bleeding, but a lower risk of reintervention and reinfarction.

(Continued)

Table 1.4 (Continued)

Title	Hypothesis	Cohort	Principal Findings	Conclusion
COR vs. MVR using DES in patients with STEMI: A Korean AMI registry-based Analysis [74].	Compare clinical outcomes of MV vs. IRA-only revascularization in patients undergoing PPCI for STEMI. Primary endpoint was incidence of MACE at 1 year.	3791 eligible STEMI patients with MVD and who underwent primary PCI using DES were collected. COR group and MVR group.	During the 1-year follow-up, 102 patients in COR group and 32 in MVR group experienced at least 1 MACE. No differences between 2 groups in rates of death, MI, or revascularization.	Although MV angioplasty during PPCI for STEMI did not reduce the MACE rate compared with COR, CR was associated with a lower rate of repeat revascularization after MV-PCI.
Complete vs. COR for patients with MVD undergoing PCI for STEMI: A systematic review and meta-analysis [75].	Meta-analysis comparing the benefits and risks of routine culprit-only PCI vs. MV-PCI in STEMI.	26 studies, 46,324 patients (7886 multivessel PCI and 38,438 culprit-only PCI).	Of the patients who received MV-PCI during index catheterization, an increase in in-hospital mortality was observed compared with patients who had COR. Patients undergoing MV-PCI as a staged procedure in-hospital, a survival benefit was observed. Combined analysis found a survival benefit with MV-PCI compared with COR.	Staged MV-PCI improved short- and long-term survival and reduced repeat PCI. Large randomized trials are still required.
Non-IRA revascularization during PPCI for STEMI: A systematic review and meta-analysis [76].	Compare outcomes of non-IRA PCI as an adjunct to PPCI in the setting of STEMI.	14 studies with 35,239 patients.	Death, MI, and revascularization were higher in same-sitting PCI group. In analyses limited to randomized controlled trials, primary end point was similar during short term and significantly lower for SS-PCI group in the long term.	SS-PCI group has higher baseline risk compared with IRA-PCI. Findings underscore need for a large, randomized controlled trial to guide therapy.
Single or MV-PCI in STEMI patients [77].	To evaluate clinical results of PCI in STEMI in patients with MVD, in relation to single or MV-PCI and to patients with SVD.	745 PCI, 346 (46%) SVD 399 (54%) MVD, among MVD patients, 156 (39%) had IRA-only treatment and 243 had MV-PCI.	At median follow-up mortality was 6.3% in SVD and 12% in MVD, new revascularization 2.9% and 9%, respectively.	MV-PCI in patients without hemodynamic compromise yields good short-term results, even if performed very early.

AMI, acute myocardial infarction; CR, coronary revascularization; COR, culprit-only revascularization; ICR, incomplete revascularization; IRA, infarct-related artery; MCS, multivessel coronary stenosis; MV, multivessel; MVD, multivessel disease; MVR, multivessel revascularization; PCI, percutaneous coronary intervention; PPCI, primary percutaneous coronary intervention; STEMI, ST-elevation myocardial infarction; SVD, single-vessel disease.

Table 1.5 Role of the intra-aortic balloon pump and counterpulsation in STEMI intervention.

Title	Hypothesis	Cohort	Principal Findings	Conclusion
Impact of IABP on long-term mortality of unselected patients with STEMI complicated by CS [78].	To assess the impact of IABP on 1-year mortality of unselected patients with STEMI presenting in CS.	Total of 51 patients; intervention ($n = 30$), controls ($n = 21$).	No difference in 30-day mortality between both groups and no impact on 1-year mortality.	No benefit of IABP on short- and long-term mortality of unselected patients with STEMI complicated by CS.
Systematic review and meta-analysis of IABP therapy in STEMI: should we change the guidelines? [79].	To assess whether IABP in STEMI with and without CS improves diastolic coronary and systemic blood flow, and reduces afterload and myocardial work.	First meta-analysis 7 randomized trials ($n = 1009$). Second meta-analysis included cohorts of STEMI patients with cardiogenic shock ($n = 10,529$).	IABP showed neither a 30-day survival benefit nor improved LVEF, with higher stroke and bleeding rates. In patients treated with thrombolysis, IABP was associated with an 18% decrease in 30-day mortality, with higher revascularization rates.	There is insufficient evidence endorsing the current guideline recommendation for the use of IABP therapy in the setting of STEMI complicated by CS.
Use and impact of IABP on mortality in patients with AMI complicated by CS: results of the Euro Heart Survey on PCI [80].	To assess use and impact on mortality of IABP in current practice of PCI in Europe.	653 patients; intervention ($n = 163$), control ($n = 490$).	In the multivariate analysis the use of IABP was not associated with an improved survival.	No beneficial effect of IABP on outcome. Large RCT urgently needed to define the role of IABP in patients with PCI for shock.
Effects of IABP on mortality of AMI [81].	Meta-analyses to analyze the relevant RCT data on the effect of IABP on mortality and occurrence of bleeding in AMI.	Total patients 2237; IABP ($n = 1112$), controls $n = 1125$).	The 6-month mortality in IABP group was not lower than in controls in the 4 RCTs that enrolled 59 AMI patients with CS. In the 4 that enrolled AMI 66 patients without CS, the data showed opposite conclusion.	IABP cannot reduce within 2-month and 6–12-month mortality of AMI patients with CS as well as within 2 months mortality of AMI patients without CS. IABP can increase the risk of bleeding.
Long-term safety and sustained LV recovery: long-term results of percutaneous LV support with Impella LP2.5 in STEMI [82].	To evaluate long-term effects of Impella LP2.5 support on the aortic valve and LVEF.	20 patients; treatment ($n = 10$), control ($n = 20$).	No differences in aortic valve abnormalities and LVEF were demonstrated between the groups. LVEF increase from baseline was greater in Impella-treated patients.	3-day support with the Impella LP2.5 is not associated with adverse effects on aortic valve at long-term follow-up. LVEF was similar in both groups. Recovery was greater in Impella group.

(*Continued*)

Table 1.5 (Continued)

Title	Hypothesis	Cohort	Principal Findings	Conclusion
Improved microcirculation in patients with an acute STEMI treated with the Impella LP2.5 percutaneous LV assist device [83].	Circulatory support during PCI in patients with STEMI aims at maintaining hemodynamic stability and organ perfusion.	6 patients; treatment group ($n = 3$), control group ($n = 3$).	Normal MC depending on both functional capillary density and flow velocity or quality as observed in healthy control, was only achieved in the Impella group and paralleled improvement in LV function.	Microcirculation assessed by sidestream dark field improved in STEMI patients treated with the Impella LP2.5 to levels observed in healthy people and remained suboptimal after 72 hours in patients without support.
The current use of Impella 2.5 in AMI complicated by CS: Results from the USpella Registry [84].	Outcomes of patients supported with Impella 2.5 pre-PCI vs. those who received post-PCI in CS complicating AMI.	63 patients received Impella 2.5 support prior to PCI and 91 patients received it post-PCI.	In pre-PCI support with Impella, more extensive revascularization with more vessels treated and more stents placed compared with Impella post-PCI. Higher survival rate in the pre-PCI group.	Early hemodynamic support is associated with more complete revascularization and improved survival in the setting of refractory CS complicating an AMI.
Randomized clinical trial to evaluate the safety and efficacy of percutaneous LV assist device vs. IABP for treatment of CS caused by MI [85].	In CS, Impella LP 2.5 may help to bridge patients to recovery compared with an IABP.	26 patients; PCI ($n = 24$), Impella ($n = 12$), IABP ($n = 13$).	The cardiac index after 30 minutes of support was significantly increased in the Impella LP2.5 group compared IABP group. 30-day mortality was 46% in both groups.	In CS caused by AMI, use of a percutaneous placed LV assist device (Impella LP 2.5) is feasible and safe, and provides superior hemodynamic support compared with standard treatment using an IABP.
Effects of mechanical LV unloading by Impella on LV dynamics in high-risk and PPCI patients [86].	To demonstrate that the Impella has beneficial effects in patients undergoing high-risk PCI and PPCI for acute STEMI.	6 patients with elective high-risk PCI, 5 patients with PPCI.	The response to increased LV unloading was not different between both groups. No change on global and systolic LV function, while diastolic function improved. There was a decrease in end-diastolic pressure, elastance, and wall stress.	LV unloading decreases end-diastolic wall stress and improves diastolic compliance dose-dependently. Beneficial LV unloading effects of Impella during high-risk and PPCI.
The PROTECT I Trial: Investigating the use of the Impella 2.5 system in patients undergoing high-risk PCI [87].	To demonstrate the hemodynamic support provided by the Impella 2.5 system when used in patients undergoing high-risk PCI.	All patients underwent PCI ($n = 14$) unprotected LMCA; ($n = 6$) on a last remaining conduit.	With increasing levels of Impella support, an increase in mean distal coronary pressure, hyperemic flow velocity, and coronary flow reserve has been observed. Significant decrease in myocardial oxygen consumption was seen.	Impella 2.5 system is safe, easy to use, and provides effective hemodynamic support during high-risk PCI.

Study	Objective	Patients/Methods	Results	Conclusion
IABP in patients with AMI complicated by CS: Results of the ALKK-PCI registry [88].	To investigate use and impact of outcome of IABP in current practice of PCI in Germany.	55,008 patients (22,039 STEMI, 32,969 NSTEMI, CS 1,435 and 478, respectively). Of total 1913 patients with shock, 487 were treated with IABP.	In-hospital mortality with and without IABP was 43.5% and 37.4%. In the multivariate analysis, use of IABP was associated with a strong trend for an increased mortality.	No benefit of IABP on outcome.
IABP in patients with AMI complicated by CS: IABP-SHOCK [89].	Whether IABP as an addition to PCI-centered therapy ameliorates MODS in patients with AMI complicated by CS.	45 consecutive patients with AMI and CS undergoing PCI were randomized to treatment with or without IABP.	Addition of IABP in CS patients was associated only with modest effects on reduction of APACHE II score, improvement of CI, reduction of inflammatory state, or BNP biomarker status were seen compared with medical therapy alone.	Addition of IABP to standard therapy did not result in a significant improvement in MODS.
IABC and infarct size in patients with acute anterior MI without shock: the CRISP-AMI randomized trial [90].	To determine whether routine IABC placement prior to reperfusion in patients with anterior STEMI without shock reduces MI size.	Initiation of IABC before PPCI (IABC plus PCI) vs. primary PCI alone.	Mean infarct size was not different. At 30 days, there were no differences between the IABC and PCI groups.	Among patients with acute anterior STEMI without shock, IABC plus primary PCI compared with PCI alone did not result in reduced infarct size.
Mortality in IABP therapy in patients with STEMI and CS: Data from nationwide inpatient sample [91].	To demonstrate that IABP therapy in patients with STEMI complicated by CS does not add any mortality benefit.	Data currently not available.	IABP therapy in patients undergoing revascularization was associated with a higher mortality than those without IABP therapy.	Routine use of IABP therapy in patients with STEMI complicated by CS does not add any mortality benefit, and may be harmful.
Hemodynamic support with Impella 2.5 vs. IABP in patients undergoing high-risk PCI: The PROTECT II Study [92].	Designed to assess whether a high-risk PCI strategy with the support of the Impella 2.5 device would result in better outcome than a revascularization strategy with IABP support.	452 patients. IABP (n = 226), Impella 2.5 (n = 226).	Impella 2.5 provided superior hemodynamic support in comparison with IABP. 30-day MACE was not different. At 90 days, a strong trend toward decreased MACE was observed in Impella 2.5.	Hemodynamic support with Impella 2.5 did not result in a superior outcome of the 30-day MACE but showed a strong trend to superior outcome at 90 days.

(Continued)

Table 1.5 (Continued)

Title	Hypothesis	Cohort	Principal Findings	Conclusion
Long-term mortality data From the BCIS-1. A randomized, controlled trial of elective BCP during high-risk PCI [93].	To find long-term mortality benefits on patients undergoing PCI assisted with IABP.	301 patients were randomly assigned to receive elective IABP insertion or to have planned PCI without IABP.	All-cause mortality at follow-up was 33% in the overall cohort, with fewer deaths occurring in the elective IABP group ($n = 42$) than in the group that underwent PCI without planned IABP support.	Elective IABP use during PCI was associated with a 34% relative reduction in all-cause mortality compared with unsupported PCI.
Early outcomes with marginal donor hearts compared with lv device support in patients with advanced heart failure [94].	To examine differences in wait list survival of patients with continuous flow LV assist devices and post-transplantation survival of patients receiving a marginal donor heart.	7298 patients; LV assist device support ($n = 2561$) and marginal donor heart ($n = 4737$).	The 30-day, 1-year, and 2-year survival was 96%, 89%, and 85%, for patients with LV assist device support on waiting list, and 97%, 89%, and 85%, respectively, for recipients of marginal donor hearts.	There was no between waiting list survival of patients with LV assist device support as bridge-to-transplant and post-transplant survival of recipients with marginal donor hearts. There could be clinical benefits for using LV assist device support as bridge-to-transplant to allow time for better allocation of optimal donor.
Intra-aortic balloon support for MI with CS [95].	Test the hypothesis that IABP, as compared with best available medical therapy alone, results in a reduction in mortality among patients with AMI complicated by CS.	600 patients; IABP group ($n = 301$), no IABP ($n = 299$).	At 30 days, 119 patients in IABP group and 123 patients in control group had died. Groups did not differ in rates of major bleeding, peripheral ischemic complications, sepsis and stroke.	Use of IABP did not reduce 30-day mortality in patients with CS complicating AMI for whom an early revascularization strategy was planned.
Comparison of hospital mortality with IABP insertion before vs. after PPCI for CS complicating AMI [96].	Insertion of IABP before PPCI might result in better survival of patients with CS compared with postponing the insertion.	Retrospectively studied 48 patients: 26 IABP before (group 1) and 22 IABP after (group 2).	Mortality, MACE and cerebrovascular events were significantly lower in group 1. Multivariate analysis identified renal failure and insertion of the IABP after PCI as the only independent predictors of in-hospital mortality.	Patients with CS complicating AMI who undergo PPCI assisted by IABP have a more favorable in-hospital outcome and lower in-hospital mortality.

Randomized comparison of intra-IABP with a percutaneous LV assist device in patients with revascularized AMI complicated by CS [97].	Mortality in CS following AMI remains unacceptably high despite PCI of IRA and use of IABP. Percutaneous LV assist device with active circulatory support might have positive hemodynamic effects and decrease mortality.	IABP ($n = 20$) or percutaneous VAD support ($n = 21$).	Hemodynamic and metabolic variables could be improved more effectively by VAD support from 0.22–0.28 W/m^2). Complications: severe bleeding or limb ischemia were found more frequently after VAD support, 30-day mortality was similar.	Hemodynamic and metabolic parameters can be reversed more effectively by VAD than by standard treatment with IABP. However, more complications were encountered.

AMI, acute myocardial infraction; APACHE II, Acute Physiology and Chronic Health Evaluation II; CS, cardiogenic shock; IABP, intra-aortic balloon pump; IRA, IRA, infarct-related artery; LV, left ventricular; LVEF, left ventricular ejection fraction; MACE, major adverse cardiac events; MI, myocardial infarction; MOSD, multiple-organ dysfunction syndrome; MVO, microvascular obstruction; PCI, percutaneous coronary intervention; STEMI, ST-elevation myocardial infarction; VAD, ventricular assist device.

References

1 Abdel-Wahab M, Toelg R, Kassner G, et al. Long-term clinical outcome of thin-strut cobalt-chromium stents in the drug-eluting stent era: results of the COBALT (Comparison of Bare-Metal Stents in All-Comers' Lesion Treatment) registry. *J Interv Cardiol*, 2011; 24(6): 496–504.

2 Sabaté M, Räber L, Heg D, et al. Comparison of newer-generation drug-eluting with bare-metal stents in patients with acute ST-segment elevation myocardial infarction. *JACC Cardiovasc Interv*, 2014; 7(1): 55–63.

3 Wallace E, Abdel-Latif A, Charnigo R, et al. Meta-analysis of long-term outcomes for drug-eluting stents versus bare-metal stents in primary percutaneous coronary interventions for ST-segment elevation myocardial infarction. *Am J Cardiol*, 2012; 109(7): 932–940.

4 Bangalore S, Amoroso N, Fusaro M, et al. Outcomes with various drug-eluting or bare metal stents in patients with ST-segment elevation myocardial infarction: a mixed treatment comparison analysis of trial level data from 34 068 patient-years of follow-up from randomized trials. *Circ Cardiovasc Interv*, 2013; 6(4): 378–390.

5 Di Lorenzo E, Sauro R, Varricchio A, et al. Benefits of drug-eluting stents as compared to bare metal stent in ST-segment elevation myocardial infarction: four year results of the paclitaxel or sirolimus-eluting stent vs bare metal stent in primary angioplasty (PASEO) randomized trial. *Am Heart J*, 2009;158(4): e43–e50.

6 Harskamp R, Kuijt W, Damman P, et al. Percutaneous coronary intervention for acute coronary syndrome due to graft failure. *Catheter Cardiovasc Interv*, 2013; 83(2): 203–209.

7 Navarese E, Tandjung K, Claessen B, et al. Safety and efficacy outcomes of first and second generation durable polymer drug eluting stents and biodegradable polymer biolimus eluting stents in clinical practice: comprehensive network meta-analysis. *BMJ*, 2013; 347: f6530. doi: 10.1136/bmj.f6530.

8 Sabaté M, Brugaletta S, Cequier A, et al. The EXAMINATION trial (everolimus-eluting stents versus bare-metal stents in ST-segment elevation myocardial infarction). *JACC Cardiovasc Interv*, 2014; 7(1): 64–71.

9 Campo G, Punzetti S, Malagù M, et al. Two-year outcomes after first- or second-generation drug-eluting stent implantation in patients with in-stent restenosis. A PRODIGY trial substudy. *Int J Cardiol*, 2014; 173(2): 343–345.

10 Garg A, Brodie B, Stuckey T, et al. New generation drug-eluting stents for ST-elevation myocardial infarction: A new paradigm for safety. *Catheter Cardiovasc Interv*, 2014; 84(6): 955–962.

11 Romano M, Buffoli F, Tomasi L, et al. Safety and effectiveness of drug eluting stent in patients with ST elevation myocardial infarction undergoing primary angioplasty. *Catheter Cardiovasc Interv*, 2008; 71(6): 759–763.

12 Brodie B, Stuckey T, Downey W, et al. Outcomes with drug-eluting stents versus bare metal stents in acute ST-elevation myocardial infarction: results from the Strategic Transcatheter Evaluation of New Therapies (STENT) Group. *Catheter Cardiovasc Interv*, 2008; 72(7): 893–900.

13 Palmerini T, Biondi-Zoccai G, Della Riva D, et al. Clinical outcomes with bioabsorbable polymer versus durable polymer-based drug-eluting and bare-metal stents. *J Am Coll Cardiol*, 2014; 63(4): 299–307.

14 De Luca G, Dirksen MT, Spaulding C, et al. Drug-eluting vs bare-metal stents in primary angioplasty. *Arch Intern Med*, 2012; 172(8): 611–621.

15 Belkacemi A, Agostoni P, Nathoe H, et al. First results of the DEB-AMI (drug eluting balloon in acute ST-segment elevation myocardial infarction) trial. *J Am Coll Cardiol*, 2012; 59(25): 2327–2337.

16 Sethi A, Bahekar A, Bhuriya R, et al. Drug-eluting stents versus bare metal stents in ST elevation myocardial infarction at a follow-up of three years or longer: a meta-analysis of randomized trials. *Exp Clin Cardiol*, 2012; 17(4): 169–174.

17 Palmerini T, Biondi-Zoccai G, Della Riva D, et al. Clinical outcomes with drug-eluting and bare-metal stents in patients with ST-segment elevation myocardial infarction. *J Am Coll Cardiol*, 2013; 62(6): 496–504.

18 Holmvang L, Kelbaek H, Kaltoft A, et al. Long-term outcome after drug-eluting versus bare-metal stent implantation in patients with ST-segment elevation myocardial infarction. *JACC Cardiovasc Interv*, 2013; 6(6): 548–553.

19 Vink M, Dirksen M, Suttorp M, et al. 5-Year follow-up after primary percutaneous coronary intervention with a paclitaxel-eluting stent versus a bare-metal stent in acute ST-segment elevation myocardial infarction. *JACC Cardiovasc Interv*, 2011; 4(1): 24–29.

20 Räber L, Kelbaek H, Ostojic M, et al. Effect of biolimus-eluting stents with biodegradable polymer vs bare-metal stents on cardiovascular events among patients with acute myocardial infarction. *JAMA*, 2012; 308(8): 777–878.

21 Singh M, Shah T, Khosla K, et al. Safety and efficacy of intracoronary adenosine administration in patients with acute myocardial infarction undergoing primary percutaneous coronary intervention: A meta-analysis of randomized controlled trials. *Ther Adv Cardiovasc Dis*, 2012; 6(3): 101–114.

22 Thiele H, Wöhrle J, Hambrecht R, et al. Intracoronary versus intravenous bolus abciximab during primary percutaneous coronary intervention in patients with acute ST-elevation myocardial infarction: a randomized trial. *Lancet*, 2012; 379(9819): 923–931.

23 Gu Y, Kampinga M, Wieringa W, et al. Intracoronary versus intravenous administration of abciximab in patients with ST-segment elevation myocardial infarction undergoing primary percutaneous coronary intervention with thrombus aspiration: the comparison of intracoronary versus intravenous abciximab administration during emergency reperfusion of ST-segment elevation myocardial infarction (CICERO) trial. *Circulation*, 2010; 122(25): 2709–2717.

24 Aung Naing K, Li L, Su Q, et al. Adenosine and verapamil for no-reflow during primary percutaneous coronary intervention in people with acute myocardial infarction. *Cochrane Database Syst Rev*, 2015; (5): CD009503. doi: 10.1002/14651858.CD009503.pub3.

25 Armstrong P, Granger C, Adams P, et al. Pexelizumab for acute ST-elevation myocardial infarction in patients undergoing primary percutaneous coronary intervention. *JAMA*, 2007; 297(1): 43–51.

26 Niccoli G, Rigattieri S, De Vita M, et al. Open-label, randomized, placebo-controlled evaluation of intracoronary adenosine or nitroprusside after thrombus aspiration during primary percutaneous coronary intervention for the prevention of microvascular obstruction in acute myocardial infarction. *JACC Cardiovasc Interv*, 2013; 6(6): 580–589.

27 Su Q, Li L, Liu Y. Short-term effect of verapamil on coronary no-reflow associated with percutaneous coronary intervention in patients with acute coronary syndrome: a systematic review and meta-analysis of randomized controlled trials. *Clin Cardiol*, 2013; 36(8): E11–E16.

28 Brener S, Maehara A, Dizon J, et al. Relationship between myocardial reperfusion, infarct size and mortality. *JACC: Cardiovasc Interv*, 2013; 6(7): 718–724.

29 De Luca G, Iorio S, Venegoni L, et al. Evaluation of intracoronary adenosine to prevent peri-procedural myonecrosis in elective percutaneous coronary intervention (from the PREVENT-ICARUS trial). *Am J Cardiol*, 2012; 109(2): 202–207.

30 Zhao YJ1, Fu XH, Ma XX, et al. Intracoronary fixed dose of nitroprusside via thrombus aspiration catheter for the prevention of the no-reflow phenomenon following primary percutaneous coronary intervention in acute myocardial infarction. *Exp Ther Med*, 2013; 6(2): 479–484.

31 Grygier M, Araszkiewicz A, Lesiak M, et al. New method of intracoronary adenosine injection to prevent microvascular reperfusion injury in patients with acute myocardial infarction undergoing percutaneous coronary intervention. *Am J Cardiol*, 2011; 107(8): 1131–1135.

32 Desmet W, Bogaert J, Dubois C, et al. High-dose intracoronary adenosine for myocardial salvage in patients with acute ST-segment elevation myocardial infarction. *Eur Heart J*, 2010; 32(7): 867–877.

33 Prati F, Petronio S, Van Boven A, et al. Evaluation of infarct-related coronary artery patency and microcirculatory function after facilitated percutaneous primary coronary angioplasty. *JACC Cardiovasc Interv*, 2010; 3(12): 1284–1291.

34 Wang J, Chen Y, Wang C, et al. The impact of pre-primary percutaneous coronary intervention β blocker use on the no-reflow phenomenon in patients with acute myocardial infarction. *Zhonghua Xin*, 2014; 42(10): 822–826.

35 Zhou H, He XY, Zhuang SW, et al. Clinical and procedural predictors of no-reflow in patients with acute myocardial infarction after primary percutaneous coronary intervention. *World J Emerg Med*, 2014; 5(2): 96–102.

36 Fokkema M, Vlaar P, Vogelzang M, et al. Effect of high-dose intracoronary adenosine administration during primary percutaneous coronary intervention in acute myocardial infarction: a randomized controlled trial. *Circ Cardiovasc Interv*, 2009; 2(4): 323–329.

37 Modolo R, Figueiredo V, Moura F, et al. Coronary artery calcification score is an independent predictor of the no-reflow phenomenon after reperfusion therapy in acute myocardial infarction. *Coronary Artery Disease*. 2015; 26(7): 562–566.

38 Amit G, Cafri C, Yaroslavtsev S, et al. Intracoronary nitroprusside for the prevention of the no-reflow phenomenon after primary percutaneous coronary intervention in acute myocardial infarction. A randomized, double-blind, placebo-controlled clinical trial. *Am Heart J*, 2006; 152(5): 887.e9–887e14.

39 Youssef A, Wu C, Hang C, et al. Impact of PercuSurge device conjugative with intracoronary administration of nitroprusside on no-reflow phenomenon following primary percutaneous coronary intervention. *Circ J*, 2006; 70(12): 1538–1542.

40 Messas N, Hess S, Adraa A, et al. Impact of manual thrombectomy on myocardial reperfusion as assessed by ST-segment resolution in STEMI patients treated by primary PCI. *Arch Cardiovasc Dis*, 2014; 107(12): 672–680.

41 Vlaar P, Svilaas T, van der Horst I, et al. Cardiac death and re-infarction after 1 year in the thrombus aspiration during Percutaneous Coronary Intervention in Acute Myocardial Infarction Study (TAPAS): A 1-year follow-up study. *Lancet*, 2008; 371(9628): 1915–1920.

42 Yokokawa T, Ujiie Y, Kaneko H, et al. Lone aspiration thrombectomy without stenting for a patient with ST-segment elevation myocardial infarction associated with coronary ectasia. *Cardiovasc Interv Ther*, 2013; 29(4): 339–343.

43 Puymirat E, Aissaoui N, Cottin Y, et al. Effect of coronary thrombus aspiration during primary percutaneous coronary intervention on one-year survival (from the FAST-MI 2010 registry). *Am J Cardiol*, 2014; 114(11): 1651–1657.

44 Mangiacapra F, Wijns W, De Luca G, et al. Thrombus aspiration in primary percutaneous coronary intervention in high-risk patients with ST-elevation myocardial infarction: a real-world registry. *Catheter Cardiovasc Interv*, 2010; 76(1): 70–76.

45 Ali A, Cox D, Dib N, et al. Rheolytic thrombectomy with percutaneous coronary intervention for Infarct size reduction in acute myocardial infarction. *J Am College Cardiol*, 2006; 48(2): 244–252.

46 Svilaas T, Vlaar P, van der Horst I, et al. Thrombus aspiration during primary percutaneous coronary intervention. *N Engl J Med*, 2008; 358(6): 557–567.

47 Garramone B, Burzotta F, De Vita M, et al. Manual thrombus-aspiration reduces microvascular obstruction after PCI in unselected STEMI patients: MCE sub-study of the randomized REMEDIA trial and insight into the pathogenesis of no-reflow. *Eur J Echocardiography*, 2005; 6: S169–S169.

48 Svilaas T, Vlaar P, van der Horst I, et al. Thrombus aspiration during primary percutaneous coronary intervention. *N Engl J Med*, 2008; 358(6): 557–567.

49 Beaudoin J, Dery J, Lachance P, et al. Impact of thrombus aspiration on angiographic and clinical outcomes in patients with ST-elevation myocardial infarction. *Cardiovasc Revasc Med*, 2010; 11(4): 218–222.

50 Jaiswal A, Kaushik M, Singh S, et al. Results of mechanical thrombectomy in ST elevation myocardial infarction: real world experience. *J Am Coll Cardiol*, 2013; 61(10 Suppl): E62.

51 Spitzer E, Heg D, Stefanini G, et al. Aspiration thrombectomy for treatment of ST-segment elevation myocardial infarction: a meta-analysis of 26 randomized trials in 11,943 patients. *Rev Esp Cardiol (Engl Ed)*, 2015; 68(9):746–52.

52 Bande M, Seth M, Menees D, et al. Manual aspiration thrombectomy (mat) does not impact short or long term survival in primary PCI: insights from the Blue Cross Blue Shield of Michigan Cardiovascular Collaborative (BMC2). *J Am Coll Cardiol*, 2014; 63(12 Suppl): A1840.

53 Kumbhani D, Bavry A, Desai M, et al. Role of aspiration and mechanical thrombectomy in patients with acute myocardial infarction undergoing primary angioplasty. *J Am Coll Cardiol*, 2013; 62(16): 1409–1418.

54 Jones D, Rathod K, Gallagher S, et al. Manual thrombus aspiration is not associated with reduced mortality in patients treated with primary percutaneous coronary intervention. *JACC Cardiovasc Interv*, 2015; 8(4): 575–584.

55 Briasoulis A, Palla M, Afonso L. Clinical outcomes of manual aspiration thrombectomy in patients with acute myocardial infarction: an updated meta-analysis. *Cardiology*, 2015; 132(2): 124–130.

56 Fröbert O, Lagerqvist B, Olivecrona G, et al. Thrombus aspiration during ST-Segment elevation myocardial infarction. *N Engl J Med*, 2013; 369(17): 1587–1597.

57 Noman A, Egred M, Bagnall A, et al. Impact of thrombus aspiration during primary percutaneous coronary intervention on mortality in ST-segment elevation myocardial infarction. *Eur Heart J*, 2012; 33(24): 3054–3061.

58 Minha S, Kornowski R, Vaknin-Assa H, et al. The impact of intracoronary thrombus aspiration on STEMI outcomes. *Cardiovasc Revasc Med*, 2012; 13(3): 167–171.

59 Zhang D, Song X, Lv S, et al. Culprit vessel only versus multivessel percutaneous coronary intervention in patients presenting with ST-segment elevation myocardial infarction and multivessel disease. *PLoS One*, 2014; 9(3): e92316.

60 Hannan EL, Samadashvili Z, Walford G, et al. Culprit vessel percutaneous coronary intervention versus multivessel and staged percutaneous coronary intervention for ST-segment elevation myocardial infarction patients with multivessel disease. *JACC Cardiovasc Interv*, 2010; 3(1): 22–31.

61 Wald D, Morris J, Wald N, et al. Randomized trial of preventive angioplasty in myocardial infarction. *N Engl J Med*, 2013; 369(12): 1115–1123.

62 Politi L, Sgura F, Rossi R, et al. A randomized trial of target-vessel versus multi-vessel revascularization in ST-elevation myocardial infarction: major adverse cardiac events during long-term follow-up. *Heart*, 2009; 96(9): 662–667.

63 Moretti C, D'Ascenzo F, Quadri G, et al. Management of multivessel coronary disease in STEMI patients: a systematic review and meta-analysis. *Int J Cardiol*, 2015; 179: 552–557.

64 Corpus R, House J, Marso S, et al. Multivessel percutaneous coronary intervention in patients with multivessel disease and acute myocardial infarction. *Am Heart J*, 2004; 148(3): 493–500.

65 Meliga E, Fiorina C, Valgimigli M, et al. Early angio-guided complete revascularization versus culprit vessel PCI followed by ischemia-guided staged PCI in STEMI patients with multivessel disease. *J Interv Cardiol*, 2011; 24(6): 535–541.

66 Toma M, Buller C, Westerhout C, et al. Non-culprit coronary artery percutaneous coronary intervention during acute ST-segment elevation myocardial infarction: insights from the APEX-AMI trial. *Eur Heart J*, 2010; 31(14): 1701–1707.

67 Chen L, Lennon R, Grantham J, et al. In-hospital and long-term outcomes of multivessel percutaneous coronary revascularization after acute myocardial infarction. *Am J Cardiol*, 2005; 95(3): 349–354.

68 Carlo D, Mara S, Flavio A, et al. Single vs multivessel treatment during primary angioplasty: results of the multicentre randomised HEpacoat™ for cuLPrit or multivessel stenting for Acute Myocardial Infarction (HELP AMI) Study. *Acute Card Care*, 2004; 6 (3–4): 128–133.

69 Kalarus Z, Lenarczyk R, Kowalczyk J, et al. Importance of complete revascularization in patients with acute myocardial infarction treated with percutaneous coronary intervention. *Am Heart J*, 2007; 153(2): 304–312.

70 Gershlick A, Khan J, Kelly D, et al. Randomized trial of complete versus lesion-only revascularization in patients undergoing primary percutaneous coronary intervention for STEMI and multivessel disease. *J Am Coll Cardiol*, 2015; 65(10): 963–972.

71 Kim MC, Jeong MH, Ahn Y, et al. What is optimal revascularization strategy in patients with multivessel coronary artery disease in non-ST-elevation myocardial infarction? Multivessel or culprit-only revascularization. *Int J Cardiol*, 2011; 153(2): 148–53.

72 Kornowski R, Mehran R, Dangas G, et al. Prognostic impact of staged versus "one-time" multivessel percutaneous intervention in acute myocardial infarction: analysis from the HORIZONS-AMI (harmonizing outcomes with revascularization and stents in acute myocardial infarction) trial. *J Am Coll Cardiol*, 2011; 58(7): 704–711.

73 Rasoul S, van Ommen V, Vainer J, et al. Multivessel revascularisation versus infarct-related artery only revascularisation during the index primary PCI in STEMI patients with multivessel disease: a meta-analysis. *Netherlands Heart J*, 2015; 23(4): 224–231.

74 Jo HS, Park JS, Sohn JW, et al. Culprit-lesion-only versus multivessel revascularization using drug-eluting stents in patients with ST-segment elevation myocardial infarction: a korean acute myocardial infarction registry-based analysis. *Korean Circ J*, 2011; 41(12): 718–725.

75 Bainey KR, Mehta SR, Lai T, et al. Complete vs culprit-only revascularization for patients with multivessel disease undergoing primary percutaneous coronary intervention for ST-segment elevation myocardial infarction: a systematic review and meta-analysis. *Am Heart J*, 2014; 167(1): 1–14.e2.

76 Bagai A, Thavendiranathan P, Sharieff W, et al. Non-infarct-related artery revascularization during primary percutaneous coronary intervention for ST-segment elevation myocardial infarction: a systematic review and meta-analysis. *Am Heart J*, 2013; 166(4): 684–693.e1.

77 Varani E, Balducelli M, Aquilina M, et al. Single or multivessel percutaneous coronary intervention in ST-elevation myocardial infarction patients. *Cathet Cardiovasc Interv*, 2008; 72(7): 927–933.

78 Dziewierz A, Siudak Z, Rakowski T, et al. Impact of intra-aortic balloon pump on long-term mortality of unselected patients with ST-segment elevation myocardial infarction complicated by cardiogenic shock. *Postepy Kardiol Interwencyjnej*, 2014; 3: 175–180.

79 Sjauw K, Engstrom A, Vis M, et al. A systematic review and meta-analysis of intra-aortic balloon pump therapy in ST-elevation myocardial infarction: should we change the guidelines?. *Eur Heart J*, 2008; 30(4): 459–468.

80 Zeymer U, Bauer T, Hamm C, et al. Use and impact of intra-aortic balloon pump on mortality in patients with acute myocardial infarction complicated by cardiogenic shock: results of the Euro Heart Survey on PCI. *EuroIntervention*, 2011; 7 (4): 437–441.

81 Ye L, Zheng M, Chen Q, et al. Effects of intra-aortic balloon counterpulsation pump on mortality of acute myocardial infarction. *PLoS ONE*, 2014; 9 (9): e108356.

82 Engström A, Sjauw K, Baan J, et al. Long-term safety and sustained left ventricular recovery: long-term results of percutaneous left ventricular support with Impella LP2.5 in ST-elevation myocardial infarction. *EuroIntervention*, 2011; 6(7): 860–865.

83 Lam K, Sjauw K, Henriques J, et al. Improved microcirculation in patients with an acute ST-elevation myocardial infarction treated with the Impella LP2.5 percutaneous left ventricular assist device. *Clin Res Cardiol*, 2009; 98(5): 311–318.

84 O'Neill W, Schreiber T, Wohns D, et al. The current use of Impella 2.5 in acute myocardial infarction complicated by cardiogenic shock: results from the USpella Registry. *J Interv Cardiol*, 2013; 27(1): 1–11.

85 Seyfarth M, Sibbing D, Bauer I, et al. A randomized clinical trial to evaluate the safety and efficacy of a percutaneous left ventricular assist device versus intra-aortic balloon pumping for treatment of cardiogenic shock caused by myocardial infarction. *J Am Coll Cardiol*, 2008; 52(19): 1584–1588.

86 Remmelink M, Sjauw K, Henriques J, et al. Effects of mechanical left ventricular unloading by Impella on left ventricular dynamics in high-risk and primary percutaneous coronary intervention patients. *Catheter Cardiovasc Interv*, 2010; 75(2): 187–194.

87 Dixon S, Henriques J, Mauri L, et al. A prospective feasibility trial investigating the use of the Impella 2.5 system in patients undergoing high-risk percutaneous coronary intervention (the PROTECT I Trial). *JACC Cardiovasc Interv*, 2009; 2(2): 91–96.

88 Zeymer U, Hochadel M, Hauptmann K, et al. Intra-aortic balloon pump in patients with acute myocardial infarction complicated by cardiogenic shock: results of the ALKK-PCI registry. *Clin Res Cardiol*, 2012; 102(3): 223–227.

89 Prondzinsky R, Lemm H, Swyter M, et al. Intra-aortic balloon counterpulsation in patients with acute myocardial infarction complicated by cardiogenic shock: The prospective, randomized IABP SHOCK Trial for attenuation of multiorgan dysfunction syndrome*. *Critical Care Med*, 2010; 38(1): 152–160.

90 Patel M, Smalling R, Thiele H, et al. Intra-aortic balloon counterpulsation and infarct size in patients with acute anterior myocardial infarction without shock. *JAMA*, 2011; 306(12): 1329–1337.

91 Pathak R, Aryal M, Karmacharya P, et al. Mortality in intra-aortic balloon pump therapy in patients with ST elevation myocardial infarction and cardiogenic shock: data from nationwide inpatient sample. *Int J Cardiol*, 2014; 176(1): 279–280.

92 Dangas G, Kini A, Sharma S, et al. Impact of hemodynamic support with Impella 2.5 versus intra-aortic balloon pump on prognostically important clinical outcomes in patients undergoing high-risk percutaneous coronary intervention (from the PROTECT II Randomized Trial). *Am J Cardiol*, 2014; 113(2): 222–228.

93 Perera D, Stables R, Clayton T, et al. Long-term mortality data from the balloon pump-assisted coronary intervention study (BCIS-1): a randomized, controlled trial of elective balloon counterpulsation during high-risk percutaneous coronary intervention. *Circulation*, 2012; 127(2): 207–212.

94 Schumer E, Ising M, Trivedi J, et al. Early outcomes with marginal donor hearts compared with left ventricular assist device support in patients with advanced heart failure. *Ann Thor Surg*, 2015; 100(2): 522–527.

95 Thiele H, Zeymer U, Neumann F, et al. Intraaortic balloon support for myocardial infarction with cardiogenic shock. *N Engl J Med*, 2012; 367(14): 1287–1296.

96 Abdel-Wahab M, Saad M, Kynast J, et al. Comparison of hospital mortality with intra-aortic balloon counterpulsation insertion before versus after primary percutaneous coronary intervention for cardiogenic shock complicating acute myocardial infarction. *Am J Cardiol*, 2010; 105(7): 967–971.

97 Thiele H, Sick P, Boudriot E, et al. Randomized comparison of intra-aortic balloon support with a percutaneous left ventricular assist device in patients with revascularized acute myocardial infarction complicated by cardiogenic shock. *Eur Heart J*, 2005; 26(13): 1276–1283.

2

European Society of Cardiology and American College of Cardiology STEMI Guidelines

Estefania Oliveros MD, Sameer Mehta MD FACC, Alexandra Ferré MD, Tracy Zhang BS, Michael Schweitzer MD, Miguel Vega Arango MD, Juanita Gonzalez Arango MD, Maria Botero Urrea MD, Maria Teresa Bedoya Reina MD, Isaac Yepes MD

Introduction

Guidelines for ST elevation myocardial infarction (STEMI) interventions have been changing dynamically since 2000. A sense of this fast-pace of updates can be gauged from the fact that, in less than a decade, the 2004 guidelines were updated twice, in 2007 and 2009. If the list of recommendations includes both the American College of Cardiology (ACC) and the European Society of Cardiology (ESC) Task Force guidelines, the task for a physician to master these essentials becomes overwhelming. The 2013 American College of Cardiology Foundation (ACCF)/American Heart Association (AHA) STEMI guideline was published with extensive collaboration from the 2011 ACCF/AHA/Society for Cardiovascular Angiography and Interventions Percutaneous Coronary Interventions writing group and numerous reviewers from different healthcare organizations. A new separation in the class III recommendation was added which includes "no benefit" or association with "harm". There is emphasis on reperfusion strategies, organization or regional systems of care, transfer algorithms, antithrombotic therapies, and secondary prevention care.

This chapter has been compiled with the straightforward aim of bringing this invaluable information together in a tabulated, easy to read format that highlights the major changes to the guidelines. We claim little credit for composing this chapter as it is essentially the outstanding work of the ACC and AHA Task Force – we have only made changes to make it easier to read. We also strongly felt that the inclusion of these guidelines in a textbook on STEMI interventions was important and that it would enable the entire information on STEMI interventions to be available to the reader in a single textbook.

Fifteen tables (Tables 2.1–2.15) have been created to facilitate this process and the authors hope that the chapter will serve as a useful tool to understand the STEMI guidelines. The tables summarize the essential information and highlight specific updates to the older guidelines. Figure 2.1 shows an algorithm for triage and transfer for percutaneous coronary intervention. Sample references have been included.

Manual of STEMI Interventions, First Edition. Edited by Sameer Mehta.
© 2017 John Wiley & Sons Ltd. Published 2017 by John Wiley & Sons Ltd.

Table 2.1 Classification of recommendations and levels of evidence.

SIZE OF TREATMENT EFFECT

Level	Class			
	I	IIa	IIb	III
	Benefit >>> Risk Procedure/treatment SHOULD be performed/administered	*Benefit >> Risk* *Additional studies with focused objectives needed;* IT IS REASONABLE to perform procedure/administer treatment	*Benefit ≥ Risk* *Additional studies with broad objectives needed; additional registry data would be helpful* Procedure/treatment MAY BE CONSIDERED	*No benefit or Harm* COR III: No benefit — Not helpful — No proven benefit COR III: Harm — Excess cost w/o benefit or harmful — Harmful to patients
A Multiple populations evaluated Data derived from multiple randomized clinical trials or meta-analysis	Recommendation that procedure or treatment is useful/effective Sufficient evidence from multiple randomized trials or meta-analyses	Recommendation in favor of treatment or procedure being useful/effective Some conflicting evidence from multiple randomized trials or meta-analyses	Recommendation's usefulness/efficacy less well established Greater conflicting evidence from multiple randomized trials or meta-analyses	Recommendation that procedure or treatment is not useful/effective an may be harmful Sufficient evidence from multiple randomized trials or meta-analyses
B Limited populations evaluated Data derived from a single randomized trial or nonrandomized studies	Recommendation that procedure or treatment is useful/effective Evidence from single randomized trial or nonrandomized studies	Recommendation in favor of treatment or procedure being useful/effective Some conflicting evidence from single randomized trial or nonrandomized studies	Recommendation's usefulness/efficacy less well established Greater conflicting evidence from single randomized trial or nonrandomized studies	Recommendation that procedure or treatment is not useful/effective an may be harmful Evidence from single randomized trial or nonrandomized studies
C Very limited populations evaluated Only consensus opinion of experts, case studies, or standard of care	Recommendation that procedure or treatment is useful/effective Only expert opinion, case studies, or standard of care	Recommendation in favor of treatment or procedure being useful/effective Only diverging expert opinion, case studies, or standard of care	Recommendation's usefulness/efficacy less well established Only diverging expert opinion, case studies, or standard of care	Recommendation that procedure or treatment is not useful/effective an may be harmful Only expert opinion, case studies, or standard of care

ESTIMATE OF CERTAINTY (PRECISION) OF TREATMENT EFFECT

			COR III: No benefit	COR III: Harm
Suggested phrases for writing recommendations	should is recommended is indicated is useful/effective/beneficial	is reasonable can be useful/effective/beneficial is probably recommended or indicated	may/might be considered may/might be reasonable usefulness/effectiveness is unknown/unclear/uncertain or not well established	is nor recommended is not indicated should not be performed/administered/other	potentially harmful causes harm associated with excess morbidity/mortality should not be performed/administered/other
Comparative effectiveness phrases	treatment/strategy A is recommended/indicated in preference to treatment B treatment A should be chosen over treatment B	treatment/strategy A is probably recommended/indicated in preference to treatment B it is reasonable to choose treatment A over treatment B			

Table 2.2 Recommendations for the use of glycoprotein IIb/IIIa receptor antagonists.

2009 Joint STEMI/PCI Focused Update Recommendations	2013 Recommendations	Level of evidence	Comments
Class IIA			
	Start intravenous GP IIb/IIIa receptor antagonist such as abciximab [1–3], high-bolus-dose tirofiban [4,5], or double-bolus eptifibatide [6] at the time of primary PCI (with or without stenting or clopidogrel pretreatment) in selected patients with STEMI who are receiving unfractionated heparin.	A, B, B	Modified: changed from IIb to IIa for tirofiban and eptifibatide.
Class IIB			
The usefulness of glycoprotein IIb/IIIa receptor antagonists (as part of a preparatory pharmacological strategy for patients with STEMI before their arrival in the cardiac catheterization laboratory for angiography and PCI) is uncertain [8,10].	Administer intravenous GP IIb/IIIa receptor antagonist in the pre-catheterization laboratory setting (e.g., ambulance, emergency department) to patients with STEMI for whom primary PCI is intended [4,7–14].	B	Modified text.
	It may be reasonable to administer intracoronary abciximab to patients with STEMI undergoing primary PCI [15–22].	B	

GP, glycoprotein; PCI, percutaneous coronary intervention.

Table 2.3 Recommendations for the use of thienopyridines.

2009 Joint STEMI/PCI Focused Update Recommendations	Level of evidence	2013 Recommendations	Level of evidence	Comments
Class I				
A loading dose of thienopyridine is recommended for STEMI patients for whom PCI is planned. Regimens should be one of the following:		A loading dose of a P2Y12 receptor inhibitor should be given as early as possible or at time of primary PCI to patients with STEMI. Options include:	B	Modified: changed text loading doses and level of evidence.
a) At least 300–600 mg of clopidogrel should be given as early as possible before or at the time of primary or nonprimary PCI.	C	a) clopidogrel 600 mg [23–25]; or		
b) Prasugrel 60 mg should be given as soon as possible for primary PCI [26,27].	B	b) prasugrel 60 mg [26]; or		
c) For STEMI patients undergoing nonprimary PCI, the following regimens are recommended:		c) ticagrelor 180 mg [27].		
(i) If the patient has received fibrinolytic therapy and has been given clopidogrel, clopidogrel should be continued as the thienopyridine of choice.	C			
(ii) If the patient has received fibrinolytic therapy without a thienopyridine, a loading dose of 300–600 mg of clopidogrel should be given as the thienopyridine of choice.	C			
(iii) If the patient did not receive fibrinolytic therapy, either a loading dose of 300–600 mg of clopidogrel should be given or, once the coronary anatomy is known and PCI is planned, a loading dose of 60 mg of prasugrel should be given promptly and no later than 1 hour after PCI [26,27].	B			
The duration of thienopyridine therapy should be as follows:		P2Y12 inhibitor therapy should be given for 1 year to patients with STEMI who receive a stent (BMS or DES) during primary PCI using the following maintenance doses:	B	Modified recommendation C to B (based on TRITON-TIMI 38), then added ticagrelor.
a) In patients receiving a stent (BMS or DES) during PCI for ACS, clopidogrel 75 mg daily [27–29] or prasugrel 10 mg daily [27] should be given for at least 12 months.	B	a) clopidogrel 75 mg daily [26,28]; or		
b) If the risk of morbidity because of bleeding outweighs the anticipated benefit afforded by thienopyridine therapy, earlier discontinuation should be considered.	C	b) prasugrel 10 mg daily [28]; or		
Continuation of clopidogrel or prasugrel beyond 15 months may be considered in patients undergoing DES placement [27].	C	c) ticagrelor 90 mg twice a day [27].		Modified: changed text.
Class III				
In STEMI patients with a prior history of stroke and transient ischemic attack for whom primary PCI is planned, prasugrel is not recommended as part of a dual antiplatelet therapy regimen.	C	Prasugrel should not be administered to patients with a history of prior stroke or transient ischemic attack [26].	B	Modified: changed text and level of evidence.

ACS, acute coronary syndrome; BMS, bare-metal stent; DES, drug-eluting stent; PCI, percutaneous coronary intervention.

Table 2.4 Recommendations for the use of parenteral anticoagulants.

2009 Joint STEMI/PCI Focused Update Recommendations	Level of evidence	2013 Recommendations	Level of evidence	Comments
Class I				
For patients proceeding to primary PCI who have been treated with ASA and a thienopyridine, recommended supportive anticoagulant regimens include the following:		For patients with STEMI undergoing primary PCI, the following supportive anticoagulant regimens are recommended:		Modified recommendation: bivalirudin was added as an acceptable anticoagulant for primary PCI; text about UFH was modified to mention activated clotting time levels. Recommendations on enoxaparin and fondaparinux were unchanged).
a) For prior treatment with UFH, additional boluses of UFH should be administered as needed to maintain therapeutic activated clotting time levels, taking into account whether GP IIb/IIIa receptor antagonists have been administered.	C	a) UFH, with additional boluses administered as needed to maintain therapeutic activated clotting time levels, taking into account whether a GP IIb/IIIa receptor antagonist has been administered; or	C	
b) Bivalirudin is useful as a supportive measure for primary PCI with or without prior treatment with UFH [9].	C	b) Bivalirudin with or without prior treatment with UFH.	B	
In STEMI patients undergoing PCI who are at high risk of bleeding, bivalirudin anticoagulation is reasonable [9].	B			
Class II				
		In patients with STEMI undergoing PCI who are at high risk of bleeding, it is reasonable to use bivalirudin monotherapy in preference to the combination of UFH and a GP IIb/IIIa receptor antagonist.	B	
Class III				
		Fondaparinux should not be used as the sole anticoagulant to support primary PCI because of the risk of catheter thrombosis.	B	

ASA, acetylsalicylic acid (aspirin); GP, glycoprotein; PCI, percutaneous coronary intervention; UFH, unfractionated heparin.

Table 2.5 Recommendations for triage and transfer for percutaneous coronary intervention.

2009 Joint STEMI/PCI Focused Update Recommendations	Level of evidence	2013 Recommendations	Level of evidence	Comments
Class I				
Each community should develop a STEMI system of care that follows standards at least as stringent as those developed for the AHA's national initiative. Mission: Lifeline, to include the following: Ongoing multidisciplinary team meetings that include emergency medical services, non–PCI-capable hospitals/STEMI referral centers, and PCI-capable hospitals/STEMI receiving centers to evaluate outcomes and quality improvement data. A process for pre-hospital identification and activation. Destination protocols for STEMI receiving centers. Transfer protocols for patients who arrive at STEMI referral centers who are primary PCI candidates, ineligible for fibrinolytic drugs, and/or in cardiogenic shock.	C	All communities should create and maintain a regional system of STEMI care that includes assessment and continuous quality improvement of EMS and hospital-based activities. Performance can be facilitated by participating in programs such as Mission: Lifeline and the D2B Alliance [29–32].	B	Modified level of evidence C to B.
		Performance of a 12-lead ECG by EMS personnel at the site of first medical contact is recommended in patients with symptoms consistent with STEMI [32–36].	B	New
		Reperfusion therapy should be administered to all eligible patients with STEMI with symptom onset within the prior 12 hours [37,38].	A	
		Primary PCI is the recommended method of reperfusion when it can be performed in a timely fashion by experienced operators [38–40].	A	
		EMS transport directly to a PCI-capable hospital for primary PCI is the recommended triage strategy for patients with STEMI, with an ideal FMC-to-device time system goal of 90 minutes or less [32,35,36].	B	Changed from D2B to FMC to device.
		Immediate transfer to a PCI-capable hospital for primary PCI is the recommended triage strategy for patients with STEMI who initially arrive at or are transported to a non-PCI-capable hospital, with an FMC-to-device time system goal of 120 minutes or less [39–42].	B	

(Continued)

Table 2.5 (Continued)

2009 Joint STEMI/PCI Focused Update Recommendations	Level of evidence	2013 Recommendations	Level of evidence	Comments
		In the absence of contraindications, fibrinolytic therapy should be administered to patients with STEMI at non-PCI-capable hospitals when the anticipated FMC-to-device time at a PCI-capable hospital exceeds 120 minutes because of unavoidable delays [37,43,44].	B	
		When fibrinolytic therapy is indicated or chosen as the primary reperfusion strategy, it should be administered within 30 minutes of hospital arrival [45].	B	
		In the absence of contraindications, fibrinolytic therapy should be given to patients with STEMI and onset of ischemic symptoms within the previous 12 hours when it is anticipated that primary PCI cannot be performed within 120 minutes of FMC [37].		
Class IIA				
It is reasonable for high-risk patients who receive fibrinolytic therapy as primary reperfusion therapy at a non–PCI-capable facility to be transferred as soon as possible to a PCI-capable facility where PCI can be performed either when needed or as a pharmacoinvasive strategy. Consideration should be given to initiating a preparatory antithrombotic (anticoagulant plus antiplatelet) regimen before and during patient transfer to the catheterization laboratory [14,15].	B	In the absence of contraindications and when PCI is not available, fibrinolytic therapy is reasonable for patients with STEMI if there is clinical and/or electrocardiographic evidence of ongoing ischemia within 12–24 hours of symptom onset and a large area of myocardium at risk or hemodynamic instability.	C	
		Reperfusion therapy is reasonable for patients with STEMI and symptom onset within the prior 12–24 hours who have clinical and/or ECG evidence of ongoing ischemia. Primary PCI is the preferred strategy in this population [36,46,47].		

Class IIB

Patients who are not at high risk who receive fibrinolytic therapy as primary reperfusion therapy at a non-PCI-capable facility may be considered for transfer as soon as possible to a PCI-capable facility where PCI can be performed either when needed or as a pharmacoinvasive strategy. Consideration should be given to initiating a preparatory antithrombotic (anticoagulant plus antiplatelet) regimen before and during patient transfer to the catheterization laboratory.

B

Modified: changed text.

Class III

Fibrinolytic therapy should not be administered to patients with ST-segment depression except when a true posterior (inferobasal) MI is suspected or when associated with ST-elevation in aVR lead [16].

B

AHA, American Heart Association; D2B, door to balloon; ECG, echocardiogram; EMC, emergency medical services; FMC, first medical contact; PCI, percutaneous coronary intervention.

Table 2.6 Recommendations for intensive glucose control in STEMI.

2009 Joint STEMI/PCI Focused Update Recommendations	Level of evidence	
Class IIA		
It is reasonable to use an insulin-based regimen to achieve and maintain glucose levels less than 180 mg/dl while avoiding hypoglycemia for patients with STEMI with either a complicated or uncomplicated course [16].	B	No changes since 2009.

Table 2.7 Recommendations for thrombus aspiration during percutaneous coronary interventions (PCI) for STEMI.

2009 Joint STEMI/PCI Focused Update Recommendations	Level of evidence	
Class IIA		
Aspiration thrombectomy is reasonable for patients undergoing primary PCI [17,18].	B	No changes since 2009.

Table 2.8 Recommendations for the use of stents in STEMI.

2009 Joint STEMI/PCI Focused Update Recommendations	Level of evidence	2013 Recommendations	Level of evidence	Comments
Class I				
		BMS should be used in patients with high bleeding risk, inability to comply with 1 year of DAPT, or anticipated invasive or surgical procedures in the next year.	C	New
It is reasonable to use a DES as an alternative to a BMS for primary PCI in STEMI [11,105].	B		A	Modified recommendation from class IIa, level of evidence B to class I, level of evidence A.
A DES may be considered for clinical and anatomic settings in which the efficacy/safety profile appears favorable [16].	B	Placement of a stent (BMS or DES) is useful in primary PCI for patients with STEMI [48,49].	B	
Class III: Harm				
		DES should not be used in primary PCI for patients with STEMI who are unable to tolerate or comply with a prolonged course of DAPT because of the increased risk of stent thrombosis with premature discontinuation of one or both agents [50–56].	B	New

BMS, bare-metal stent; DAPT, dual antiplatelet therapy; DES, drug-eluting stent; PCI, percutaneous coronary intervention

Table 2.9 Recommendation for angiography in patients with chronic kidney disease.

2009 Joint STEMI/PCI Focused Update Recommendations	Level of evidence	2013 Recommendations	Level of evidence	Comments
Class I				
In chronic kidney disease patients undergoing angiography, isosmolar contrast agents are indicated and are preferred.	A	In patients with chronic kidney disease undergoing angiography who are not having chronic dialysis, either an isosmolar contrast medium. (level of evidence A) or a low molecular weight contrast medium other than ioxaglate or iohexol is indicated [19].	B	Modified: changed text.

Table 2.10 Recommendations for the use of fractional flow reserve.

2009 PCI Focused Update Recommendation	Level of evidence	Comments
Coronary pressure (FFR) or Doppler velocimetry can be useful to determine whether PCI of a specific coronary lesion is warranted. FFR or Doppler velocimetry can also be useful as an alternative to performing noninvasive functional testing (e.g., when the functional study is absent or ambiguous) to determine whether an intervention is warranted. It is reasonable to use intracoronary physiological measurements (coronary pressure, FFR) [20] or Doppler velocimetry in the assessment of the effects of intermediate coronary stenoses (30–70% luminal narrowing) in patients with symptoms of angina.	A, C	Modified recommendation: level of evidence changed from B to A for FFR; C for Doppler.
Routine assessment with intracoronary physiological measurements such as coronary pressure (FFR) or Doppler ultrasound to assess the severity of angiographic disease in concordant vascular distribution in patients with angina and a positive, unequivocal noninvasive functional study is not recommended.	C	Modified recommendation.

FFR, fractional flow reserve; PCI, percutaneous coronary intervention

Table 2.11 Recommendations for percutaneous coronary interventions (PCI) for unprotected left main coronary artery disease.

2009 Joint STEMI/PCI Focused Update Recommendations	Level of evidence	
Class IIB		
PCI of the left main coronary artery with stents as an alternative to coronary artery bypass graft may be considered in patients with anatomic conditions that are associated with a low risk of PCI procedural complications and clinical conditions that predict an increased risk of adverse surgical outcomes [21].	B	New

Table 2.12 Antiplatelet therapy to support primary percutaneous coronary interventions (PCI) for STEMI.

European Society of Cardiology	2013	Level of evidence
Class I		
Aspirin 150–300 mg initially	Aspirin 162–325 mg should be given before primary PCI [25,57,58].	B
	After PCI, aspirin should be continued indefinitely [59,60].	A
Class IIA		
After PCI, aspirin 100 mg a day	It is reasonable to use 81 mg of aspirin/day in preference to higher maintenance doses after primary PCI [25,59,61,62].	B

Table 2.13 Antiplatelet and anticoagulant therapy discussed in the 2013 American Heart Association (AHA) and European Society of Cardiology (ESC) guidelines to support percutaneous coronary interventions in STEMI.

Recommendations	ACC/AHA	ESC
Aspirin	IB	IB
Thienopyridines:	IB	IB
prasugrel	IB	IB
ticagrelor	IB	IC
clopidogrel		
Anti-GP IIb/IIIa if there is massive thrombus in angiography, slow, no-reflow, or thrombotic complications		IIaC
Anti-GP IIb/IIIa inhibitor with UFH	IIA	IIbB
Pre-hospital anti-GP IIb/IIa:	IIaA	IIbA
abciximab	IIaB	IIbB
eptifibatide	IIaB	IIbB
tirofiban		
Bivalirudin	IB	IB
Enoxaparin	–	IIbB
UFH	IC	IC
Fondaparinux	IIIB	IIIB

GP, glycoprotein; UFH, unfractionated heparin.

Table 2.14 Evaluation and management of patients with STEMI and out-of-hospital cardiac arrest.

2013 Recommendations	Level of evidence	
Class IB		
Therapeutic hypothermia should be started as soon as possible in comatose patients with STEMI and out-of-hospital cardiac arrest caused by ventricular fibrillation or pulseless ventricular tachycardia, including patients who undergo primary PCI [63,64].	B	New
Immediate angiography and PCI when indicated should be performed in resuscitated out-of-hospital cardiac arrest patients whose initial EKG shows STEMI [65–70].		

EKG, electrocardiogram; PCI, percutaneous coronary intervention.

Table 2.15 Primary percutaneous coronary interventions and STEMI.

2013 Recommendations	Level of evidence	
Class I		
Primary PCI should be performed in patients with STEMI and ischemic symptoms of less than 12 hours' duration [38,71,72].	A	New
Primary PCI should be performed in patients with STEMI and ischemic symptoms of less than 12 hours' duration who have contraindications to fibrinolytic therapy, irrespective of the time delay from first medical contact [73,74].	B	
Primary PCI should be performed in patients with STEMI and cardiogenic shock or acute severe heart failure, irrespective of time delay from MI onset [75–80].	B	
Class IIA		
Primary PCI is reasonable in patients with STEMI if there is clinical and/or EKG evidence of ongoing ischemia between 12 and 24 hours after symptom onset [46,47].	B	New
Class III		
PCI should not be performed in a non-infarct artery at the time of primary PCI in patients with STEMI who are hemodynamically stable [79–81].	B	New

MI, myocardial infarction; PCI, percutaneous coronary intervention.

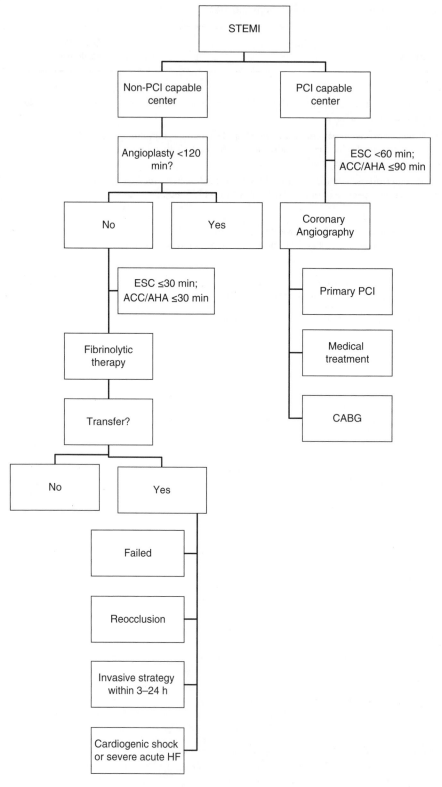

Figure 2.1 Triage and transfer for PCI.

References

1 Brener SJ, Barr LA, Burchenal JE, et al. Randomized, placebo-controlled trial of platelet glycoprotein IIb/IIIa blockade with primary angioplasty for acute myocardial infarction. ReoPro and Primary PTCA Organization and Randomized Trial (RAPPORT) Investigators. *Circulation*, 1998; 98(8): 734–741.

2 Stone GW, Grines CL, Cox DA, et al. Comparison of angioplasty with stenting, with or without abciximab, in acute myocardial infarction. *N Engl J Med*, 2002; 346(13): 957–966.

3 Montalescot G, Barragan P, Wittenberg O, et al. Platelet glycoprotein IIb/IIIa inhibition with coronary stenting for acute myocardial infarction. *N Engl J Med*, 2001; 344(25): 1895–1903.

4 ten Berg JM, van't Hof AW, Dill T, et al. Effect of early, pre-hospital initiation of high bolus dose tirofiban in patients with ST-segment elevation myocardial infarction on short- and long-term clinical outcome. *J Am Coll Cardiol*, 2010; 55(22): 2446–2455.

5 Valgimigli M, Campo G, Percoco G, et al. Comparison of angioplasty with infusion of tirofiban or abciximab and with implantation of sirolimus-eluting or uncoated stents for acute myocardial infarction: the MULTISTRATEGY randomized trial. *JAMA*, 2008; 299(15): 1788–1799.

6 Akerblom A, James SK, Koutouzis M, et al. Eptifibatide is noninferior to abciximab in primary percutaneous coronary intervention: results from the SCAAR (Swedish Coronary Angiography and Angioplasty Registry). *J Am Coll Cardiol*, 2010; 56(6): 470–475.

7 Ellis SG, Armstrong P, Betriu A, et al. Facilitated percutaneous coronary intervention versus primary percutaneous coronary intervention: design and rationale of the Facilitated Intervention with Enhanced Reperfusion Speed to Stop Events (FINESSE) trial. *Am Heart J*, 2004; 147(4): E16.

8 Ellis SG, Tendera M, de Belder MA, et al. 1-year survival in a randomized trial of facilitated reperfusion: results from the FINESSE (Facilitated Intervention with Enhanced Reperfusion Speed to Stop Events) trial. *JACC Cardiovasc Interv*, 2009; 2(10): 909–916.

9 Montalescot G, Borentain M, Payot L, et al. Early vs late administration of glycoprotein IIb/IIIa inhibitors in primary percutaneous coronary intervention of acute ST-segment elevation myocardial infarction: a meta-analysis. *JAMA*, 2004; 292(3): 362–366.

10 Maioli M, Bellandi F, Leoncini M, et al. Randomized early versus late abciximab in acute myocardial infarction treated with primary coronary intervention (RELAx-AMI Trial). *J Am Coll Cardiol*, 2007; 49(14): 1517–1524.

11 Keeley EC, Boura JA, Grines CL. Comparison of primary and facilitated percutaneous coronary interventions for ST-elevation myocardial infarction: quantitative review of randomised trials. *Lancet*, 2006; 367(9510): 579–588.

12 Van't Hof AW, Ten Berg J, Heestermans T, et al. Prehospital initiation of tirofiban in patients with ST-elevation myocardial infarction undergoing primary angioplasty (On-TIME 2): a multicentre, double-blind, randomised controlled trial. *Lancet*, 2008; 372(9638): 537–546.

13 El Khoury C, Dubien PY, Mercier C, et al. Prehospital high-dose tirofiban in patients undergoing primary percutaneous intervention. The AGIR-2 study. *Arch Cardiovasc Dis*, 2010; 103(5): 285–292.

14 G DEL, Bellandi F, Huber K, et al. Early glycoprotein IIb-IIIa inhibitors in primary angioplasty-abciximab long-term results (EGYPT-ALT) cooperation: individual patient's data meta-analysis. *J Thromb and Haemost*, 2011; 9(12): 2361–2370.

15 Stone GW, Maehara A, Witzenbichler B, et al. Intracoronary abciximab and aspiration thrombectomy in patients with large anterior myocardial infarction: the INFUSE-AMI randomized trial. *JAMA*, 2012; 307(17): 1817–1826.

16 Mehilli J, Kastrati A, Schulz S, et al. Abciximab in patients with acute ST-segment-elevation myocardial infarction undergoing primary percutaneous coronary intervention after clopidogrel loading: a randomized double-blind trial. *Circulation*, 2009; 119(14): 1933–1940.

17 Bellandi F, Maioli M, Gallopin M, et al. Increase of myocardial salvage and left ventricular function recovery with intracoronary abciximab downstream of the coronary occlusion in patients with acute myocardial infarction treated with primary coronary intervention. *Catheter Cardiovasc Interv*, 2004; 62(2): 186–192.

18 Romagnoli E, Burzotta F, Trani C, et al. Angiographic evaluation of the effect of intracoronary abciximab administration in patients undergoing urgent PCI. *Int J Cardiol*, 2005; 105(3): 250–255.

19 Iversen A, Galatius S, Jensen JS. The optimal route of administration of the glycoprotein IIb/IIIa receptor antagonist abciximab during percutaneous coronary intervention; intravenous versus intracoronary. *Curr Cardiol Rev*, 2008; 4(4): 293–299.

20 Kakkar AK, Moustapha A, Hanley HG, et al. Comparison of intracoronary vs. intravenous administration of abciximab in coronary stenting. *Catheter Cardiovasc Interv*, 2004; 61(1): 31–34.

21 Wohrle J, Grebe OC, Nusser T, et al. Reduction of major adverse cardiac events with intracoronary compared with intravenous bolus application of abciximab in patients with acute myocardial infarction or unstable angina undergoing coronary angioplasty. *Circulation*, 2003; 107(14): 1840–1843.

22 Bertrand OF, Rodes-Cabau J, Larose E, et al. Intracoronary compared to intravenous abciximab and high-dose bolus compared to standard dose in patients with ST-segment elevation myocardial infarction undergoing transradial primary percutaneous coronary intervention: a two-by-two factorial placebo-controlled randomized study. *Am J Cardiol*, 2010; 105(11): 1520–1527.

23 Investigators CO, Mehta SR, Bassand JP, et al. Dose comparisons of clopidogrel and aspirin in acute coronary syndromes. *N Engl J Med*, 2010; 363(10): 930–942.

24 Patti G, Barczi G, Orlic D, et al. Outcome comparison of 600- and 300-mg loading doses of clopidogrel in patients undergoing primary percutaneous coronary intervention for ST-segment elevation myocardial infarction: results from the ARMYDA-6 MI (Antiplatelet therapy for Reduction of MYocardial Damage during Angioplasty-Myocardial Infarction) randomized study. *J Am Coll Cardiol*, 2011; 58(15): 1592–1599.

25 Mehta SR, Tanguay JF, Eikelboom JW, et al. Double-dose versus standard-dose clopidogrel and high-dose versus low-dose aspirin in individuals undergoing percutaneous coronary intervention for acute coronary syndromes (CURRENT-OASIS 7): a randomized factorial trial. *Lancet*, 2010; 376(9748): 1233–1243.

26 Wiviott SD, Braunwald E, McCabe CH, et al. Prasugrel versus clopidogrel in patients with acute coronary syndromes. *N Engl J Med*, 2007; 357(20): 2001–2015.

27 Steg PG, James S, Harrington RA, et al. Ticagrelor versus clopidogrel in patients with ST-elevation acute coronary syndromes intended for reperfusion with primary percutaneous coronary intervention: a platelet inhibition and patient outcomes (PLATO) trial subgroup analysis. *Circulation*, 2010; 122(21): 2131–2141.

28 Montalescot G, Wiviott SD, Braunwald E, et al. Prasugrel compared with clopidogrel in patients undergoing percutaneous coronary intervention for ST-elevation myocardial infarction (TRITON-TIMI 38): double-blind, randomised controlled trial. *Lancet*, 2009; 373(9665): 723–731.

29 Aguirre FV, Varghese JJ, Kelley MP, et al. Rural interhospital transfer of ST-elevation myocardial infarction patients for percutaneous coronary revascularization: the Stat Heart Program. *Circulation*, 2008; 117(9): 1145–1152.

30 Henry TD, Sharkey SW, Burke MN, et al. A regional system to provide timely access to percutaneous coronary intervention for ST-elevation myocardial infarction. *Circulation*. 2007; 116(7): 721–728.

31 Jollis JG, Roettig ML, Aluko AO, et al. Implementation of a statewide system for coronary reperfusion for ST-segment elevation myocardial infarction. *JAMA*, 2007; 298(20): 2371–2380.

32 Le May MR, So DY, Dionne R, et al. A citywide protocol for primary PCI in ST-segment elevation myocardial infarction. *N Engl J Med*, 2008; 358(3): 231–240.

33 Dieker HJ, Liem SS, El Aidi H, et al. Pre-hospital triage for primary angioplasty: direct referral to the intervention center versus interhospital transport. *JACC Cardiovasc Interv*, 2010; 3(7): 705–711.

34 Diercks DB, Kontos MC, Chen AY, et al. Utilization and impact of pre-hospital electrocardiograms for patients with acute ST-segment elevation myocardial infarction: data from the NCDR (National Cardiovascular Data Registry) ACTION (Acute Coronary Treatment and Intervention Outcomes Network) Registry. *J Am Coll Cardiol*, 2009; 53(2): 161–166.

35 Rokos IC, French WJ, Koenig WJ, et al. Integration of pre-hospital electrocardiograms and ST-elevation myocardial infarction receiving center (SRC) networks: impact on Door-to-Balloon times across 10 independent regions. *JACC Cardiovasc Interv*, 2009; 2(4): 339–346.

36 Sorensen JT, Terkelsen CJ, Norgaard BL, et al. Urban and rural implementation of pre-hospital diagnosis and direct referral for primary percutaneous coronary intervention in patients with acute ST–elevation myocardial infarction. *Eur Heart J*, 2011; 32(4): 430–436.

37 Indications for fibrinolytic therapy in suspected acute myocardial infarction: collaborative overview of early mortality and major morbidity results from all randomised trials of more than 1000 patients. Fibrinolytic Therapy Trialists' (FTT) Collaborative Group. *Lancet*, 1994; 343(8893): 311–322.

38 Keeley EC, Boura JA, Grines CL. Primary angioplasty versus intravenous thrombolytic therapy for acute myocardial infarction: a quantitative review of 23 randomised trials. *Lancet*, 2003; 361(9351): 13–20.

39 Andersen HR, Nielsen TT, Vesterlund T, et al. Danish multicenter randomized study on fibrinolytic therapy versus acute coronary angioplasty in acute myocardial infarction: rationale and design of the DANish trial in Acute Myocardial Infarction-2 (DANAMI-2). *Am Heart J*, 2003; 146(2): 234–241.

40 Dalby M, Bouzamondo A, Lechat P, Montalescot G. Transfer for primary angioplasty versus immediate thrombolysis in acute myocardial infarction: a meta-analysis. *Circulation*. 2003; 108(15): 1809–1814.

41 Andersen HR, Nielsen TT, Rasmussen K, et al. A comparison of coronary angioplasty with fibrinolytic therapy in acute myocardial infarction. *N Engl J Med*, 2003; 349(8): 733–742.

42 Nielsen PH, Terkelsen CJ, Nielsen TT, et al. System delay and timing of intervention in acute myocardial infarction (from the Danish Acute Myocardial Infarction-2 [DANAMI-2] trial). *Am J Cardiol*, 2011; 108(6): 776–781.

43 Nallamothu BK, Bates ER. Percutaneous coronary intervention versus fibrinolytic therapy in acute myocardial infarction: is timing (almost) everything? *Am J Cardiol*, 2003; 92(7): 824–826.

44 Pinto DS, Kirtane AJ, Nallamothu BK, et al. Hospital delays in reperfusion for ST-elevation myocardial infarction: implications when selecting a reperfusion strategy. *Circulation*, 2006; 114(19): 2019–2025.

45 Boersma E, Maas AC, Deckers JW, et al. Early thrombolytic treatment in acute myocardial infarction: reappraisal of the golden hour. *Lancet*, 1996; 348(9030): 771–775.

46 Schomig A, Mehilli J, Antoniucci D, et al. Mechanical reperfusion in patients with acute myocardial infarction presenting more than 12 hours from symptom onset: a randomized controlled trial. *JAMA*, 2005; 293(23): 2865–2872.

47 Gierlotka M, Gasior M, Wilczek K, et al. Reperfusion by primary percutaneous coronary intervention in patients with ST-segment elevation myocardial infarction within 12 to 24 hours of the onset of symptoms (from a prospective national observational study [PL-ACS]). *Am J Cardiol*, 2011; 107(4): 501–508.

48 Nordmann AJ, Hengstler P, Harr T, et al. Clinical outcomes of primary stenting versus balloon angioplasty in patients with myocardial infarction: a meta-analysis of randomized controlled trials. *Am J Med*, 2004; 116(4): 253–262.

49 Zhu MM, Feit A, Chadow H, et al. Primary stent implantation compared with primary balloon angioplasty for acute myocardial infarction: a meta-analysis of randomized clinical trials. *Am J Cardiol*, 2001; 88(3): 297–301.

50 Spertus JA, Kettelkamp R, Vance C, et al. Prevalence, predictors, and outcomes of premature discontinuation of thienopyridine therapy after drug-eluting stent placement: results from the PREMIER registry. *Circulation*, 2006; 113(24): 2803–2809.

51 Kaluza GL, Joseph J, Lee JR, et al. Catastrophic outcomes of noncardiac surgery soon after coronary stenting. *J Am Coll Cardiol*, 2000; 35(5): 1288–1294.

52 Grines CL, Bonow RO, Casey DE, Jr., et al. Prevention of premature discontinuation of dual antiplatelet therapy in patients with coronary artery stents: a science advisory from the American Heart Association, American College of Cardiology, Society for Cardiovascular Angiography and Interventions, American College of Surgeons, and American Dental Association, with representation from the American College of Physicians. *Circulation*, 2007; 115(6): 813–818.

53 Park DW, Park SW, Park KH, et al. Frequency of and risk factors for stent thrombosis after drug-eluting stent implantation during long-term follow-up. *Am J Cardiol*, 2006; 98(3): 352–356.

54 Jeremias A, Sylvia B, Bridges J, et al. Stent thrombosis after successful sirolimus-eluting stent implantation. *Circulation*, 2004; 109(16): 1930–1932.

55 Pfisterer M, Brunner-La Rocca HP, Buser PT, et al. Late clinical events after clopidogrel discontinuation may limit the benefit of drug-eluting stents: an observational study of drug-eluting versus bare-metal stents. *J Am Coll Cardiol*, 2006; 48(12): 2584–2591.

56 Nasser M, Kapeliovich M, Markiewicz W. Late thrombosis of sirolimus-eluting stents following noncardiac surgery. *Catheter Cardiovasc Interv*, 2005; 65(4): 516–519.

57 Jolly SS, Pogue J, Haladyn K, et al. Effects of aspirin dose on ischaemic events and bleeding after percutaneous coronary intervention: insights from the PCI-CURE study. *Eur Heart J*, 2009; 30(8): 900–907.

58 Barnathan ES, Schwartz JS, Taylor L, et al. Aspirin and dipyridamole in the prevention of acute coronary thrombosis complicating coronary angioplasty. *Circulation*, 1987; 76(1): 125–134.

59 Antithrombotic Trialists C. Collaborative meta-analysis of randomised trials of antiplatelet therapy for prevention of death, myocardial infarction, and stroke in high risk patients. *BMJ*, 2002; 324(7329): 71–86.

60 Schomig A, Neumann FJ, Kastrati A, et al. A randomized comparison of antiplatelet and anticoagulant therapy after the placement of coronary-artery stents. *N Engl J Med*, 1996; 334(17): 1084–1089.

61 Steinhubl SR, Bhatt DL, Brennan DM, et al. Aspirin to prevent cardiovascular disease: the association of aspirin dose and clopidogrel with thrombosis and bleeding. *Ann Intern Med*, 2009; 150(6): 379–386.

62 Serebruany VL, Steinhubl SR, Berger PB, et al. Analysis of risk of bleeding complications after different doses of aspirin in 192,036 patients enrolled in 31 randomized controlled trials. *Am J Cardiol*, 2005; 95(10): 1218–1222.

63 Bernard SA, Gray TW, Buist MD, et al. Treatment of comatose survivors of out-of-hospital cardiac arrest with induced hypothermia. *N Engl J Med*, 2002; 346(8): 557–563.

64 Hypothermia after Cardiac Arrest Study G. Mild therapeutic hypothermia to improve the neurologic outcome after cardiac arrest. *N Engl J Med*, 2002; 346(8): 549–556.

65 Nichol G, Aufderheide TP, Eigel B, et al. Regional systems of care for out-of-hospital cardiac arrest: A policy statement from the American Heart Association. *Circulation*, 2010; 121(5): 709–729.

66 Bendz B, Eritsland J, Nakstad AR, et al. Long-term prognosis after out-of-hospital cardiac arrest and primary percutaneous coronary intervention. *Resuscitation*, 2004; 63(1): 49–53.

67 Borger van der Burg AE, Bax JJ, Boersma E, et al. Impact of percutaneous coronary intervention or coronary artery bypass grafting on outcome after nonfatal cardiac arrest outside the hospital. *Am J Cardiol*, 2003; 91(7): 785–789.

68 Gorjup V, Radsel P, Kocjancic ST, et al. Acute ST-elevation myocardial infarction after successful cardiopulmonary resuscitation. *Resuscitation*, 2007;72(3):379–385.

69 Bulut S, Aengevaeren WR, Luijten HJ, et al. Successful out-of-hospital cardiopulmonary resuscitation: what is the optimal in-hospital treatment strategy? *Resuscitation*, 2000; 47(2): 155–161.

70 Werling M, Thoren AB, Axelsson C, Herlitz J. Treatment and outcome in post-resuscitation care after out-of-hospital cardiac arrest when a modern therapeutic approach was introduced. *Resuscitation*, 2007; 73(1): 40–45.

71 Zijlstra F, Hoorntje JC, de Boer MJ, et al. Long-term benefit of primary angioplasty as compared with thrombolytic therapy for acute myocardial infarction. *N Engl J Med*, 1999; 341(19): 1413–1419.

72 A clinical trial comparing primary coronary angioplasty with tissue plasminogen activator for acute myocardial infarction. The Global Use of Strategies to Open Occluded Coronary Arteries in Acute Coronary Syndromes (GUSTO IIb) Angioplasty Substudy Investigators. *N Engl J Med*, 1997; 336(23): 1621–1628.

73 Grzybowski M, Clements EA, Parsons L, et al. Mortality benefit of immediate revascularization of acute ST-segment elevation myocardial infarction in patients with contraindications to thrombolytic therapy: a propensity analysis. *JAMA*, 2003; 290(14): 1891–1898.

74 Zahn R, Schuster S, Schiele R, et al. Comparison of primary angioplasty with conservative therapy in patients with acute myocardial infarction and contraindications for thrombolytic therapy. Maximal Individual Therapy in Acute Myocardial Infarction (MITRA) Study Group. *Catheter Cardiovasc Interv*, 1999; 46(2): 127–133.

75 Hochman JS, Sleeper LA, Webb JG, et al. Early revascularization in acute myocardial infarction complicated by cardiogenic shock. SHOCK Investigators. Should We Emergently Revascularize Occluded Coronaries for Cardiogenic Shock. *N Engl J Med*, 1999; 341(9): 625–634.

76 Hochman JS, Lamas GA, Buller CE, et al. Coronary intervention for persistent occlusion after myocardial infarction. *N Engl J Med*, 2006; 355(23): 2395–2407.

77 Thune JJ, Hoefsten DE, Lindholm MG, et al. Simple risk stratification at admission to identify patients with reduced mortality from primary angioplasty. *Circulation*, 2005; 112(13): 2017–2021.

78 Wu AH, Parsons L, Every NR, et al., Second National Registry of Myocardial I. Hospital outcomes in patients presenting with congestive heart failure complicating acute myocardial infarction: a report from the Second National Registry of Myocardial Infarction (NRMI–2). *J Am Coll Cardiol*, 2002; 40(8): 1389–1394.

79 Hannan EL, Samadashvili Z, Walford G, et al. Culprit vessel percutaneous coronary intervention versus multivessel and staged percutaneous coronary intervention for ST-segment elevation myocardial infarction patients with multivessel disease. *JACC Cardiovasc Interv*, 2010; 3(1): 22–31.

80 Toma M, Buller CE, Westerhout CM, et al. Non-culprit coronary artery percutaneous coronary intervention during acute ST-segment elevation myocardial infarction: insights from the APEX-AMI trial. *Eur Heart J*, 2010; 31(14): 1701–1707.

81 Vlaar PJ, Mahmoud KD, Holmes DR, Jr., et al. Culprit vessel only versus multivessel and staged percutaneous coronary intervention for multivessel disease in patients presenting with ST-segment elevation myocardial infarction: a pairwise and network meta-analysis. *J Am Coll Cardiol*, 2011; 58(7): 692–703.

3

The Role of Thrombolytic Therapy in the Era of STEMI Interventions

Nestor Mercado MD, Theodore L. Schreiber MD, Cindy L. Grines MD

Introduction

Primary percutaneous coronary intervention (PCI) for ST-segment elevation myocardial infarction (STEMI) is defined as a strategy of emergent angiography followed by mechanical revascularization of the infarct-related artery (IRA) with a thrombectomy device or balloon catheter (with or without the subsequent placement of a coronary stent), without prior administration of thrombolytic therapy [1]. This approach is currently recommended by the American College of Cardiology Foundation/American Heart Association (ACCF/AHA) STEMI guidelines [2] as the preferred reperfusion strategy for STEMI patients within 12 hours of onset of symptoms when performed by an experienced team in a primary PCI-capable hospital in a timely fashion within 90 minutes from first medical contact. Primary PCI is performed in approximately 85% of STEMI cases that undergo coronary reperfusion in the United States; thrombolytic therapy in 9% and the combination of thrombolysis with primary PCI in 4% of STEMI cases [3]. Thrombolysis still has an important role in the predominant era of primary PCI, as this treatment strategy cannot be delivered to all STEMI patients within the recommended time frames, as a result of different logistic barriers.

In this chapter, we review the randomized clinical trial evidence supporting the use of primary PCI as the preferred treatment strategy for STEMI patients. We discuss the clinical benefit, risks and contraindications of thrombolytic therapy in STEMI and explore the clinical impact of time to reperfusion when selecting a reperfusion strategy and the potential limitations to the implementation of primary PCI as a universal reperfusion strategy for STEMI patients. Finally, we provide an evidence-based approach regarding the role of thrombolysis and the pharmacoinvasive approach in the current era of widespread primary PCI for STEMI treatment.

Thrombolytic Therapy: Clinical Benefit, Risks and Contraindications

There are four thrombolytic agents approved for clinical use in the United States (Table 3.1) [4,5]. These agents have been extensively studied over the past decades with GISSI-1 (Gruppo Italiano per lo Studio della Sopravvivenza nell'Infarto miocardico) and ISIS-2 (International Study of Infarct Survival) being the major landmark trials. These trials demonstrated a 26%

Table 3.1 Characteristics of thrombolytic therapy agents.

Agent	Streptokinase	Alteplase	Reteplase	Tenecteplase
Source	Group C streptococci	Recombinant, human	Recombinant, human	Recombinant, human
Molecular weight (kDA)	47	63–70	39	57
Metabolism	Hepatic	Hepatic	Renal	Hepatic
Mode of action	Activator complex	Direct	Direct	Direct
Antigenicity	Yes	No	No	No
Plasma half-life (minutes)	–	3.5	14	17
Plasma clearance (ml/minute)	–	572	283	151
Administration	Infusion 30–60 minutes	Bolus + infusion 90 minutes	Double bolus 90 minutes apart	Single bolus
Weight-adjusted dosing	No	Yes	No	No
Dose	1.5 mega units	<100 mg[a]	10 units + 10 units	30–50 mg[b]
Fibrin specificity[c]	None	++	+	+++
TIMI 3 at 90 minutes (% of patients)	32	54	60	63
Cost/dose (USD)	$300–613	$2,200–2,974	$2,200–2,750	$2,200–2,833

[a] Bolus 15 mg, infusion of 0.75 mg/kg for 30 minutes (maximum 50 mg), then 0.5 mg/kg not to exceed 35 mg over the next 60 minutes, to an overall maximum of 100 mg.
[b] 30 mg for weight < 60 kg; 35 mg for 60–69 kg; 40 mg for 70–79 kg; 45 mg for 80–89 kg; 50 mg for > 90 kg.
[c] Semiquantitative scale based on depletion of fibrinogen and other measures of systemic anticoagulation.

reduction in 30-day mortality among patients treated with streptokinase compared with placebo [6–8]. Streptokinase remains the most frequently used thrombolytic agent worldwide. However, since the GUSTO-1 (Global Use of Streptokinase and Tissue Plasminogen Activator for Occluded Coronary Arteries) trial demonstrated a further mortality reduction by accelerated or front-loaded (100 mg infusion over 90 minutes, with over half of the dose within 30 minutes) compared with streptokinase, front-loaded tissue plasminogen activator (tPA) became the gold standard for pharmacological reperfusion therapy [9]. An angiographic substudy demonstrated the relation between the patency of the initially occluded coronary artery and outcome [10]. During the 1990s, several wild-type tPA mutants were developed with less high-affinity fibrin capacity, a longer half-life, and therefore a greater thrombolytic potency. In phase II trials, the bolus injection of reteplase (rPA) was associated with more rapid and complete vessel patency than front-loaded tPA [11–13]. Subsequently, large phase III mortality trials failed to show superiority with rPA and demonstrated equivalent results with tenecteplase (TNK) when compared with tPA [14]. Altogether, the introduction of bolus thrombolytic agents did not result in a net clinical benefit. This said, the major advantage is that, today, thrombolytic agents are available with a similar efficacy and safety profile to that of front-loaded tPA, but are easier to administer as a bolus. Selection for thrombolysis in major hospitals is usually based on cost and drug availability, given the lack of significant differences in terms of safety and clinical efficacy of the four approved agents. Regardless of which thrombolytic agent used, aspirin, clopidogrel, and an anticoagulant such as heparin, enoxaparin, or fondaparinux are recommended (Table 3.2) [4].

Table 3.2 Guidelines recommending antithrombotic therapy with thrombolytic therapy.

Recommendation	Class	Level of Evidence
Antiplatelet therapy		
Aspirin:		
162–325 mg loading dose	I	A
81–325 mg daily maintenance dose (indefinite)	I	A
81 mg daily is the preferred maintenance dose	IIa	B
P2Y12 receptor inhibitors:		
Clopidogrel	I	A
Age ≤ 75 years: 300 mg loading dose		
Followed by 75 mg daily for at least 14 days and up to 1 year in absence of bleeding	I	A (14 days)
		C (up to 1 year)
Age > 75 years: no loading dose, give 75 mg	I	A
Followed by 75 mg daily for at least 14 days and up to 1 year in the absence of bleeding	I	A (14 days)
		C (up to 1 year)
Anticoagulant therapy		
UFH:		
Weight-based IV bolus and infusion adjusted to obtain aPTT of 1.5–2 times control for 48 hours or until revascularization. IV bolus of 60 units/kg (maximum 4000 units) followed by an infusion of 12 units/kg/hour (maximum 1000 units) initially, adjusted to maintain aPTT at 1.5–2 times control (approximately 50–70 seconds) for 48 hours or until revascularization	I	C
Enoxaparin:		
If age < 75 years: 30-mg IV bolus, followed in 15 minutes by 1 mg/kg subcutaneously every 12 hours (maximum 100 mg for the first 2 doses)	I	A
If age ≥ 75 years: no bolus, 0.75 mg/kg subcutaneously every 12 hours (maximum 75 mg for the first 2 doses)		
Regardless of age, if creatinine clearance < 30 ml/minute: 1 mg/kg subcutaneously every 24 hours		
Duration: For the index hospitalization, up to 8 days or until revascularization		
Fondaparinux:	I	B
Initial dose 2.5 mg IV, then 2.5 mg subcutaneously daily starting the following day, for the index hospitalization up to 8 days or until revascularization		
Contraindicated if creatinine clearance < 30 ml/minute		

aPTT, activated partial thromboplastin time; IV, intravenous.

The risks of thrombolysis are primarily related to bleeding complications or the subsequent development of intracranial hemorrhage. In a meta-analysis, the use of bolus thrombolytic agents was associated with an increased incidence of intracranial hemorrhage [15]. However, this increased risk was not evident in the group of patients treated with TNK-tPA or rPA compared with front-loaded tPA [16]. The intensity of anti-thrombin treatment also seems to be a confounding factor [16].

The risk of intracranial hemorrhage can be assessed before administering thrombolysis, using a multivariate model that incorporates clinical variables (older age, female gender, weight less than 70 kg, systolic blood pressure greater than 160 mmHg or diastolic blood pressure greater than 95 mmHg, prior stroke, international normalized ratio greater than 4 and use of tPA) that are predictive of intracranial hemorrhage [17]. It is generally accepted that patients with a high risk of intracranial hemorrhage should be treated with primary PCI [2]. Intracranial hemorrhage manifests clinically as an acute change in neurological status during the first 24 hours after treatment. Emergency non-contrast computed tomography of the head should be performed and if the diagnosis is confirmed, appropriate treatment with fresh frozen plasma, plasma and protamine should be considered, together with a neurological evaluation and other measures aimed to reduce the intracranial pressure.

Absolute Contraindications to Thrombolytic Therapy

The absolute contraindications to thrombolysis are any prior intracranial hemorrhage, known structural cerebral vascular lesion (such a s arteriovenous malformation), known malignant intracranial neoplasm (primary or metastatic), ischemic stroke within 4.5 hours (except acute ischemic stroke within 4.5 hours), suspected aortic dissection, active bleeding, or bleeding diathesis (excluding menses), significant closed head or facial trauma within 3 months, intracranial or intraspinal surgery within 2 months, severe uncontrolled hypertension (unresponsive to emergency therapy) and, for streptokinase, prior treatment within the previous 6 months.

Relative Contraindications to Thrombolytic Therapy

The absolute contraindications to thrombolysis are a history of chronic, severe, poorly controlled hypertension, significant hypertension on presentation (systolic blood pressure greater than 180 mmHg or diastolic blood pressure greater than 110 mmHg), history of prior ischemic stroke over 3 months, dementia, known intracranial pathology not covered in absolute contraindications, traumatic or prolonged (over 10 minutes) cardiopulmonary resuscitation, major surgery (less than 3 weeks), recent (within 2–4 weeks) internal bleeding, non-compressible vascular punctures, pregnancy, active peptic ulcer and oral anticoagulant therapy.

Primary PCI: Overview of Randomized Clinical Trials

Although thrombolytic therapy saves lives, it has limited efficacy at opening the vessel, with increased risk of intracranial bleeding, and many patients are considered ineligible for thrombolytics. Conversely, primary PCI has few contraindications, does not cause intracranial bleeding and opens over 90% of infarct-related arteries. In 2003, we performed a comprehensive meta-analysis of 23 randomized trials comparing primary PCI with balloon angioplasty or bare-metal stents (BMS) compared with thrombolysis for STEMI patients 18 (Figure 3.1). In this overview, primary PCI was associated with a lower short-term mortality (5% compared with 7%), lower incidence of nonfatal reinfarction (3% compared with 7%) and lower incidence of stroke (1% compared with 2%). Compared with thrombolytic therapy, primary PCI showed a 27% reduction in short-term mortality (an estimated survival benefit of 21 lives saved per 1000 patients treated). Primary PCI was also associated with a dramatically lower incidence of intracranial hemorrhage than thrombolysis (0.05% compared with 1.1%), but the overall risk of major bleeding (mostly related to access-site bleeding) was higher with PCI (7% compared with 5%). A lower risk of bleeding was noted in the 13 most recent trials, attributable to lower doses of intravenous heparin, smaller sheath sizes, and improved operator technique. The relative treatment effect appears to be similar across all subgroups of patients. Based on several trials, the current guidelines state that primary PCI is the preferred reperfusion strategy (Figure 3.1).

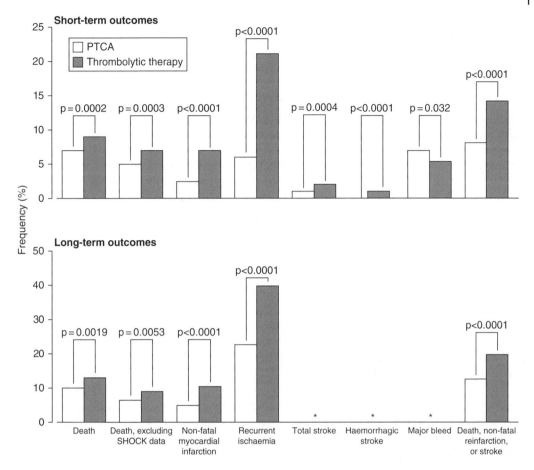

Figure 3.1 Short- and long-term clinical outcomes in patients treated with primary percutaneous coronary intervention or thrombolytic therapy. Reproduced with permission from *Lancet*, 2003; 361: 13–20 [18] (PTCA, percutaneous transluminal coronary angioplasty).

Clinical Impact of Time to Reperfusion

In animal studies, the relationship between the duration of coronary artery occlusion and extent of myocardial necrosis is unequivocal [19]. Accordingly, the main goal of reperfusion therapy is to restore blood flow in the IRA as early as possible, to salvage jeopardized myocardium, limit infarct size, preserve ventricular function and improve survival. Data from a number of randomized trials of thrombolysis have confirmed this notion [20,21]. In aggregate, these studies suggest that the mortality benefit of thrombolysis is strongly time dependent, with the greatest response observed in those patients presenting early after symptom onset [22].

A meta-analysis of six randomized controlled trials of pre-hospital versus in-hospital thrombolysis that included 6434 STEMI patients showed a significant reduction in all-cause mortality among patients treated with pre-hospital compared with in-hospital therapy (odds ratio, OR, 0.83; 95% confidence interval, CI, 0.70–0.98) [23]. The estimated times to thrombolysis were 104 and 164 minutes for the pre-hospital and in-hospital groups, respectively. The 2013 STEMI guidelines [2] recognize the benefits of this strategy but also the potential limitations, such as lack of resources and trained personnel, and endorse the need for additional research regarding implementation of pre-hospital strategies aimed at reducing the total ischemic time.

In contrast, the relationship between time to treatment and clinical outcomes for patients undergoing primary PCI appears to be less time dependent. Boersma and colleagues performed a patient-level meta-analysis of 22 studies; 6763 patients were randomized to primary PCI ($n = 3380$) or thrombolysis ($n = 3383$) [24]. Time to treatment was categorized into presentation delay (time from symptom onset to randomization). At 30 days, primary PCI was associated with a lower mortality compared with thrombolysis (5.3% vs. 7.9%; $P < 0.001$). Primary PCI was also superior to thrombolysis irrespective of the presentation delay. Mortality reduction by primary PCI widened from 1.3% in patients randomized in the first hour after symptom onset to 4.2% for those randomized over 6 hours but the absolute mortality rates for primary PCI increased with increasing presentation delay and PCI-related delay.

This effect may be explained in part by the findings of a pooled analysis of four trials of primary or rescue PCI, in which the primary endpoint was infarct size [25]. In this analysis of 1234 patients, a longer duration from symptom onset to first balloon inflation was strongly predictive of a greater infarct size, with both presentation delay and PCI-related delay contributing to a larger infarct size. Infarct size was smaller when reperfusion was accomplished within 2 hours of symptom onset, intermediate with reperfusion between 2–3 hours, and large when first balloon inflation was performed over 3 hours of symptom onset, with little impact of further delays beyond 3 hours. These data affirm current recommendations for patient transport to STEMI tertiary centers as soon after symptom onset as possible, and to try to minimize door-to-balloon times, with 90 minutes as a suitable benchmark [2]. Finally, one National Registry of Myocardial Infarction (NRMI) study of 192,509 patients at 645 hospitals showed that the time at which the odds of death in those treated with with primary PCI were equal to those treated with thrombolysis occurred when the PCI-related time delay was close to 120 minutes [26]. Accordingly, STEMI guidelines [2] suggest the use of thrombolytic therapy (administered within 30 minutes of arrival) when the anticipated delay to primary PCI exceeds 120 minutes (Figure 3.2).

Facilitated PCI and the Pharmacoinvasive Strategy

The rationale of facilitated PCI (pharmacological reperfusion with thrombolysis alone, glycoprotein IIB/IIIA inhibitors alone or the combination of reduced dose TT and glycoprotein IIB/IIIA inhibitors followed by immediate coronary angiography and PCI) is based on two premises: First, STEMI patients undergoing primary PCI with thrombolysis in myocardial infarction (TIMI) flow 2 or 3 have a better prognosis that patients with TIMI 1 or 0 of the IRA; and second, primary PCI cannot be delivered to all STEMI patients within the recommended time frames as a result of different logistic barriers. In 2006, we performed another meta-analysis of 17 randomized trials of facilitated PCI compared with primary PCI for STEMI patients [27]. Facilitated PCI was associated with a higher short-term mortality (5% vs. 3%), higher incidence of nonfatal reinfarction (3% vs. 2%), stroke (1% vs. 0.3%), hemorrhagic stroke (0.7% vs. 0.1%) and urgent target-vessel revascularization (4% vs. 1%).

The Facilitated Intervention with Enhanced Reperfusion Speed to Stop Events (FINESSE) trial randomized STEMI patients undergoing PCI to combination-facilitated PCI (half-dose reteplase plus abciximab pretreatment), abciximab-facilitated PCI (abciximab pretreatment) or primary PCI (abciximab started at the time of PCI) [28]. The results showed no differences in mortality (5.2%, 5.5% and 4.5%, respectively), or the composite clinical end point of all-cause mortality, ventricular fibrillation within 48 hours, and new-onset congestive heart failure

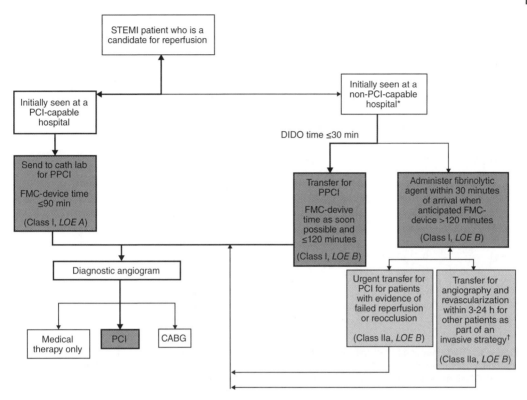

Figure 3.2 Reperfusion therapy for patients with STEMI. * Patients with cardiogenic shock or severe heart failure initially seen at a non-percutaneous coronary intervention (PCI)-capable hospital should be transferred for cardiac catheterization and revascularization as soon as possible, irrespective of time delay from onset of myocardial infarction (class I, level of evidence (LOA): B). † Angiography and revascularization should not be performed within the first 2–3 hours after administration of fibrinolytic therapy. CABG, coronary artery bypass graft; cath lab, catheterization laboratory; DIDO, door in, door out; FMC, first medical contact (reproduced with permission from *J Am Coll Cardiol*, 2013; 61: e78–e140 [2]).

(9.8%, 10.5% and 10.7%, respectively) between the treatment groups and a stepwise increase in bleeding complications, intracranial hemorrhage and blood transfusions. An updated meta-analysis (including the FINESSE trial) corroborated these findings [29]. As a result of these studies, current STEMI guidelines discourage the use of the facilitated PCI approach of very early catheterization (within 2–3 hours) and recommend that PCI immediately after thrombolysis should be limited to rescue PCI for failed thrombolysis [2].

The fundamental difference of the pharmacoinvasive strategy compared to facilitated PCI is based on the notion that thrombolysis is administered as the primary reperfusion therapy when primary PCI is not available within the first 120 minutes of first medical contact. This approach is followed by systematic early (3–24 hours after thrombolysis to avoid bleeding complications) invasive coronary angiography and PCI to treat incomplete reperfusion and reca-nalization of the IRA. Two meta-analysis demonstrated that the pharmacoinvasive strategy of thrombolytic therapy followed by PCI in high-risk STEMI patients significantly reduced reinfarction and recurrent ischemia, compared with thrombolytic therapy alone (Figure 3.3) [30,31]. There was no significant increase in bleeding complications, and these beneficial effects were still present at 12 months of follow-up. However, the studies proved the pharma-coinvasive approach was better than thrombolysis, but the trials did not use pre-hospital

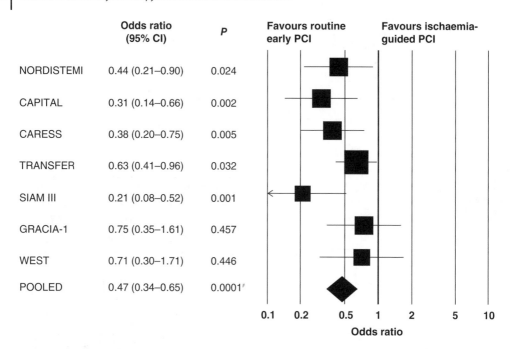

Figure 3.3 Thirty-day combined endpoint of mortality, reinfarction and ischemia with odds ratio (95% confidence interval, CI) favoring routine early percutaneous coronary intervention (PCI) following thrombolytic therapy (*P* < 0.0001, significant; reproduced with permission from *Eur Heart J*, 2011; 32: 972–982 [31]).

thrombolysis, and no trial compared the pharmacoinvasive approach to primary PCI. Accordingly, the Strategic Reperfusion Early After Myocardial Infarction (STREAM) trial randomized STEMI patients within 3 hours of onset of symptoms who were unable to undergo PCI within 60 minutes of onset of symptoms to pre-hospital thrombolysis with full-dose TNK followed by routine coronary angiography within 6–24 hours compared with primary PCI [32]. The results showed no differences in the composite end point of all-cause mortality, shock, congestive heart failure, or reinfarction between the two treatment groups (12.4% for pre-hospital thrombolysis versus 14.3% for primary PCI). Furthermore more strokes occurred with pre-hospital thrombolysis with full-dose TNK compared with primary PCI (1.6% vs. 0.5%) driven primarily by more episodes of intracranial hemorrhage in the elderly (1.0% vs. 0.2%) at the beginning of the study. This led to a protocol amendment that mandated a 50% reduction in the dose of TNK given to patients over 75 years of age, with no additional differences in intracranial hemorrhage rates between the groups (0.5% vs. 0.3%). Although STREAM was a negative trial, given the lack of immediate access to primary PCI in parts of the world, the pharmacoinvasive approach is now considered reasonable.

Conclusions

Primary PCI is a superior treatment strategy compared to thrombolysis for STEMI patients when it can be delivered in a timely fashion. Current evidence support the pharmacoinvasive strategy as an attractive treatment modality in carefully selected high-risk STEMI patients presenting to hospitals without on-site PCI capabilities or those patients in which the anticipated PCI-related time delay is greater than 120 minutes. Alternatively, thrombolytic therapy alone remains an important strategy when cost, logistics or other issues prevent an invasive approach.

References

1 Keeley EC, Grines CL. Primary coronary intervention for acute myocardial infarction. *JAMA*, 2004; 291: 736–739.

2 O'Gara PT, Kushner FG, Ascheim DD, et al. 2013 ACCF/AHA guideline for the management of ST-elevation myocardial infarction: A report of the American College of Cardiology Foundation/American Heart Association Task Force on Practice Guidelines. *J Am Coll Cardiol*, 2013; 61: e78–e140.

3 Grines CL, Schreiber T. Primary percutaneous coronary intervention: The deception of delay. *J Am Coll Cardiol*, 2013; 61: 1696–1697.

4 Granger CB, Califf RM, Topol EJ. Thrombolytic therapy for acute myocardial infarction. A review. Drugs. 1992;44:293–325.

5 Turcasso NM, Nappi JM. Tenecteplase for treatment of acute myocardial infarction. *Ann Pharmacother*, 2001; 35: 1233–1240.

6 Effectiveness of intravenous thrombolytic treatment in acute myocardial infarction. Gruppo italiano per lo studio della streptochinasi nell'infarto miocardico (gissi). *Lancet*, 1986; 1: 397–402.

7 ISIS-2 (Second International Study of Infarct Survival) Collaborative Group. Randomised trial of intravenous streptokinase, oral aspirin, both, or neither among 17,187 cases of suspected acute myocardial infarction: Isis-2. *Lancet*, 1988; 2: 349–360.

8 Boersma E, Simoons ML. Reperfusion strategies in acute myocardial infarction. *Eur Heart J*, 1997; 18: 1703–1711.

9 GUSTO Investigators. An international randomized trial comparing four thrombolytic strategies for acute myocardial infarction. *N Engl J Med*, 1993; 329: 673–682.

10 GUSTO Angiographic Investigators. The effects of tissue plasminogen activator, streptokinase, or both on coronary–artery patency, ventricular function, and survival after acute myocardial infarction. *N Engl J Med*, 1993; 329: 1615–1622.

11 Smalling RW, Bode C, Kalbfleisch J, et al. More rapid, complete, and stable coronary thrombolysis with bolus administration of reteplase compared with alteplase infusion in acute myocardial infarction. RAPID investigators. *Circulation*, 1995; 91: 2725–2732.

12 Bode C, Smalling RW, Berg G, et al. Randomized comparison of coronary thrombolysis achieved with double-bolus reteplase (recombinant plasminogen activator) and front-loaded, accelerated alteplase (recombinant tissue plasminogen activator) in patients with acute myocardial infarction. The RAPID II investigators. *Circulation*, 1996; 94: 891–898.

13 Cannon CP, Gibson CM, McCabe CH, Adgey AA, Schweiger MJ, Sequeira RF, Grollier G, Giugliano RP, Frey M, Mueller HS, Steingart RM, Weaver WD, Van de Werf F, Braunwald E. TNK-tissue plasminogen activator compared with frontloaded alteplase in acute myocardial infarction: Results of the TIMI 10b trial. Thrombolysis in myocardial infarction (TIMI) 10b investigators. *Circulation*, 1998; 98: 2805–2814.

14 GUSTO III investigators. A comparison of reteplase with alteplase for acute myocardial infarction. The global use of strategies to open occluded coronary arteries. *N Engl J Med*, 1997; 337: 1118–1123.

15 Mehta SR, Eikelboom JW, Yusuf S. Risk of intracranial haemorrhage with bolus versus infusion thrombolytic therapy: A metaanalysis. *Lancet*, 2000; 356: 449–454.

16 Armstrong PW, Granger C, Van de Werf F. Intracranial haemorrhage with bolus thrombolytic agents. *Lancet*, 2000; 356: 1849; author reply 1850.

17 Simoons ML, Maggioni AP, Knatterud G, et al. Individual risk assessment for intracranial haemorrhage during thrombolytic therapy. *Lancet*, 1993; 342: 1523–1528.

18 Keeley EC, Boura JA, Grines CL. Primary angioplasty versus intravenous thrombolytic therapy for acute myocardial infarction: A quantitative review of 23 randomised trials. *Lancet*, 2003; 361: 13–20.

19 Reimer KA, Lowe JE, Rasmussen MM, et al. The wavefront phenomenon of ischemic cell death. 1. Myocardial infarct size vs duration of coronary occlusion in dogs. *Circulation*, 1977; 56: 786–794.

20 Newby LK, Rutsch WR, Califf RM, et al. Time from symptom onset to treatment and outcomes after thrombolytic therapy. GUSTO-1 investigators. *J Am Coll Cardiol*, 1996; 27: 1646–1655.

21 Goldberg RJ, Mooradd M, Gurwitz JH, et al. Impact of time to treatment with tissue plasminogen activator on morbidity and mortality following acute myocardial infarction (the Second National Registry of Myocardial Infarction). *Am J Cardiol*, 1998; 82: 259–264.

22 Boersma E, Maas AC, Deckers JW, et al. Early thrombolytic treatment in acute myocardial infarction: Reappraisal of the golden hour. *Lancet*, 1996; 348: 771–775.

23 Morrison LJ, Verbeek PR, McDonald AC, et al. Mortality and prehospital thrombolysis for acute myocardial infarction: A meta-analysis. *JAMA*, 2000; 283: 2686–2692.

24 Boersma E, and the Primary Coronary Angioplasty vs Thrombolysis Group. Does time matter? A pooled analysis of randomized clinical trials comparing primary percutaneous coronary intervention and in-hospital fibrinolysis in acute myocardial infarction patients. *Eur Heart J*, 2006; 27: 779–788.

25 Stone GW, Dixon SR, Grines CL, et al. Predictors of infarct size after primary coronary angioplasty in acute myocardial infarction from pooled analysis from four contemporary trials. *Am J Cardiol*, 2007; 100: 1370–1375.

26 Pinto DS, Kirtane AJ, Nallamothu BK, et al. Hospital delays in reperfusion for ST-elevation myocardial infarction: Implications when selecting a reperfusion strategy. *Circulation*, 2006; 114: 2019–2025.

27 Keeley EC, Boura JA, Grines CL. Comparison of primary and facilitated percutaneous coronary interventions for ST-elevation myocardial infarction: Quantitative review of randomised trials. *Lancet*, 2006; 367: 579–588.

28 Ellis SG, Tendera M, de Belder MA, et al. Facilitated PCI in patients with ST-elevation myocardial infarction. *N Engl J Med*, 2008; 358: 2205–2217.

29 De Luca G, Marino P. Facilitated angioplasty with combo therapy among patients with ST-segment elevation myocardial infarction: A meta-analysis of randomized trials. *Am J Emerg Med*, 2009; 27: 683–690.

30 Borgia F, Goodman SG, Halvorsen S, et al. Early routine percutaneous coronary intervention after fibrinolysis vs. Standard therapy in ST-segment elevation myocardial infarction: A meta-analysis. *Eur Heart J*, 2010; 31: 2156–2169.

31 D'Souza SP, Mamas MA, Fraser DG, et al. Routine early coronary angioplasty versus ischaemia-guided angioplasty after thrombolysis in acute ST-elevation myocardial infarction: A meta-analysis. *Eur Heart J*, 2011; 32: 972–982.

32 Armstrong PW, Gershlick A, Goldstein P, et al. The strategic reperfusion early after myocardial infarction (stream) study. *Am Heart J*, 2010; 160: 30–35 e31.

4

Anticoagulants in STEMI Interventions

Vincenzo Vizzi MD, Thomas W. Johnson BSc MBBS MD FRCP, Andreas Baumbach MD

Introduction

The main goal of ST-elevation myocardial infarction (STEMI) treatment is the prompt recanalization of the infarct-related artery to reduce myocardial damage and improve prognosis. With the establishment of infarct networks and rapid access to revascularization, the role of ancillary anticoagulant therapy has become crucial. In this chapter, we focus our attention exclusively on the anticoagulation strategy in STEMI patients undergoing an invasive strategy. We provide a comprehensive overview of the treatment options currently available.

Anticoagulants

Three different classes of anticoagulant are administered in addition to oral antiplatelet drugs in the context of primary percutaneous coronary intervention (PPCI): unfractionated heparin, low molecular weight heparins (including enoxaparin and fondaparinux) and bivalirudin, an intravenous reversible direct thrombin inhibitor (Tables 4.1 and 4.2).

Unfractionated Heparin

Unfractionated heparin is an indirect inhibitor of the factor Xa and thrombin (factor IIa). For heparin to work, it needs to bind to antithrombin III and, from a pharmacokinetic point of view, its action is unpredictable. Current guidelines recommend a dose of 70–100 iu/kg for PPCI, which can be administered intracoronarily or intravenously. Because of its unpredictable pharmacokinetic profile, the activated clotting time should be monitored regularly during the procedure to obtain a value between 250 and 350 seconds. There has been no trial evaluating unfractionated heparin against placebo in the setting of PPCI but, in view of the large body of experience with this agent, it is widely used and achieves a class I recommendation in the most recent guidelines [1–3].

Fondaparinux and Enoxaparin

Fondaparinux is a synthetic pentasaccharide that inhibits activated factor X. Its use in the setting of acute STEMI was tested in the OASIS-6 trial [4]. In the 3788 patients of the entire cohort undergoing PPCI, fondaparinux did not confer any benefit in comparison with

Manual of STEMI Interventions, First Edition. Edited by Sameer Mehta.
© 2017 John Wiley & Sons Ltd. Published 2017 by John Wiley & Sons Ltd.

Table 4.1 Selection of the most important studies on anticoagulants in STEMI patients undergoing primary percutaneous coronary intervention (PPCI). The ischemic endpoint was the main ischemic endpoint at 30 days available in the study results. The bleeding endpoint was the main definition used for major/severe bleeding in each trial.

Study	Drug(s)	Dose	Glycoprotein IIb/IIIa (%)	Hazard ratio (range)		
				Ischemia	Bleeding	Mortality
OASIS-6 (PPCI group) [4]	Fondaparinux	2.5 mg or 5 mg	n/a	1.20 (0.91–1.57)	1.18 (0.63–2.22)	1.16 (0.85–1.58)
	Heparin (UF ± GP IIb/IIIa)	65–100 iu/kg				
ATOLL [5]	Enoxaparin	0.5 mg/kg iv	n/a	0.59 (0.38–0.91)[a]	0.92 (0.51–1.66)	0.60 (0.33–1.07)
	Heparin (UF)	70–100 iu/kg				
HORIZONS-AMI [6]	Bivalirudin (± GP IIb/IIIa)	Bolus 0.75 mg/kg Infusion 1.75 mg/kg/h (stopped after PCI)	7.2	1.00 (0.75–1.32)	0.60 (0.46–0.77)[a]	0.66 (0.44–1.00)[a]
	Heparin (UF ± GP IIb/IIIa)	60 iu/kg + GP IIb/IIIa (up to 12 hours or 18 hours after PCI)	97.7			
EUROMAX [10,11]	Bivalirudin	Bolus 0.75 mg/kg Infusion 1.75 mg/kg/h (continued after PCI at full or reduced dose)	11.5	1.38 (0.90–2.13) bivalirudin vs. routine GP IIb/IIIa	0.44 (0.27–0.71)[a]	1.27 (0.69–2.33)
	Heparin (UF or LMW) ± GP IIb/IIIa	UF 60–100iu LMW 0.5 mg/kg ± GP IIb/IIIa	69.1	0.83 (0.56–0.68)[a] bivalirudin vs. routine GP IIb/IIIa	0.41 (0.25–0.68)[a]	0.71 (0.41–1.24)
HEAT-PPCI [12]	Bivalirudin (± GP IIb/IIIa)	Bolus 0.75 mg/kg Infusion 1.75 mg/kg/h (stopped after PCI)	13	1.52 (1.09–2.13)[a]	0.93 (0.73–1.18)	1.18 (0.78–1.79)
	Heparin (UF ± GP IIb/IIIa)	70iu/kg	15			

Study	Treatment	Dose				
BRAVE-4 [20]	Bivalirudin + prasugrel	Bolus 0.75 mg/kg Infusion 1.75 mg/kg/h (stopped after PCI but could be continued as thrombotic bailout)	3	1.09 (0–1.79)	1.18 (0.74–1.88)	1.02 (0.31–3.37)
	Heparin + clopidogrel	70 iu/kg	6.1			
BRIGHT [13]	Bivalirudin (± GP IIb/IIIa)	Bolus 0.75 mg/kg Infusion 1.75 mg/kg/h (continued after PCI)	4.4	0.87 (0.57–1.34) bivalirudin vs. heparin alone	0.54 (0.35–0.83)[a] bivalirudin vs. heparin alone	0.99 (0.46–2.1) bivalirudin vs. heparin alone
				1.02 (0.65–1.56) bivalirudin vs. heparin + GP IIb/IIIa	0.33 (0.22–0.49)[a] bivalirudin vs. heparin + GP IIb/IIIa	0.86 (0.41–1.8) bivalirudin vs. heparin + GP IIb/IIIa
	Heparin	100 iu/kg	5.6			
	Heparin (± GP IIb/IIIa)	60 iu/kg	100			

[a] $P < 0.05$ (95% confidence interval).

GP, glycoprotein; h, hour; HR, hazard ratio; iv, intravenously; LMW, low molecular weight; UF, unfractionated.

Table 4.2 Dose, contraindications, advantages and disadvantages of the main anticoagulant drugs available for STEMI patients undergoing primary percutaneous coronary intervention.

Anticoagulant	Dose	Contraindication	Advantages	Disadvantages
Unfractionated heparin	70–100 iu/kg 60 iu/kg if glycoprotein IIb/IIIa inhibitors	Known heparin-induced thrombocytopenia	Well tested. No need for dose adjustment in chronic kidney disease. Cheap.	Heparin-induced thrombocytopenia. Unpredictable pharmacokinetics (needs frequent monitoring for activated clotting).
Bivalirudin	0.75 mg/kg bolus 1.75 mg/kg/h infusion (1.4 mg/kg/h in moderate chronic kidney disease)	Severe chronic kidney disease	Well tested. Fewer bleeding complications compared with unfractionated heparin and concomitant glycoprotein IIb/IIIa inhibitor administration. Predictable pharmacokinetic and short half-life.	Expensive. Higher risk of stent thrombosis if infusion stopped at the end of the procedure. Dose adjustment necessary in moderate chronic kidney disease.
Enoxaparin	0.5 mg/kg intravenously	Known heparin-induced thrombocytopenia	Predictable pharmacokinetics. Cheap.	Limited evidence (single randomized study and for enoxaparin only). No clear advantages in comparison with unfractionated heparin.

unfractionated heparin with regard to death and myocardial infarction at 30 days or severe bleeding events. Fondaparinux was also associated with a significantly higher risk of guiding catheter-associated thrombosis (22 vs. 0, $P < 0.01$) and a higher risk of coronary complications (abrupt coronary artery closure, new angiographic thrombus, catheter thrombus, no-reflow, dissection, or perforation: 270 vs. 225, $P = 0.04$). In the light of these results, fondaparinux is not recommended in patients with acute STEMI undergoing revascularization.

The ATOLL (Acute STEMI Treated with primary angioplasty and intravenous enoxaparin Or unfractionated heparin to Lower ischemic and bleeding events at short- and Long-term follow-up) trial has compared intravenous enoxaparin or unfractionated heparin in patients undergoing PPCI [5]. The lower incidence of the primary endpoint in the enoxaparin group (composite of death, complication of myocardial infarction, procedure failure, or major bleeding at 30 days) failed to reach statistical significance (28% vs. 34%; relative risk, RR, 0.83, 95% confidence interval, CI, 0.68–1.01, $P = 0.06$). However, enoxaparin significantly reduced the ischemic endpoint of death, recurrent myocardial infarction/acute coronary syndrome or urgent revascularization by 41% (RR 0.59, 95% CI 0.38–0.91), with a trend toward a reduction in mortality (RR 0.60, 95% CI 0.33–1.07), which was significant when considering the combination of death and resuscitated cardiac arrest ($P = 0.049$). Interestingly, the benefit conferred by the enoxaparin related to the ischemic endpoints rather than a reduction in bleeding events.

Bivalirudin

Bivalirudin is an intravenous direct inhibitor of thrombin, with a rapid onset and short half-life.

With four large, randomized studies available, it is the most extensively investigated anticoagulant in acute STEMI treatment. In the HORIZONS-AMI trial [6] 3602 STEMI patients undergoing invasive angiography were randomized to receive bivalirudin alone or unfractionated heparin and glycoprotein (GP) IIb/IIIa inhibitors. The two primary endpoints of the study were major bleeding and net clinical events, defined as the combination of major bleeding or major adverse cardiovascular events, including death, reinfarction, target-vessel revascularization for ischemia, and stroke. Bivalirudin reduced the 30-day rate of net adverse clinical events (9.2% vs. 12.1%, RR 0.76, 95% CI 0.63–0.92, $P = 0.005$). This result was driven by a lower rate of major bleeding (4.9% vs. 8.3%, RR 0.60, 95% CI 0.46–0.77; $P < 0.001$) and persisted on long-term follow-up [7,8]. Serious concerns were raised, however, by the significantly higher number of acute (<24 hours) stent thrombosis in the bivalirudin group in comparison with the unfractionated heparin plus GP IIb/IIIa group (1.3 vs. 0.3%, $P < 0.001$). The administration of a heparin bolus before the randomization and of a loading dose of clopidogrel 600 mg reduced, respectively, the incidence of acute and subacute stent thrombosis [9].

In the EUROMAX trial [10] bivalirudin administered in STEMI patients during their transport to the catheterization laboratory significantly reduced the incidence of a composite of death or major bleeding, not associated with coronary artery bypass graft, at 30 days, in comparison with unfractionated heparin and optional GP IIb/IIIa inhibitors (5.1% vs. 8.5%, RR 0.60, 95% CI 0.43–0.82; $P = 0.001$). This benefit was mainly driven by a reduction of major bleeding (2.6% vs. 6.0%, RR 0.43, 95% CI 0.28–0.66; $P < 0.001$). In keeping with HORIZONS-AMI, there was a significant increase in acute stent thrombosis observed in the bivalirudin group (1.1% vs. 0.2%, RR 6.11, 95% CI 1.37–27.24, $P = 0.007$). A pre-specified analysis of EUROMAX [11] has specifically looked at the three different anticoagulant strategies adopted in the study (bivalirudin alone vs. unfractionated heparin plus GP IIb/IIIa vs. unfractionated heparin with bailout GP IIb/IIIa) and confirmed that bivalirudin monotherapy is superior in reducing the incidence of the primary composite endpoint of death or major bleeding. Again, there was a trend toward a higher rate of acute stent thrombosis in the bivalirudin group, albeit not statistically significant. It should be noted that, to reflect current practice, the EUROMAX study protocol allowed the administration of GP IIb/IIIa inhibitors as a bailout strategy in the bivalirudin arm and either as a routine combination or bailout in the unfractionated heparin arm of the study. The use of GP IIb/IIIa inhibitors differed significantly between groups (overall, 11.5% in the bivalirudin group vs. 69.1% in the control group received the drug), which might have influenced the study outcome.

The HEAT-PPCI trial [12] was a single UK center-based study where 1,829 STEMI patients were randomized to bivalirudin monotherapy versus heparin monotherapy. The study protocol allowed the use of GP IIb/IIIa inhibitors only as bailout therapy. A major strength of the study was the "all-comer" design, with the majority of patients presenting to the catheterization laboratory being included (1829/1917 patients). The rate of radial access was high (>80%), as was the use of potent oral antiplatelet agents (>90% received either prasugrel or ticagrelor). In accordance with the study protocol, the bivalirudin infusion was stopped at the end of the PCI. GP IIb/IIIa inhibitors were administered in 13% of the bivalirudin group and in 15% of the heparin group.

The use of bivalirudin (as compared with heparin) in the HEAT-PPCI trial was associated with a higher incidence of the primary efficacy outcome (composite of all-cause mortality, cerebrovascular accident, reinfarction, or unplanned target lesion revascularization at 28 days): 8.7% vs. 5.7% (absolute risk difference 3.0%, RR 1.52, 95% CI 1.09–2.13, $P = 0.01$). Similar to HORIZONS and EUROMAX, a higher rate of stent thrombosis was observed with the use of bivalirudin compared with heparin (3.4% vs. 0.9%, absolute risk difference 2.6%, RR 3.91, 95% CI 1.61–9.52, $P = 0.001$). Surprisingly, contrary to HORIZONS-AMI and EUROMAX, bivalirudin did not guarantee any protection in terms of bleeding events, with a similar incidence of major bleeding (primary safety endpoint): 3.5% in the bivalirudin group and 3.1% in the heparin group (absolute risk difference 0.4%, RR 1.15, 95% CI 0.70–1.89, $P = 0.59$).

Interestingly, the higher incidence of stent thrombosis observed in the above-mentioned trials was not replicated in the more recent BRIGHT study [13], a multicenter randomized trial conducted in China. The investigators enrolled 2194 patients with STEMI undergoing PPCI ($n = 1,925$) or with high-risk non-STEMI (NSTEMI) undergoing emergency PCI ($n = 269$) and randomized them to receive bivalirudin, heparin alone, or heparin plus tirofiban. In the bivalirudin group, the infusion was continued at the maintenance dose for at least 30 minutes and up to 4 hours post PCI. The bailout administration of GP IIb/IIIa inhibitors in the heparin and bivalirudin randomization arms was minimal: 5.6% in the heparin group and 4.4% in the bivalirudin group. The study showed that patients randomized to bivalirudin experienced a significantly lower incidence of net adverse cardiac events at 30 days: a composite of major adverse cardiac or cerebral events (all-cause death, reinfarction, ischemia-driven target-vessel revascularization, or stroke) or any bleeding as defined by the Bleeding Academic Research Consortium definition (grades 1–5). The primary endpoint occurred in 8.8% of the patients in the bivalirudin group, in 13.2% of the heparin group (RR 0.67, 95% CI 0.50 to 0.90, difference −4.3%; 95% CI −7.5% to −1.1%; $P = 0.008$) and in the 17% of the heparin + tirofiban group (RR for bivalirudin vs. heparin plus tirofiban, 0.52; 95% CI, 0.39 to 0.69; difference, −8.1%; 95% CI, −11.6% to −4.7%; $P < 0.001$). Bivalirudin also significantly reduced the risk of bleeding and, for the first time, it did not increase the risk of stent thrombosis.

Discussion

Bivalirudin and unfractionated heparin are the most tested anticoagulant drugs in the setting of primary PCI. At a first glance, the choice among them seems very hard in view of the conflicting results coming from the data available (Table 4.1). A critical analysis should therefore take into account two different aspects: the safety profile in terms of bleeding and the protection from ischemic events.

The Bleeding Risk

The reduction of bleeding observed with bivalirudin in the HORIZONS-AMI trial [6], leading to a lower incidence of death, is an endpoint that is hard to ignore. Accordingly, for many years, bivalirudin has been the anticoagulant of choice in the context of STEMI, owing to its better safety profile. Taking into account that the HORIZONS-AMI trial was conducted nearly 10 years ago, the current practice has significantly changed since then. A major criticism of the study design relates to the routine use of GP IIb/IIIa inhibitors in addition to heparin. The evidence for this seems to be equivocal and was never supported by strong data, with the exception of an historical meta-analysis regarding abciximab [14]. Even fewer data exist for eptifibatide and tirofiban. Furthermore, the arrival of more potent oral antiplatelet drugs, such as ticagrelor and prasugrel, may eliminate the need for acute GP IIb/IIIa inhibitor administration.

Recent guidelines reflect the change of practice and reserve GP IIb/IIIa use for selected cases [1,2,10]. The key question is therefore: does bivalirudin still protect from bleeding complications when a GP IIb/IIIa inhibitor is not used?

In both the HEAT-PPCI [12] and BRIGHT [13] studies, GP IIb/IIIa inhibitors were administered as bailout and in a small percentage of patients, but the two studies gave conflicting results. Indeed, in the HEAT-PPCI study population, the bivalirudin did not confer any advantage in terms of bleeding rates versus heparin, while in the BRIGHT study it did. The two studies were different in terms of design and these differences have been used to explain the contrasting findings [15]:

- The healthcare systems and study populations were dissimilar: BRIGHT was a multicenter study entirely conducted in China, whereas HEAT-PPCI a single-center study conducted in Liverpool, United Kingdom.
- Different heparin doses were employed: 70 iu/kg in HEAT-PPCI and 100 iu/kg in BRIGHT.
- Different syndromes were studied: high-risk NSTEMI patients were part of the BRIGHT study population, while HEAT-PPCI included only exclusively STEMI patients.
- The management of the bivalirudin infusion post-PCI was different.
- The time of administration of the study drugs was different: anticoagulation started before the arrival in the catheterization laboratory in HEAT-PPCI and after the arrival in BRIGHT.
- Novel oral antiplatelet drugs (prasugrel and ticagrelor) were not used in BRIGHT.

The Risk of Stent Thrombosis

A consistent finding among the HORIZONS-AMI, EUROMAX and HEAT-PPCI trials was that bivalirudin increases the risk of stent thrombosis. This seems to be true even if prasugrel or ticagrelor are used, as in the HEAT-PPCI study. A recent meta-analysis including these three trials has confirmed this finding and that bivalirudin is associated with a four times higher risk of acute stent thrombosis [16]. As detailed earlier, the BRIGHT study contradicts this finding, and the lower incidence of stent thrombosis observed is most likely related to the prolonged infusion of bivalirudin beyond the end of PPCI procedure.

Our group has demonstrated a significant delay in effective platelet inhibition achieved with pre-procedural loading of prasugrel, with high residual platelet activity observed in 75% of patients at 1 hour and 24% of patients at 2 hours post-procedure. The combined use of the HORIZONS protocol for bivalirudin administration was associated with a high rate of acute stent thrombosis and all events occurred within 2 hours of bivalirudin cessation [17]. Similarly, it has been demonstrated by Parodi and colleagues that, in patients undergoing PPCI, at 2 hours after the oral loading dose, there was a high residual platelet reactivity in 44% of those receiving prasugrel and 60% of dose receiving ticagrelor [18]. With the emphasis on minimizing the time from arrival in hospital to recanalization of the occluded coronary artery, the observed delay in platelet inhibition with oral antiplatelet loading, combined with rapid reversal of bivalirudin's antithrombotic effect, secondary to its short half-life, potentially exposes patients to a period of elevated thrombotic risk. Whereas the use of unfractionated heparin, with its more prolonged and less predictable half-life, may provide protection against acute thrombotic complications while the oral antiplatelet agents achieve therapeutic levels. The results of the BRIGHT study support this concept, as bivalirudin was continued beyond the termination of the PPCI procedure (median infusion time post-PCI 180 minutes).

In light of these findings, many centers have started routinely to prolong the infusion of bivalirudin. Obviously, this has had significant impact in terms of costs, and it could significantly impact on the proved cost-effectiveness of bivalirudin versus heparin and GP IIb/IIIa inhibitor in the lifelong time horizon [19].

How to Choose: The Eternal Dilemma Between Bleeding and Ischemic Risk

An ideal anticoagulant drug (or combination of drugs) should guarantee an optimal antithrombotic efficacy without significantly increasing the risk of bleeding (Figure 4.1). Unfortunately, such a drug has yet to be found.

After the change in guideline recommendation [1], the protocol adopted in our institution has been amended accordingly (Figure 4.2). The majority of our patients undergo PPCI using the radial approach and they receive a prasugrel or ticagrelor loading dose as soon as they arrive in the catheterization laboratory. We recently moved from a routine use of bivalirudin monotherapy to heparin and we reserve the use of bivalirudin for patients with high bleeding risk (i.e. planned femoral approach, chronic kidney disease, history of previous bleeding). GP IIb/IIIa inhibitors are used in case of high thrombotic burden or thrombotic complications (angiographically visible thrombus after stent deployment and slow flow/no-reflow phenomena).

We acknowledge that an antithrombotic/antiplatelet regimen that neutralizes the thrombotic process underlying STEMI, without exposing the patient to the risk of bleeding does not exist. However, our strategy reflects a "personalized" approach, tailoring the antithrombotic strategy according to the patient's thrombotic and bleeding profile, minimizing their risk of an adverse outcome.

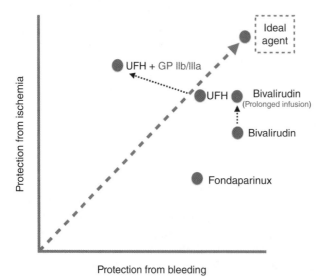

Figure 4.1 Different efficacy of the available anticoagulant drugs, according to the data coming from the primary percutaneous coronary intervention (PPCI) studies. The ideal agent should offer the best efficacy in reducing ischemic events, giving at the same time an optimal protection from bleeding complications. The picture shows that adding glycoprotein IIb/IIIa inhibitors to unfractionated heparin improves the antithrombotic efficacy, but at the cost of a significantly increased risk of thrombosis. Prolonging the bivalirudin infusion after PPCI would overcome this problem.

PPCI anticoagulant therapy

Heparin 10,000 units must be available on all PPCI trolleys

Heparin 70–100 units/kg IV bolus dose*

Check activated clotting time (ACT) within 15 minutes of bolus dose

Give further doses of heparin to maintain ACT >250 seconds
Recheck ACT every 15 mins

Check final ACT at the end of the case

Weight (kg)	Recommended heparin loading dose (70 units/kg)
40	2800
50	3500
60	4200
70	4900
80	5600
90	6300
100	7000
110	7700
120	8400
130	9100
140	9800

If heparin contraindicated, use bivalirudin 0.75 mg/kg IV bolus dose followed by IV infusion of 1.75 mg/kg/hr for up to 4 hours post procedure

*Reduce loading dose of heparin to 50–70 kg if glycoprotein IIb/IIIa inhibitor required.

Figure 4.2 Anticoagulant protocol for patients undergoing primary percutaneous coronary intervention adopted by the Bristol Heart Institute, Bristol, United Kingdom.

References

1 Windecker S, Kolh P, Alfonso F, et al. 2014 ESC/EACTS guidelines on myocardial revascularization: The Task Force on Myocardial Revascularization of the European Society of Cardiology (ESC) and the European Association for Cardio-Thoracic Surgery (EACTS) Developed with the special contribution of the European Association of Percutaneous Cardiovascular Interventions (EAPCI). *Eur Heart J*, 2014; 35(37): 2541–2619.

2 O'Gara PT, Kushner FG, Ascheim DD, et al. 2013 ACCF/AHA Guideline for the Management of ST-Elevation Myocardial Infarction: A Report of the American College of Cardiology Foundation/American Heart Association Task Force on Practice Guidelines. *Circulation*, 2013; 127(4): e362–e425.

3 Steg PG, James SK, Atar D, et al. ESC Guidelines for the management of acute myocardial infarction in patients presenting with ST-segment elevation. *Eur Heart J*, 2012; 33(20): 2569–2619.

4 Yusuf S, Mehta SR, Chrolavicius S, et al. Effects of fondaparinux on mortality and reinfarction in patients with acute ST-segment elevation myocardial infarction: the OASIS-6 randomized trial. *JAMA*, 2006; 295(13): 1519–1530.

5 Montalescot G, Zeymer U, Silvain J, et al. Intravenous enoxaparin or unfractionated heparin in primary percutaneous coronary intervention for ST-elevation myocardial infarction: the international randomised open-label ATOLL trial. *Lancet*, 2011; 378(9792): 693–703.

6 Stone GW, Witzenbichler B, Guagliumi G, et al. Bivalirudin during primary PCI in acute myocardial infarction. *N Engl J Med*, 2008; 358(21): 2218–2230.

7 Mehran R, Lansky AJ, Witzenbichler B, et al. Bivalirudin in patients undergoing primary angioplasty for acute myocardial infarction (HORIZONS-AMI): 1-year results of a randomised controlled trial. *Lancet*, 2009; 374(9696): 1149–1159.

8 Stone GW, Witzenbichler B, Guagliumi G, et al. Heparin plus a glycoprotein IIb/IIIa inhibitor versus bivalirudin monotherapy and paclitaxel-eluting stents versus bare-metal stents in acute myocardial infarction (HORIZONS-AMI): final 3-year results from a multicentre, randomised controlled trial. *Lancet*, 2011; 377(9784): 2193–2204.

9 Dangas GD, Caixeta A, Mehran R, et al. Frequency and predictors of stent thrombosis after percutaneous coronary intervention in acute myocardial infarction. *Circulation*, 2011; 123(16): 1745–1756.

10 Steg PG, van't Hof A, Hamm CW, et al. Bivalirudin started during emergency transport for primary PCI. *N Engl J Med*, 2013; 369(23): 2207–2217.

11 Zeymer U, van't Hof A, Adgey J, et al. Bivalirudin is superior to heparins alone with bailout GP IIb/IIIa inhibitors in patients with ST-segment elevation myocardial infarction transported emergently for primary percutaneous coronary intervention: a pre-specified analysis from the EUROMAX trial. *Eur Heart J*, 2014; 35(36): 2460–2467.

12 Shahzad A, Kemp I, Mars C, et al. Unfractionated heparin versus bivalirudin in primary percutaneous coronary intervention (HEAT-PPCI): an open-label, single centre, randomised controlled trial. *Lancet*, 2014; 384(9957): 1849–1858.

13 Han Y, Guo J, Zheng Y, et al. Bivalirudin vs heparin with or without tirofiban during primary percutaneous coronary intervention in acute myocardial infarction: the BRIGHT randomized clinical trial. *JAMA*, 2015; 313(13): 1336–1346.

14 De Luca G, Suryapranata H, Stone GW, et al. Abciximab as adjunctive therapy to reperfusion in acute ST-segment elevation myocardial infarction: a meta-analysis of randomized trials. *JAMA*, 2005; 293(14): 1759–1765.

15 Cavender MA, Faxon DP. Can BRIGHT restore the glow of bivalirudin? *JAMA*, 2015; 313(13): 1323–1324.

16 Cavender MA, Sabatine MS. Bivalirudin versus heparin in patients planned for percutaneous coronary intervention: a meta-analysis of randomised controlled trials. *Lancet*, 2014; 384(9943): 599–606.

17 Johnson TW, Mumford A, Mundell S, et al. A study of platelet inhibition, using a "point of care" platelet function test, following primary percutaneous coronary intervention for ST-elevation myocardial infarction (PINPOINT-PPCI). *Eur Heart J*, 2014; 35(Abstract Suppl): 995.

18 Parodi G, Valenti R, Bellandi B, et al. Comparison of prasugrel and ticagrelor loading doses in ST-segment elevation myocardial infarction patients: RAPID (Rapid Activity of Platelet Inhibitor Drugs) primary PCI study. *J Am Coll Cardiol*, 2013; 61(15): 1601–1606.

19 Schwenkglenks M, Toward TJ, Plent S, et al. Cost-effectiveness of bivalirudin versus heparin plus glycoprotein IIb/IIIa inhibitor in the treatment of acute ST-segment elevation myocardial infarction. *Heart*, 2012; 98(7): 544–551.

20 Schulz S, Richardt G, Laugwitz KL, et al. Prasugrel plus bivalirudin vs. clopidogrel plus heparin in patients with ST-segment elevation myocardial infarction. *Eur Heart J*, 2014; 35(34): 2285–2294.

5

New Oral and Intravenous Adenosine Diphosphate Blockers in STEMI Intervention

James J. Ferguson III MD

Introduction

This chapter summarizes our current clinical understanding of newer-generation adenosine diphosphate (ADP) receptor blockers as adjunctive therapy in the treatment of patients presenting with ST-elevation myocardial infarction (STEMI) who undergo coronary intervention. A brief description of the role of platelets in coagulation, and a general overview of current antiplatelet agents, provides a conceptual framework on which to position these new agents as adjunctive therapy. A review of the clinical data on both old and new ADP blockers in acute coronary syndrome (ACS) follows, recognizing that a great deal of our understanding of the utility of these agents for STEMI is derived or inferred from subgroups within larger ACS studies, and even other percutaneous coronary intervention (PCI) studies outside the STEMI setting. The relatively few trials focusing solely on STEMI intervention are highlighted. Other more general issues on the use of newer-generation ADP blockers are discussed, such as impaired oral absorption of drugs in the setting of STEMI, duration of therapy post intervention, and the use of ADP blockers in conjunction with oral anticoagulants in STEMI patients on warfarin or the newer oral anticoagulants. Finally, future directions in ADP therapy are highlighted, including studies of ADP blockers without background aspirin therapy and potential reversal strategies.

Physiology

STEMI and the Pro-Thrombotic State

Plaque rupture frequently initiates pathophysiologic processes that culminate in occlusion of a coronary artery and clinical manifestations of STEMI [1]. Thrombus formation at the site of plaque rupture results in obstruction of coronary blood flow, leading to subsequent myocardial necrosis. More than 90% of patients presenting with STEMI have evidence of coronary thrombus formation at the site of plaque disruption [2–5]. To prevent myocardial cell death and subsequent ventricular remodeling, reperfusion therapy (by either catheter-based or pharmacological approaches) is undertaken in patients presenting with STEMI to rapidly and completely re-establish coronary blood flow. Ancillary therapy with antithrombin and anti-platelet agents to inhibit coagulation is also important to both facilitate reperfusion and maintain infarct-related artery patency. The formation of a new clot during PCI or thrombolysis has been independently associated with both lower rates of reperfusion and increased incidence of abrupt vessel closure [6].

Manual of STEMI Interventions, First Edition. Edited by Sameer Mehta.
© 2017 John Wiley & Sons Ltd. Published 2017 by John Wiley & Sons Ltd.

Platelets and Coagulation

Plaque rupture leads to the release of tissue factor and the exposure of both the underlying collagen endothelial cellular matrix of the injured vessel and the highly thrombogenic lipid–collagen content of the ruptured atherosclerotic plaque. Platelets adhere to exposed collagen via glycoprotein (GP) Ib and Ia/IIa, and proceed to activate, aggregate and degranulate. The release of thromboxane, serotonin, epinephrine, ADP and thrombin by the platelet leads to further platelet activation, and at the site of injury, the generation and further accumulation of thrombin. Platelet activation also results in complex changes in the phospholipid composition of the platelet membrane. In its activated form, the platelet membrane provides an optimal surface for the function of key coagulation enzymes and participates as an important cofactor in several of the major enzymatic steps necessary for the ultimate formation of cross-linked fibrin [7].

A number of newer platelet-related aspects of coagulation should be mentioned. There is emerging appreciation of the role of meizothrombin (generated without participation of the catalytic platelet membrane) and its augmentation of the effects of protein C in the distal vasculature, and other aspects of vascular thrombin–thrombomodulin regulation [8]. Additionally, while we have appreciated the significant interactions of platelets with white blood cells, more recent attention has focused on the emerging role of neutrophil extracellular traps, which not only participate in immune responses to foreign bacterial pathogens, but also contribute to thrombotic progression at the site of injury in ways that create new frameworks to which platelets can bind and activate [9]. There have also been significant advances in our understanding of the role of "procoagulant" platelets (also known as "balloon" platelets), which have features distinct from normal "activated" platelets in that the IIb/IIIa integrin is NOT activated but their spread, ballooned, surface still serves as a site for coagulation factor binding to accelerate the formation of thrombus [10,11].

Overview of Antiplatelet Agents

Coagulation can be practically viewed as a four-step process of platelet activation, platelet aggregation, thrombin generation and thrombin activity (Figure 5.1), since all current therapies act on one or more of these steps. Antiplatelet agents can obviously affect the first two direct

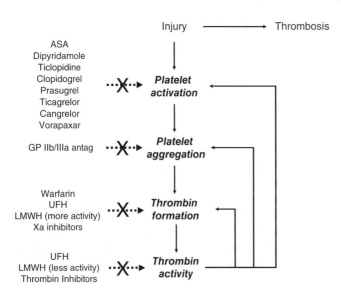

Figure 5.1 The process of coagulation viewed as four key steps. All available anticoagulant and antiplatelet agents work at one or more of the steps, as illustrated. GP, glycoprotein; LMWH, low molecular weight heparin; UFH, unfractionated heparin.

Table 5.1 P2Y$_{12}$ Inhibitors.

	Ticlopidine	Clopidogrel	Prasugrel	Ticagrelor	Cangrelor
Drug class	Thienopyridine	Thienopyridine	Thienopyridine	CPTP	ATP analog
Receptor blockade	Irreversible	Irreversible	Irreversible	Reversible	Reversible
Pro-drug	Yes	Yes	Yes	No	No
Administration	Oral	Oral	Oral	Oral	IV
Onset of action	2–3 hours	2–6 hours	30 minutes	30 minutes	2 minutes
Duration of pharmacodynamic effect	Approx. 1 week	3–10 days	7–10 days	3–5 days	1–2 hours
Mechanism of recovery	Manufacture of new platelets	Manufacture of new platelets	Manufacture of new platelets	Falling plasma levels	Falling plasma levels
Half-life (active moiety)	Active moiety not identified; presumably similar to other thienopyridines	30–60 minutes	30–60 minutes	6–12 hours	5–10 minutes
Indication	Stroke (coronary artery stenting)	ACS PCI in stable coronary artery disease	PCI in ACS	ACS Prior MI	PCI in patients with or without ACS
ENT-1 effect	No	No	No	Yes	Weak (metabolite)
Withdrawal before surgery	10–14 days	5 days	7 days	5 days	1 hour

ACS, acute coronary syndrome; ATP, adenosine triphosphate; IV, intravenous; MI, myocardial infarction; PCI, percutaneous coronary intervention.

platelet steps, but may also impact the latter stages, given the substantial dependence of thrombin generation on the presence of an activated platelet membrane, and the feedback actions of thrombin on further platelet activation. The following section outlines the major categories of antiplatelet therapy considered in STEMI patients undergoing coronary intervention (Table 5.1).

Aspirin

Aspirin (acetylsalicylic acid) irreversibly inhibits the platelet enzyme cyclooxygenase-1 (COX-1), preventing the oxygenation of arachidonic acid and interfering with the synthesis of thromboxane-A2 (TXA2). TXA2 is important because it is a mediator of platelet activation via platelet TXA2 receptors and an important amplification mechanism. A single activated platelet, as it releases TXA2, can activate other adjacent platelets, which can then activate even more local platelets. The effects of aspirin on TXA2-induced activation are largely dose-independent; giving higher doses of aspirin does not generally increase the degree of platelet inhibition in response to TXA2. In addition to its COX-dependent actions, aspirin has other, non-COX-mediated effects which are more dose dependent [12].

Thienopyridines

The ADP-receptor antagonists ticlopidine and clopidogrel are pro-drugs that, when activated, bind to the platelet $P2Y_{12}$ receptor, inhibiting ADP binding and subsequent ADP-induced platelet aggregation (Figure 5.2). Adverse effects of ticlopidine include neutropenia and thrombotic thrombocytopenic purpura. Although rare, these adverse effects occur sufficiently frequently that hematologic monitoring is advised. Although thrombocytopenia and neutropenia can also be seen with clopidogrel, they are much less frequent than with ticlopidine, and hematologic monitoring is not routinely necessary with clopidogrel [13]. In light of its favorable adverse-effect profile, the lack of need for laboratory monitoring and once-daily dosing, clopidogrel has emerged as the preferred and more extensively used agent in the setting of PCI. Clopidogrel has become part of routine adjunctive pharmacology in the setting of PCI, and is widely used in the management of ACS. However, concerns regarding variability in the antiplatelet effect in individual patients, potential drug–drug interactions, and warnings from the US Food and Drug Administration (FDA) regarding genetic predispositions toward clopidogrel "non-responsiveness" have prompted increased interest in effective alternatives [14].

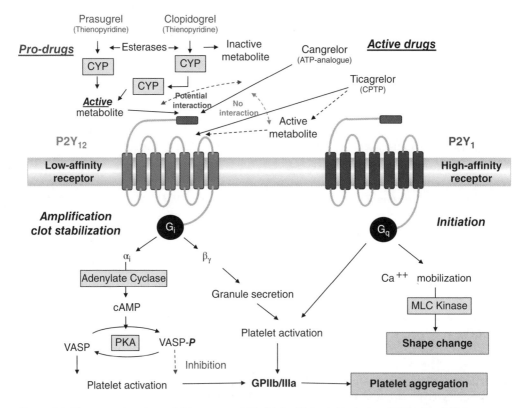

Figure 5.2 There are two primary P2Y receptors, $P2Y_1$ (high affinity; initiation) and $P2Y_{12}$ (low affinity; amplification and clot stabilization); $P2Y_{12}$ inhibitors include pro-drugs (thienopyridines clopidogrel and prasugrel) and active drugs (adenosine triphosphate, ATP, analog cangrelor and cyclo-pentyl-triazolo-pyrimidine, CPTP, ticagrelor). There are potential interactions between the binding of cangrelor and thienopyridines; no such interactions have been noted between cangrelor and ticagrelor. G-protein-coupled signaling of the P2Y receptors culminates in platelet shape change, activation and aggregation. cAMP, cyclic adenosine monophosphate; MLC, myosine light chain; PKA, protein kinase A; VASP, vasodilator-stimulated phosphoprotein.

Prasugrel is a newer thienopyridine, which differs from clopidogrel in its metabolism and activation, with greater potency and faster onset of activity [15,16]. Prasugrel is approximately ten- to one hundred-fold more potent than clopidogrel, and peak plasma concentrations of the active metabolite are reached approximately 30 minutes after administration. Prasugrel is cleared both by the liver and the kidney: about 68% of the prasugrel dose is excreted in the urine and 27% in the feces, as inactive metabolites. The half-life for the active metabolite of prasugrel is approximately 7.4 hours. Prasugrel may help to overcome some of the lack of responsiveness that may arise in identified populations that do not metabolize clopidogrel well [17]. Other new non-thienopyridine ADP-receptor blockers include cangrelor and ticagrelor.

Cangrelor

Cangrelor is an intravenous, rapidly reversible $P2Y_{12}$ antagonist recently approved as adjunctive pharmacotherapy during PCI. It is a non-thienopyridine adenosine triphosphate (ATP) analog, available in an intravenous formulation. Unlike clopidogrel, it does not require metabolic activation and its effects are rapidly reversible with a short half-life of 3–5 minutes [18]. Doses of 2–4 µg/kg/minute provide rapid, virtually complete inhibition of ADP-stimulated platelet aggregation, with an acceptable safety profile [19,20]. One unique feature of cangrelor is its rapid speed of offset following cessation of therapy, which is a function of its structural similarity to ATP. The half-life of cangrelor is 3–5 minutes; following drug discontinuation, platelet function returns to normal in 30–60 minutes.

Ticagrelor

Ticagrelor belongs to the chemical class of cyclo-pentyl-triazolo-pyrimidines (CPTPs). It is the first direct-acting, reversibly binding oral ADP receptor antagonist [21,22]. Ticagrelor provides a more rapid onset, and more extensive and more consistent degree of platelet inhibition than clopidogrel. Ticagrelor (in physiologically relevant concentrations) has also been shown to inhibit the uptake of adenosine via a blockade of the equilibrative nucleoside transporter-1, and, clinically, has been shown to have effects on adenosine-mediated dyspnea, endothelial function, and coronary blood flow [23–26]. In addition to its $P2Y_{12}$ inhibitory effect, ticagrelor may also interfere with $P2Y_{13}$ signaling, but in a way that does not interfere with pro-platelet formation by megakaryocytes. $P2Y_{13}$, like $P2Y_{12}$, is a purinergic Gi-coupled purinergic receptor which appears to have a potential physiologic role in ATP release from red blood cells, bone remodeling, pro-platelet formation, reverse cholesterol transport, and neuropathic pain [27]. Data from 2015 have also suggested that ticagrelor may increase recruitment of endothelial progenitor cells to sites of injury [28].

Ticagrelor is not a pro-drug and does not require metabolic activation. After oral drug administration, ticagrelor is absorbed in the small intestine with detectable plasma levels in 15 minutes. Peak plasma concentrations and steady state are dose proportional and occur between 1.5 and 3 hours. Ticagrelor has a rapid onset of activity (a maximum inhibition of platelet aggregation of 88% at 2 hours post administration) and a significantly faster offset of activity than the irreversibly bound thienopyridines. The inhibition of platelet aggregation 24 hours after stopping ticagrelor (58%) is higher than that measured with clopidogrel, but 3 days after stopping ticagrelor it has fallen to a level equivalent to that seen 5 days after stopping clopidogrel. In contrast to thienopyridines, where the return of platelet function is dependent on the manufacture of new platelets to replace those to whom the thienopyridines are irreversibly bound, return of platelet function of ticagrelor appears to be directly related to falling plasma levels of active drug and an active metabolite. Ticagrelor is predominantly metabolized by CYP3A4/5 in the liver; less than 1% is excreted in the urine. The half-life of ticagrelor is 8–10 hours.

Other Available Antiplatelet Agents

Glycoprotein IIb/IIIa Inhibitors

Glycoprotein IIb/IIIa (GP IIb/IIIa) serves as the final common pathway for platelet aggregation. Ligands such as dimeric fibrinogen and multimeric von Willebrand factor bind to GP IIb/IIIa receptors on platelets, and act to cross-link adjacent platelets. GP IIb/IIIa inhibitors interfere with this binding, effectively preventing the accumulation of a critical mass of activated platelet membranes (a necessary cofactor for coagulation) at the site of injury. Three intravenous GP IIb/IIIa inhibitors are currently available: abciximab, tirofiban, and eptifibatide. Abciximab is a chimeric human–murine monoclonal antibody fragment that targets the GP IIb/IIIa receptor, while tirofiban (non-peptide) and eptifibatide (non-immunogenic cyclic heptapeptide with an active pharmacophore) are high-affinity, competitive, non-antibody GP IIb/IIIa receptor inhibitors that mimic the active recognition moiety of fibrinogen [29].

Protease-Activated Receptor-1 Antagonists

Another recently approved class of antiplatelet agents is the protease-activated receptor-1 (PAR-1) antagonists [30]. Protease-activated receptors are G-protein-coupled receptors with a unique proteolytic activation mechanism. They are activated by thrombin (and other coagulation and inflammatory proteases) found at sites of tissue injury. They play a particularly important role in the pathogenesis of clinical disorders characterized by chronic inflammation or smoldering activation of the coagulation cascade. PAR-1 (in conjunction with PAR-4) appears to play an important role in linking to the initiation of inflammatory signaling pathways [31,32]. One oral PAR-1 antagonist (vorapaxar) was recently approved by the FDA to reduce thrombotic cardiovascular events in patients with a history of myocardial infarction or peripheral arterial disease; however, it is not currently approved for acute STEMI treatment [33].

Aspirin in STEMI

Oral antiplatelet therapy with aspirin has become a foundational part of STEMI care, dating back to the early days of fibrinolytic therapy. The Second International Study of Infarct Survival Study evaluated the role of aspirin during thrombolysis with streptokinase in 17,187 patients randomized to streptokinase alone, aspirin alone, streptokinase plus aspirin, and placebo [34]. Patients treated with aspirin alone had a 2.4% absolute reduction in the incidence of vascular mortality compared with placebo (9.4% vs. 11.8%, $P < 0.00001$). The combination of aspirin plus streptokinase resulted in a 5.2% absolute reduction in 5-week vascular mortality compared with placebo alone (8.0% vs. 13.2%, $P < 0.00001$). Roux et al. published a meta-analysis on 32 studies evaluating concurrent thrombolysis and aspirin therapy, and demonstrated an absolute reduction of 14% in the angiographic incidence of infarct-related artery reocclusion in patients receiving aspirin compared with patients not receiving aspirin therapy (11% vs. 25%, $P < 0.001$), as well as a reduction in recurrent ischemic events from 41% to 25% ($P < 0.001$). [35]. The benefit of aspirin in preventing infarct-related coronary artery reocclusion and subsequent vascular death appears to be independent of either thrombolysis or thrombolytic agent used. Since aspirin is such an integral part of adjunctive pharmacology for PCI, no trials have randomized patients undergoing PCI to aspirin or placebo. The significant independent benefit of aspirin on improving outcomes in STEMI patients has resulted in aspirin therapy within 24 hours of symptom onset becoming the standard of care for all patients presenting with STEMI, regardless of reperfusion strategy.

ADP Blockers in ACS, PCI and STEMI Intervention

Older Agents (Table 5.2)

In the early era of percutaneous balloon coronary intervention, ticlopidine was part of the general antithrombotic armamentarium that included dipyridamole, aspirin, low molecular weight dextran, and very high doses of unfractionated heparin. As attention turned to longer-term therapy, particular with the emergence of coronary stents, clopidogrel rapidly supplanted ticlopidine because of its favorable adverse-effect profile [36], and the fact that it did not require testing for the dreaded, potentially fatal, adverse effect of neutropenia. Several trials subsequently evaluated the role of clopidogrel (as the de facto standard of care in addition to aspirin) in patients presenting with non-STEMI ACS. The Clopidogrel in Unstable Angina to Prevent Recurrent Events (CURE) trial randomized 12,562 patients with ACS (without STEMI) presenting within 24 hours after symptom onset to clopidogrel (300 mg load, followed by 75 mg once daily) or placebo [37]. All patients were treated with aspirin and received either clopidogrel or placebo for 3–12 months. It is worth noting, however, that this trial was carried out at a time when a conservative, wait-and-watch approach for non-ST-elevation acute coronary syndrome (NSTEACS) was much more common. The primary endpoint, a composite of cardiovascular death, nonfatal myocardial infarction and stroke, was reduced from 11.4% to 9.3% in patients receiving dual antiplatelet therapy ($P < 0.001$). However, there was an increase in major bleeding in patients treated with clopidogrel compared with placebo (3.7% vs. 2.7%, $P = 0.001$), without a significant increase in life-threatening bleeding or hemorrhagic strokes.

An important substudy focused on patients in CURE who underwent PCI; it included a total of 2658 patients with PCI (of the total cohort of 12,562) who were randomized to receive clopidogrel or placebo. PCI was performed during the initial hospitalization took place a median of 6 days after starting therapy and a median of 10 days after starting therapy in the overall study, reflecting the more conservative treatment standards at the time [38]. Following PCI, both groups of patients received open-label thienopyridine treatment for 4 weeks, after which initial randomized therapy with clopidogrel or placebo was restarted for the duration of subsequent follow-up. The primary endpoint of this substudy (a composite of cardiovascular death, myocardial infarction, and urgent target-vessel revascularization, TVR, within 30 days of PCI) was significantly reduced in the clopidogrel group (4.5% vs. 6.4%, $P = 0.03$). Long-term treatment with clopidogrel compared with placebo resulted in a relative risk reduction of 31% in cardiovascular death and myocardial infarction, including events before and after PCI ($P = 0.001$), with no significant difference in major bleeding at follow-up.

Another study of clopidogrel in patients undergoing PCI (not in the setting of myocardial infarction) was the Clopidogrel for the Reduction of Events During Observation trial, which randomized 2116 patients undergoing elective PCI to clopidogrel (300 mg loading dose, followed by 75 mg daily for 12 months) or placebo [39]. Patients in the placebo group received 75 mg of clopidogrel daily for 28 days after PCI. The primary endpoints were the composite of death, myocardial infarction, and stroke at 1 year, and the incidence of death, myocardial infarction, and urgent TVR at 28 days. Treatment with clopidogrel resulted in a relative risk reduction of 26.9% in the primary composite endpoint at one year (8.5% vs. 11.5%, $P = 0.02$). There was no significant difference between treatment groups in the reduction of death, myocardial infarction or urgent TVR at 28 days ($P = 0.23$). A pre-specified subgroup analysis of patients receiving clopidogrel ≥ 6 hours prior to PCI and, compared with placebo-matched patients, demonstrated a non-significant relative risk reduction of 38.6% in the combined 28-day endpoint ($P = 0.51$). There was no reduction in the endpoint in patients receiving clopidogrel < 6 hours prior to PCI. Risk of thrombolysis in myocardial infarction (TIMI) major bleeding was higher in patients receiving clopidogrel at 1 year (8.8% vs. 6.7%, $P = 0.07$).

Table 5.2 Ticlopidine and clopidogrel studies.

Trial	Study Population	Patients (n)	Treatment Groups	Duration	Primary Endpoints	Results
CLASSICS [36]	Successful stent placement	1,020	Clopidogrel 300 mg/75 mg Clopidogrel no load/75 mg Ticlopidine no load/250 mg twice daily	28 days	Composite (safety/tolerability) Major bleeding Neutropenia, thrombocytopenia, early drug discontinuation for non-cardiac adverse effects (at 28 days)	Significant ↓ Clopidogrel combined 4.6% Ticlopidine 9.1%
CAPRIE [37]	3 groups History of ischemic stroke (≥1 week, ≤6 months) History of MI (≤35 days) PAD	19,185	Clopidogrel 75 mg Aspirin 325 mg	1–3 years Mean 1.91 years	Composite Vascular death, MI, stroke	Significant ↓ Clopidogrel 5.32% Aspirin 5.83% (per year)
CURE [38]	Non-STEACS	12,562	Clopidogrel + aspirin vs. aspirin	3–12 months (mean 9 months)	Composite CV death, MI, stroke	Significant ↓ Clopidogrel + aspirin 9.3% Aspirin 11.4%
CREDO [39]	Elective PCI	2,116	Clopidogrel 300 mg/75 mg (x 12 months) 75 mg load/75 mg (x 28 days)	1 year	Composite Death, MI, stroke (at 1 year)	Significant ↓ 300/75 8.5% 75/75 11.5%
CURRENT-OASIS 7 [40]	ACS patients managed with an early invasive strategy	25,087	2 x 2 Clopidogrel 600 mg/150 mg (7 days)/75 mg vs. 300 mg/75 mg Aspirin 300–325 mg/day vs. 75–100 mg/day	30 days	Composite CV death, MI, stroke (at 30 days)	Clopidogrel arms: No significant difference Aspirin arms: No significant difference

CLARITY – TIMI 28 [41]	STEMI Thrombolytic drug	3,491	Clopidogrel 300/mg75 mg Placebo	Composite Death, Rec MI (prior to angiography) Infarct artery occlusion on angiography	Up to time of angiography (done at 48–192 hours (median 84 hours)	Significant ↓ Clopidogrel 15.0% Placebo 21.7%
COMMIT-CCS-2 [42]	Suspected MI (primary PCI excluded)	45,852	Clopidogrel 75 mg/day Placebo	Composite All-cause mortality, MI, Stroke	Until discharge or up to 4 weeks (whichever came first) Mean 15 days	Significant ↓ Clopidogrel 9.2% Placebo 10.1%
CHARISMA [102]	Clinically evident CV disease or multiple risk factors	15,603	Clopidogrel 75 mg/day Placebo (background aspirin in all)	Composite CV death, MI, stroke	Median 28-month follow-up	No significant difference Clopidogrel 6.8% Placebo 7.3%

ACS, acute coronary syndrome; CV, cardiovascular; MI, myocardial infarction; PAD, peripheral artery disease; PCI, percutaneous coronary intervention; ↓ = reduction.

The CURRENT-OASIS 7 trial assessed the efficacy of a higher loading and maintenance dose of clopidogrel (600 mg, then 150 mg for 7 days, then 75 mg daily) compared with the standard dosing regimen (300 mg, then 75 mg), as well as comparing high-dose (300–325 mg daily) to low-dose (75–100 mg daily) aspirin therapy in patients presenting with ACS (unstable angina/non-STEMI) and STEMI managed with an early invasive strategy [40]. The study randomized 25,087 patients, of whom 70.8% presented with ACS and 29.2% presented with STEMI. Coronary angiography was performed on 24,769 patients; 17,232 (70%) of the study patients actually underwent PCI. Of the patients who did not undergo PCI, 1809 were referred for coronary artery bypass graft (CABG), 2430 with occlusive coronary artery disease were treated medically, and 3616 had no significant coronary artery disease. The primary efficacy outcome was the composite of cardiovascular death, myocardial infarction, and stroke at 30 days. The primary safety outcome was major bleeding. There were no significant differences in outcomes seen in patients randomized to high-dose or low-dose aspirin therapy, despite a trend to increased gastrointestinal bleeding in patients treated with high-dose aspirin (0.38 vs. 0.24, $P = 0.051$). In patients undergoing PCI, high-dose clopidogrel was associated with a statistically significant decrease in the combined primary endpoint (3.9% vs. 4.5%, $P = 0.036$), the incidence of myocardial infarction (2.6% vs. 2.0%, $P = 0.012$), and the incidence of stent thrombosis (2.3% vs. 1.6%, $P = 0.002$). In patients who presented with STEMI, there was a similar decrease in both the incidence of the combined primary endpoint, and the incidence of stent thrombosis and myocardial infarction in patients treated with high-dose clopidogrel relative to standard dosing (4.2% vs. 5.0%, and 2.8% vs. 4.0%, respectively; P-values not reported). The incidences of TIMI major bleeding, fatal bleeding and CABG-related bleeding were similar in patients treated with higher dosing and standard dosing of clopidogrel. Patients who did not undergo PCI had no difference in the combined primary endpoint, irrespective of randomization to high-dose or standard dose clopidogrel (4.9% vs. 4.2% $P = 0.14$).

Several studies have examined the use of clopidogrel in STEMI patients undergoing thrombolysis. The CLARITY-TIMI 28 [41] and COMMIT/CCS-2 [42] trials showed significant benefit of clopidogrel pretreatment in patients presenting with STEMI and treated with thrombolytic therapy. The CLARITY-TIMI 28 trial evaluated 3491 patients with STEMI who presented within 12 hours of symptom onset who were treated with thrombolysis, aspirin and, when indicated, unfractionated heparin, and randomized them to receive either clopidogrel (300 mg load and 75 mg once daily) or placebo [41]. All patients underwent angiography; the primary efficacy endpoint was the composite of death, recurrent myocardial infarction prior to angiography, and presence of infarct-related artery occlusion (TIMI flow grade 0 or 1) on angiography. Dual antiplatelet therapy with aspirin and the addition of clopidogrel resulted in a 6.7% absolute reduction of the primary efficacy endpoint compared with aspirin and placebo (15.0% vs. 21.7%, $P < 0.001$). At 30 days, patients treated with clopidogrel had a continued relative risk reduction in the primary endpoint of cardiovascular death, recurrent myocardial infarction and urgent TVR compared with patients treated with placebo (11.6% vs. 14.1 %, $P = 0.03$).

COMMIT/CCS-2 evaluated 45,852 patients within 24 hours of suspected acute myocardial infarction onset and randomized patients to clopidogrel (75 mg daily) or placebo [42]. All patients received aspirin; 93% of those enrolled had ST-segment elevation or left bundle branch block pattern on initial electrocardiogram. Treatment with clopidogrel was continued until hospital discharge or up to 4 weeks in patients with prolonged hospitalizations. The mean duration of therapy in survivors was 15 days. The primary endpoints were the composite of all-cause mortality, recurrent myocardial infarction, and stroke. Patients treated with clopidogrel had a significant decrease in death, recurrent myocardial infarction, and stroke compared with placebo (9.2% vs. 10.1%, $P = 0.002$), as well as a decrease in all-cause mortality

(7.5% vs. 8.1%, $P = 0.03$). Clopidogrel-treated patients had similar rate of bleeding compared with placebo-treated patients with respect to the combined incidence of intracranial hemorrhage, fatal bleeding, and transfusions (0.58% vs. 0.55%, $P = 0.59$).

Newer Agents

Prasugrel (Table 5.3)

The Therapeutic Outcomes by Optimizing Platelet Inhibition with Prasugrel – Thrombolysis in Myocardial Infarction 38 (TRITON-TIMI 38) trial compared prasugrel with clopidogrel in 13,608 patients with moderate-to-high-risk ACS, including 3534 STEMI patients > 12 hours after onset of symptoms or within 14 days of medical treatment of STEMI [43]. Prasugrel was given as a 60 mg loading dose, followed by 10 mg daily. Clopidogrel was administered as a 300 mg loading dose and then daily for 75 mg. Study drug therapy was given for 6–15 months (median duration 14.5 months). The combined primary endpoint included death from cardiovascular causes, nonfatal myocardial infarction, and nonfatal stroke. The key safety endpoint was TIMI major and minor bleeding. The incidence of the primary endpoint was lower in patients treated with prasugrel compared with clopidogrel (9.9% vs. 12.1%, $P < 0.001$). A reduction in the combined primary efficacy endpoint was also seen in the subgroup of patients with STEMI treated with prasugrel. Compared with clopidogrel-treated patients, prasugrel-treated patients had lower rates of myocardial infarction (7.4% vs. 9.7%, $P < 0.001$), urgent TVR (2.5% vs. 3.7%, $P < 0.001$), and stent thrombosis (1.1% vs. 2.4%, $P < 0.001$). The incidence of major bleeding was increased in patients treated with prasugrel (2.4% vs. 1.8%, $P = 0.03$). The rate of life-threatening bleeding (1.4% vs. 0.9%, $P = 0.01$), nonfatal bleeding (1.1% vs. 0.9%; HR 1.25; $P = 0.23$), fatal bleeding (0.4% vs. 0.1%, $P = 0.002$) and CABG-related TIMI major bleeding (13.4% vs. 3.2%; $P < 0.001$) were all significantly increased in patients treated with prasugrel.

The STEMI substudy of TRITON-TIMI 38 evaluated the findings in 3534 STEMI patients (1760 prasugrel, 1765 clopidogrel) in TRITON-TIMI 38 undergoing PCI. This analysis included both patients undergoing immediate revascularization ("primary" PCI, $n = 2,340$) and patients undergoing delayed revascularization (so-called "secondary" PCI, $n = 1085$) [44]. In the total STEMI population, at 30 days, 6.5% of patients receiving prasugrel had met the primary endpoint compared with 9.5% who received clopidogrel ($P = 0.0017$), and this effect continued out to 15 months (10.0% v 12.4%, $P = 0.0221$). The secondary endpoint of cardiovascular death, myocardial infarction, or urgent target-vessel revascularization was also significantly reduced with prasugrel at 30 days ($P = 0.0205$) and 15 months ($P = 0.0250$), as was stent thrombosis ($P = 0.0084$). Treatments did not differ with respect to TIMI major bleeding unrelated to CABG at 30 days ($P = 0.3359$) and 15 months ($P = 0.6451$). TIMI major bleeding after CABG was significantly increased with prasugrel ($P = 0.0033$).

TRILOGY ACS was a study of 9326 ACS patients who were medically managed and did not undergo revascularization [45]. Patients were randomized to receive either prasugrel or clopidogrel (in addition to aspirin) for up to 30 months. Prasugrel patients over 75 years of age received 5 mg per day instead of the usual daily dose of 10 mg. The mean duration of study drug treatment was 17 months. The primary endpoint, the composite of cardiovascular death, myocardial infarction or stoke in the 7243 patients less than 75 years of age was not significantly different in the two treatment group (13.9% with prasugrel, 16.0% with clopidogrel; $P = 0.21$), with similar results in the overall study population (18.7% with prasugrel, 20.3% with clopidogrel; $P = 0.45$). Major bleeding (GUSTO severe non-CABG and TIMI major non-CABG) was also not significantly different between the two treatment arms. There was no significant statistical interaction between history of prior myocardial infarction and outcomes between treatment groups.

Table 5.3 Prasugrel studies.

Trial	Study population	Patients (n)	Treatment		Primary endpoints	Duration	Results
			Groups				
TRITON-TIMI 38 [43,44]	ACS patients undergoing PCI (no prior thienopyridine)	13,608	60 mg/10 mg prasugrel 300 mg/75 mg clopidogrel (background aspirin)		Composite CV death, MI, stroke	6–15 months Median 14.5 months	Significance ↓ Prasugrel 9.9% Clopidogrel 12.1%
TRILOGY ACS [45]	Medically managed ACS (not undergoing PCI)	9,326	Prasugrel 10 mg (5 mg if >75 years) Clopidogrel 75 mg		Composite CV death, MI, stroke (In patients <75)	Up to 30 months (mean 17 months)	No significant difference Prasugrel 13.9% Clopidogrel 16.0%
ACCOAST [46]	Troponin (+) ACS	4,033	Pretreatment: 30 mg prior If PCI, additional 30 mg, then 10 mg/day No pretreatment: If PCI, 60 mg load, then 10 mg/day		Composite CV death, MI, stroke Urgent revascularization (at 7 days)	Up to 7 days	No significant difference Pretreatment 10.0% No pretreatment 9.8%

ACS, acute coronary syndrome; CV, cardiovascular; MI, myocardial infarction; PCI, percutaneous coronary intervention; ↓ = reduction.

The ACCOAST study included 4033 patients with troponin (plus) NSTEACS undergoing angiography and possible PCI [46]. Participating subjects were randomized to receive pretreatment with either 30 mg of prasugrel or placebo prior to angiography (median time from initial study drug to angiography was 4.2–4.4 hours). If PCI was performed, the prasugrel pretreatment arm received an additional 30 mg of prasugrel; placebo-preloaded patients received a 60-mg loading dose of prasugrel prior to PCI. The primary endpoint, the composite of cardiovascular death, myocardial infarction, stroke, urgent revascularization, or GP IIb/IIIa bailout out to 7 days did not differ between the two treatment arms (10.0% with prasugrel pretreatment, 9.8% with no pretreatment; $P = 0.81$). TIMI major bleeding (and bleeding assessed with multiple other bleeding scales) was significantly higher in the prasugrel pretreatment arm. Similar outcomes for both efficacy and bleeding were noted at 30 days.

Ticagrelor (Table 5.4)

The Platelet Inhibition and Patient Outcomes (PLATO) study was a large phase III clinical trial which enrolled 18,624 hospitalized patients with ACS and randomized them to either ticagrelor (180 mg loading dose, followed by 90 mg twice daily; $n = 9,333$) or clopidogrel (300–600 mg loading dose, or continued prior therapy, followed by 75 mg/day; $n = 9291$) [47]. Therapy was continued for 6–12 months; all patients were treated with concomitant aspirin. The primary endpoint was the composite of cardiovascular death, myocardial infarction, or stroke at 1 year. In the overall study, primary outcome events were significantly lower with ticagrelor (9.8% vs. 11.7% with clopidogrel; $P < 0.001$). This benefit was present not only within the first 30 days (4.8% vs. 5.4% with clopidogrel; $P = 0.045$), but also from day 31 onwards (5.3% vs. 6.6% with clopidogrel; $P < 0.001$). Moreover, there was a significant reduction in both cardiovascular death (4.0% vs. 5.1% with clopidogrel; $P = 0.001$) and total mortality (4.5% vs. 5.9% with clopidogrel; $P < 0.001$). Study-defined major bleeding did not differ between groups (11.6% vs. 11.2% with clopidogrel; $P = NS$). Total TIMI major bleeding was also not significantly different between groups (7.9% vs. 7.7% with clopidogrel; $P = NS$); however non-CABG TIMI major bleeding was significantly higher with ticagrelor (2.8% vs. 2.2%; $P = 0.03$). The incidence of dyspnea was significantly higher with ticagrelor (13.8% vs. 7.8% with clopidogrel; $P < 0.001$), and transient increases in creatinine and serum uric acid while on study treatment with ticagrelor were noted, but resolved at follow-up.

In an analysis of the 7544 STEACS and new patients with left bundle branch block in PLATO who were intended for primary PCI [48], primary outcomes were non-significantly lower with ticagrelor (9.4% with ticagrelor vs. 10.8% with clopidogrel; $P = 0.07$), consistent with the overall PLATO results. Myocardial infarction (4.7% with ticagrelor vs. 5.8% with clopidogrel; $P = 0.03$), total mortality (5.0% with ticagrelor vs. 6.1% with clopidogrel; $P = 0.05$), and definite stent thrombosis (1.6% with ticagrelor vs. 2.4% with clopidogrel; $P = 0.03$) were all individually significantly lower with ticagrelor. Stroke, although low, was significantly higher with ticagrelor (1.7% vs 1.0%; $P = 0.02$), while there were no significant differences between ticagrelor and clopidogrel in PLATO major bleeding (9.0% with ticagrelor vs. 9.2% with clopidogrel; $P = 0.76$) or TIMI major bleeding (6.1% with ticagrelor vs. 6.4% with clopidogrel; $P = 0.66$).

The ATLANTIC study [49] examined the question of whether the use of pre-hospital ticagrelor could improve coronary perfusion or clinical outcomes in STEMI patients undergoing primary PCI. A total of 1862 STEMI patients were randomized within 6 hours of pain onset to receive either pre-hospital loading with ticagrelor, administered in the ambulance, or loading with ticagrelor in the catheterization laboratory at the time of the procedure. The co-primary endpoints were the percent of patients who did not have > 70% ST-segment resolution

Table 5.4 Ticagrelor studies.

Trial	Study population	Treatment			Primary Endpoints	Results
		Patients (n)	Groups	Duration		
PLATO [47]	UA/NSTEMI managed invasively or conservatively STEMI undergoing primary PCI	18,624	Ticagrelor 180 mg/90 mg twice daily Clopidogrel 300 mg or 600 mg/75 mg (background aspirin)	Median 277 days	Composite CV death, MI, stroke	Significant ↓ Ticagrelor 9.8% Clopidogrel 11.7%
PEGASUS – TIMI 54 [50]	1–3 years post-MI (STE or NSTE)	21,162	Ticagrelor 60 mg Ticagrelor 90 mg Placebo (background aspirin)	Median 33 months	Composite CV death, MI, stroke	Significant ↓ Ticagrelor 90 7.85% Ticagrelor 60 7.77% Placebo 9.04%
ATLANTIC [49]	STEMI undergoing primary PCI	1,862	Pre-hospital load versus in-hospital load of 180 mg ticagrelor	Prior to PCI	% of patients with >70% ST-segment resolution plus % patients without TIMI grade 3 flow	No significant difference One or both endpoints: Pre-hospital 94.2% In-hospital 94.5% Both endpoints: Pre-hospital 72.7% In-hospital 73.5%

ACS, acute coronary syndrome; CV, cardiovascular; MI, myocardial infarction; PCI, percutaneous coronary intervention; STE, ST-elevation; UA, unstable angina; ↓ = reduction.

before PCI and the proportion of patients who did not achieve TIMI grade 3 flow at the time of initial angiography. Secondary endpoints included the incidence of stent thrombosis (Academic Research Consortium definite) and major adverse clinical events. There were no significant differences between pre-hospital and in-hospital loading in either of the two co-primary endpoints (ST-segment resolution and TIMI grade 3 flow). There were also no differences between groups in the percentage of patients not achieving at least 70% ST-segment resolution following PCI, and no difference between groups in major adverse cardiovascular clinical events. There was, however, a significant reduction in definite stent thrombosis in the pre-hospital loading group (0% vs. 0.8% in the first 24 hours and 0.2% vs. 1.2% at 30 days). No significant differences were noted between groups in major bleeding events. Two important points to consider in evaluating the results of ATLANTIC trial are the differences in administration times between the pre-hospital loaded group and the in-hospital loaded group (a median of 38 minutes) and the time from randomization to angiography (a median of 41 minutes).

The PEGASUS study included 21,162 patients who were enrolled 1–3 years following an index myocardial infarction event (STEMI or NSTEMI; median of 1.7 years post event) [50]. Qualifying patients were randomized to either ticagrelor 90 mg twice daily, ticagrelor 60 mg twice daily, or placebo twice daily, on a background of low-dose (75–150 mg) aspirin. The primary efficacy endpoint was the composite of cardiovascular death, myocardial infarction, or stroke. The primary safety endpoint was TIMI major bleeding. Patients were followed for a median of 33 months on therapy. Primary composite endpoints occurred significantly less frequently with ticagrelor: 7.85% in the 90-mg group ($P < 0.008$ vs. placebo), 7.77% in the 60-mg group ($P = 0.004$ vs. placebo) than in the placebo group (9.04%). Individual components of the primary endpoint (cardiovascular death, myocardial infarction, and stroke) occurred in 2.44%, 4.40%, and 1.61% of the 90-mg group, 2.86%, 4.53%, and 1.47% of the 60-mg group, and 3.39%, 5.25% and 1.94% of the placebo group. TIMI major bleeding was more frequent with Ticagrelor: in 2.60% of the 90-mg group ($P < 0.001$ vs. placebo), 2.30% of the 60-mg group ($P < 0.001$ vs. placebo) and 1.06% in the placebo group. Dyspnea was reported more frequently with ticagrelor: in 18.93% of the 90-mg group ($P < 0.001$ vs. placebo), 15.84% of the 60-mg group ($P < 0.001$ vs. placebo) and 6.38% of the placebo group.

Cangrelor (Table 5.5)

In the CHAMPION-PCI trial, cangrelor was compared with clopidogrel in 8716 patients presenting with ACS and treated with PCI [51]. The primary efficacy end point was the composite of death from any cause, myocardial infarction, or ischemia-driven revascularization at 48 hours. There was no statistical difference between cangrelor vs. clopidogrel with respect to the incidence of the primary composite end point (7.5% vs. 7.1%, $P = 0.59$). The rate of major bleeding (using ACUITY criteria) was higher with cangrelor, a difference that approached statistical significance (3.6% vs. 2.9%, $P = 0.06$). The incidence of TIMI major bleeding or TIMI and GUSTO severe or life-threatening bleeding, however, was similar between cangrelor and clopidogrel. A secondary exploratory endpoint of death from any cause, Q-wave myocardial infarction, or ischemia-driven revascularization, showed a trend toward a reduction with cangrelor, which did not approach statistical significance (0.6% vs. 0.9%, $P = 0.14$).

The efficacy of cangrelor to reduce the incidence of ischemic events following PCI was also evaluated in 5362 patients who were not pretreated with clopidogrel in the CHAMPION-PLATFORM trial [52]. Patients were randomized to either the study drug or placebo at the time of PCI, followed by 600 mg of clopidogrel. The primary end point was the composite of death, myocardial infarction, or ischemia-driven revascularization at 48 hours. Enrollment was prematurely stopped for futility following an interim analysis of the data

Table 5.5 Cangrelor studies.

Trial	Study population	Patients (n)	Treatment Groups	Duration	Primary Endpoints	Results
CHAMPION PCI [51]	ACS undergoing PCI	8,716	Cangrelor arm: 30 μg/kg bolus; 4 μg/kg/minute infusion for > 2 hours or the duration of the procedure (whichever longer) 600 mg clopidogrel after the infusion Clopidogrel arm: Placebo bolus and infusion Clopidogrel 600 mg immediately after the procedure	48 hours	Composite All-cause mortality, MI Ischemia-driven revascularization (at 48 hours)	No significant difference Cangrelor 7.5% Clopidogrel 7.1%
CHAMPION PLATFORM [52]	PCI patients not pretreated with clopidogrel	5,362	Cangrelor arm 30 μg/kg bolus; 4 μg/kg/minute infusion for > 2 hours or the duration of the procedure 600 mg clopidogrel after the infusion Clopidogrel arm Placebo bolus and infusion Clopidogrel 600 mg immediately after the procedure	48 hours	Composite Death, MI Ischemia-driven revascularization (at 48 hours)	No significant difference Cangrelor 7.0% Clopidogrel 8.0% (trial halted prematurely for futility)
CHAMPION PHOENIX [53]	Urgent or elective PCI	11,145	Cangrelor 30 μg/kg bolus; 4 μg/kg/minute infusion for > 2 hours or the duration of the procedure 600 mg clopidogrel after the infusion Clopidogrel 300 mg or 600 mg on-table	48 hours	Composite All-cause mortality, MI Ischemia-driven revascularization Stent thrombosis (including intra-procedural) (at 48 hours)	Significant reduction Cangrelor 4.7% Clopidogrel 5.9%

ACS, acute coronary syndrome; MI, myocardial infarction; PCI, percutaneous coronary intervention.

that strongly suggested that the trial could not demonstrate the superiority of cangrelor for the primary end point. The primary end point occurred in 7% of patients receiving cangrelor and 8.0% of patients treated with placebo ($P = 0.17$). The occurrence of two pre-specified endpoints, the incidence of stent thrombosis and the rate of all-cause mortality were reduced in patients treated with cangrelor relative to placebo (0.6% vs. 0.2%, $P = 0.02$; 0.7% vs. 0.2%, $P = 0.02$, respectively). With respect to bleeding, there was no significant increase in the need for blood transfusions (1.0% vs. 0.6%, $P = 0.13$); however, there was an increase in the incidence of arteriotomy-related bleeding in patients treated with cangrelor (3.5% vs. 5.5%, $P < 0.001$).

The CHAMPION PHOENIX study randomized 11,145 patients undergoing either urgent or elective PCI to receive cangrelor (30 µg/kg bolus followed by an infusion of 4 µg/kg/minute for at least 2 hours) or a loading dose of 600 mg or 300 mg of clopidogrel after the coronary anatomy was defined by angiography [53]. Because of interactions with cangrelor and thienopyridines (described below), the protocol specified that clopidogrel was administered after the end of the cangrelor infusion. The primary efficacy outcome endpoint was the composite of all-cause mortality, myocardial infarction, ischemia-driven revascularization, or stent thrombosis (including the new category of intraprocedural stent thrombosis) at 48 hours in the MITT population ($n = 10,942$). Most patients (63.4%) received their loading dose immediately prior to the PCI procedure; 6.4% received the loading dose during the procedure, 30.1% received the loading dose within 1 hour of the procedure, and a few patients (0.1%) received their loading dose later than 1 hour after the procedure. There was no relationship between the timing of the loading dose and clinical outcomes (P interaction = 0.99).

The presenting diagnosis was STEMI in 18.2%, NSTEACS in 27.5% (including unstable angina in 5.7%), and stable angina in 56.1%. The median time from admission to PCI was 4.4 hours (interquartile range 1.9–21 hours). The primary safety endpoint was non-CABG GUSTO severe bleeding. Cangrelor-treatment significantly reduced the incidence of primary efficacy events (4.7% vs. 5.9%; p = 0.005), with no significant increase in major bleeding events (0.16% vs. 0.11%; $P = 0.44$). Definite stent thrombosis (including intraprocedural stent thrombosis) was also significantly reduced (0.8% vs. 1.4%; $P = 0.01$). The benefits of cangrelor on primary outcomes in STEMI patients (3.5% vs. 4.4%) were similar to those in NSTEACS patients and stable angina patients (5.8% vs. 7.4%; P interaction = 0.98), although numerically more benefit was noted in the stable patients. Transient dyspnea was noted more frequently with cangrelor (1.2% vs. 0.3%; $P < 0.001$).

Cangrelor was approved by the European Medicines Agency in March 2015 for the reduction of thrombotic cardiovascular events in adult patients with coronary artery disease undergoing PCI who have not received an oral $P2Y_{12}$ inhibitor prior to the PCI procedure and in whom oral therapy with $P2Y_{12}$ inhibitors is not feasible or desirable [54] and by the US Food and Drug Administration in June, 2015 as an adjunct for PCI for reducing the risk of periprocedural myocardial infarction, repeat coronary revascularization and stent thrombosis in patients who have not been treated with a $P2Y_{12}$ platelet inhibitor and are not being given a GP IIb/IIIa inhibitor [55].

There are interactions between cangrelor binding and thienopyridine binding [56–58], and the transition from cangrelor to oral agents depends on the drug to which the patient is being transitioned. If patients transition from cangrelor to clopidogrel or prasugrel, a loading dose of the oral agent should be administered only after stopping cangrelor. In patients transitioning to ticagrelor, a loading dose of the oral agent can be given at any time during the cangrelor infusion, or immediately following it [59].

Other Important Issues

Nonprimary Percutaneous Coronary Intervention

One group of patients that has not been widely studied are STEMI patients undergoing delayed PCI (nonprimary reperfusion). The TRITON-TIMI 38 study described earlier included both "primary" PCI patients (within 12 hours of pain onset, $n = 2340$) and an additional 1085 "secondary" PCI patients in their STEMI subgroup analysis [60]. Secondary interventions were defined as PCI procedures occurring later than 12 hours (and up to 14 days) from symptom onset, either as part of routine medical management, or with demonstrated recurrent ischemia. The primary endpoint of the overall study was the composite of cardiovascular death, myocardial infarction, and stroke at 18 months. Because of ascertainment issues surrounding periprocedural myocardial infarctions in the acute STEMI setting, additional analyses excluded periprocedural myocardial infarction. Of note, prior clopidogrel use was an exclusion criterion for TRITON-TIMI 38, even in the secondary PCI STEMI patients. The median time from symptom onset to revascularization in the primary PCI group was 3.7 hours; in the secondary PCI group it was 47.3 hours. The improvement in 30-day primary outcomes with prasugrel tended to be somewhat more prominent in the secondary PCI group (primary 6.7% vs. 8.3%; secondary 6.5% vs. 12.4%: P interaction = 0.06), driven mostly by myocardial infarction (primary 5.1% vs. 5.6%; secondary 5.0% vs. 10.9%; P interaction = 0.01) and especially periprocedural myocardial infarction (primary 4.0% vs. 3.4%; secondary 4.5% vs. 8.2%; P interaction = 0.02).

At 15 months, similar trends were noted in primary endpoints (primary 10.3% vs. 11.6%; secondary 9.6% vs. 14.2%; P interaction = 0.15), total myocardial infarction (primary 7.1% vs. 7.9%; secondary 6.7% vs. 11.9%; P interaction = 0.05) and periprocedural myocardial infarction (primary 4.0% vs. 3.5%; secondary 4.5% vs. 8.2%; P interaction = 0.02). Conversely, non-procedural myocardial infarction outcomes appeared similar between primary and secondary myocardial infarction interventions at both 30 days (primary 1.2% vs. 2.3%; secondary 0.7% vs. 2.7%; P interaction = 0.29) and 15 months (primary 3.3% vs. 4.5%; secondary 2.4% vs. 4.1%; P interaction = 0.57). The authors concluded that the efficacy of prasugrel compared with clopidogrel in STEMI patients undergoing PCI was consistent for both primary and secondary PCI, especially from the perspective of reducing events outside of periprocedural myocardial infarction.

Oral Absorption in STEMI

Earlier literature [61] had suggested that when clopidogrel pharmacokinetics and pharmacodynamics were compared in STEMI patients compared with healthy controls, STEMI patients had lower drug levels of clopidogrel (and its active metabolite), with lower C_{max}, higher T_{max} and lower area under the curve (AUC), as well lower levels of platelet inhibition. Additionally, Osmancik and co-workers documented that hemodynamically unstable STEMI patients has lesser degrees of platelet inhibition than in stable STEMI patients, an effect they attributed, at least in part, to impaired gut function [62]. The effects of narcotics (frequently used in STEMI) on gastric absorption of orally administered medications has been well documented [63], and has also been shown to have a significant effect on orally administered clopidogrel [64].

More recently, Alexopoulos et al. [65] measured platelet function in 55 STEMI patients randomized to ticagrelor or prasugrel. Measurements of platelet reactivity (VerifyNow® system and Multiplate® analyzer) were obtained at baseline, at 1, 2, 6, and 24 hours, and at 5 days after randomization. The primary endpoint, VerifyNow measurements at 1 hour, did not differ significantly between agents, but the authors did note a substantial rate of high on-treatment platelet reactivity (defined as a platelet reactivity unit, PRU, > 208): 46.2% of the ticagrelor group and 34.6% of the prasugrel group. This was one of the first studies documenting delayed onset of antiplatelet activity with new orally administered antiplatelet agents in the setting of STEMI.

This was corroborated by Parodi and co-workers in the Rapid Activity of Platelet Inhibitor Drugs trial [66] In this study, 50 STEMI patients undergoing primary PCI were randomized to either ticagrelor or prasugrel; platelet reactivity (VerifyNow) was measured at baseline, and at 2, 4, 8 and 12 hours after dosing. The investigators observed no difference in platelet reactivity at 2 hours, but also documented high on-treatment reactivity (defined as a PRU > 240) at the 2-hour time point: 60% of ticagrelor patients and 44% of prasugrel patients. They also made the important observation that morphine use was an independent predictor of high on-treatment reactivity, in addition to baseline PRU. A number of other studies have also noted similar effects of morphine [67,68]. Franchi et al. [69] have shown that morphine significantly affects the onset pharmacokinetics and pharmacodynamics of ticagrelor in STEMI patients, with delayed drug absorption and less platelet inhibition after an oral loading dose of ticagrelor in STEMI patients treated with morphine. The same group has shown that increasing oral loading doses of ticagrelor does not overcome this poor absorption [70]. The potential clinical importance of this was highlighted in the above-mentioned ATLANTIC study, in which the subgroup of patients not treated with morphine were noted to have significant better TIMI perfusion at the time of angiography; there was no such difference noted in patients who did receive morphine [49] Kubica et al. [71] have also shown that morphine significantly reduced both the speed of onset and the total exposure to ticagrelor in STEMI patients.

Crushed Tablets

Crushing ticagrelor tablets before oral or nasogastric tube administration has been shown to increase bioavailability [72]. Teng et al. performed a bioavailability study comparing crushed ticagrelor tablets, administered orally or via a nasogastric tube, to orally administered intact ticagrelor tablets in 36 healthy volunteers. Subjects were treated in a triple-crossover design protocol (with a minimum of 7 days between treatments) with single 90-mg tablets and serial blood sampling for pharmacokinetic measurement of plasma ticagrelor and its active metabolite AR-C124910XX concentrations at multiple post-dosing time points [73]. The investigators noted higher initial plasma concentrations with the nasogastric tube and oral crushed tablets at 30 minutes post-dosing (264.6 ng/ml, 148.6 ng/ml and 33.3 ng/ml, respectively), and a shorter T_{max} with crushed compared with intact tablets. (1 hour vs. 2 hours). All AUC and C_{max} mean ratios between treatments fell within pre-specified bioequivalence limits (80–125% for both ticagrelor and the primary active metabolite).

The MOJITO study [74] examined whether administering crushed ticagrelor tablets in patients with myocardial infarction might result in more rapid inhibition of platelet aggregation. A total of 82 STEMI patients were randomized to receive either two crushed ticagrelor tablets (180 mg total) or two intact tablets before primary PCI. Platelet function testing (VerifyNow) was performed at baseline and a 1, 2, 4, and 8 hours after study drug administration. The primary endpoint was the PRU measurement at 1 hour. High platelet reactivity was defined as a PRU greater than 208. At 1 hour, the median PRU was 169 in the crushed-tablet group and 252 in the intact-tablet group ($P < 0.006$). There were no differences in PRU between groups at subsequent time points. Morphine use was found to be an independent predictor of increased high platelet reactivity at 1 hour, even in the crushed-tablet group.

Alexopoulos et al. performed a small study in which 20 STEMI patients undergoing primary PCI were randomized to receive either a standard 180 mg ticagrelor dose (two whole 90-mg tablets) or two crushed, dispersed 90-mg tablets [75]. Blood samples for pharmacokinetics and pharmacodynamics were obtained, and demonstrated that serum levels/exposure of ticagrelor were significantly higher at 1 hour in patients receiving crushed tablets., and the time to maximal plasma concentration was significantly shorter [75].

Duration of Therapy

Dual Antiplatelet Therapy

The Dual Antiplatelet Therapy (DAPT) trial was an international multicenter study comparing the risks and benefits of 30 vs. 12 months of thienopyridine therapy (in addition to aspirin) in patients following coronary stenting with either a bare-metal (BMS) or a drug-eluting stent (DES). The overall study combined five smaller individual studies into a single uniform randomized trial. The DES arm of the study enrolled 9661 patients who received a drug-eluting stent [76]. In order to qualify for the study, patients had to have successfully completed 12 months of thienopyridine therapy (with no intervening clinical or bleeding events), including both clopidogrel and prasugrel, plus aspirin. Patients were randomized to either continue their thienopyridine, or to receive placebo, both on a background of maintenance aspirin therapy. Study drug treatment was continued for 18 months following randomization. The co-primary outcome endpoints were stent thrombosis (definite or probable) and major adverse cardiovascular and cerebrovascular events (MACCE) inkling cardiovascular death, myocardial infarction, and stroke over the time interval from 12–30 months after the original intervention. Results were reported as 18-month Kaplan–Meier event rates. The primary safety endpoint was GUSTO moderate or severe bleeding. Approximately 10.5% of the enrolled patients were STEMI interventions, and approximately 15.5% were NSTEMI interventions. The extended treatment group had significantly lower rates of stent thrombosis (0.4% vs. 1.4%; $P < 0.001$) and MACCE (4.3% vs. 5.9%; $P < 0.001$). The individual endpoint of myocardial infarction was also significantly lower with extended treatment (2.1% vs. 4.1%; $P < 0.001$), while all-cause mortality was marginally significantly higher with extended treatment (2.0% vs. 1.5%; $P = 0.05$). GUSTO moderate or severe bleeding was also significantly higher in the extended therapy group.

Yeh et al. [77] published an additional analysis which looked more closely at 3526 patients with myocardial infarction and 8072 with non-myocardial infarction in the total cohort of 11,648 patients (9961 DES and 1687 BMS) in DAPT. Of the 3576 patients with myocardial infarction, 1680 (47%) underwent their original revascularization in the setting of a STEMI, while the remaining 1896 (53%) were revascularized for a NSTEMI. The effects of extended thienopyridine treatment on clinical outcomes (stent thrombosis and MACCE) and bleeding were similar in myocardial infarction and non-myocardial infarction patients, although, as a whole, stent thrombosis (definite or probable) was more frequent in myocardial infarction patients (1.2% vs. 0.7%; $P = 0.01$), as was the individual outcome endpoint of myocardial infarction (3.7% vs. 2.8%; $P = 0.001$). In patients receiving extended thienopyridine therapy, the co-primary outcome of MACCE was reduced more prominently in myocardial infarction patients (3.9% with extended therapy vs. 6.8%; $P < 0.001$) than in those without myocardial infarction (4.4% with extended therapy vs. 5.3%; $P = 0.08$; P interaction $= 0.03$).

As previously noted, the PEGASUS study showed that adding ticagrelor (either 90 mg or 60 mg twice daily) to aspirin for an extended period of time provided clinical benefit in patients with a history of an myocardial infarction in the prior 1–3 years, with an increase in non-CABG major bleeding [50]. Recently, the 60-mg twice daily dose of ticagrelor was approved by the FDA for use (in addition to low-dose aspirin) in patients with a prior history of myocardial infarction, with no restrictions on timing. The dosing recommendation is to load (180 mg) in the acute ACS setting, treat for up to 1 year with 90 mg twice daily, and then from 1 year onwards to use 60 mg twice daily [78].

A number of meta-analyses have also looked at this issue from varying perspectives. In general, shorter DAPT duration is associated with lower rates of clinically significant bleeding, and higher rates of stent thrombosis, especially so with first-generation DES. Interestingly, all-cause mortality tended to be higher with prolonged DAPT – significantly so in some, but not all analyses, even ones using data from the same studies [79–81].

Udell and co-workers [82] examined the duration of DAPT therapy in the specific circumstance following myocardial infarction in a meta-analysis of more than 33,000 patients from the CHARISMA, PRODIGY, ARCTIC-Interruption, DAPT, DES-LATE and PEGASUS trials. The primary endpoint of this analysis – the composite of cardiovascular death, myocardial infarction or stroke – was significantly reduced (6.4% with extended DAPT vs. 7.5% with aspirin alone; $P < 0.001$). Individual endpoints of cardiovascular death, myocardial infarction, stoke, and definite/probable stent thrombosis were all significantly lower with extended DAPT in post-myocardial infarction patients. Not surprisingly, major bleeding was significantly higher (1.9% with extended DAPT vs. 1.1% with aspirin alone; $P = 0.004$) [82].

Use with Oral Anticoagulants
The WOEST study [83] was an open-label multicenter trial performed in the Netherlands and Belgium that randomized a total of 573 patients on oral anticoagulants undergoing PCI to receive either clopidogrel plus aspirin (in addition to their baseline oral anticoagulation, OAC, triple therapy), or clopidogrel alone (in addition to their baseline OAC, double therapy). Approximately one-quarter of the cases were done via a radial approach; approximately one-third of patients were taking a PPI, and only 25–30% of patients were ACS patients. The primary endpoint was any bleeding event at 1 year; this occurred in 19.4% of the double therapy group and 44.4% of the triple-therapy group ($P < 0.0001$). The incidence of multiple bleeding events and transfusion were also significantly lower in the double therapy group. A secondary outcome endpoint of the composite of death, myocardial infarction, stroke, TVR and stent thrombosis was also significantly lower in the double therapy group, even after correcting for imbalances in baseline characteristics. This was largely driven by differences in all-cause mortality (2.5% in the double therapy group and 6.3% in the triple-therapy group).

Saraffoff et al. [84] examined a consecutive series of 377 patients undergoing DES placement who were also treated with oral anticoagulants following stenting. A total of 356 received clopidogrel, and 21 received prasugrel, in addition to background therapy with aspirin and their usual oral anticoagulant. Prasugrel patients had a higher risk profile and most had high platelet reactivity to clopidogrel. Overall, ischemic endpoints in these patients were similar in clopidogrel- and prasugrel-treated patients, but bleeding was substantially more frequent with prasugrel treatment (28.6% with prasugrel vs. 6.7% with clopidogrel). At present, there are no large-scale data with ticagrelor triple therapy, and no dual therapy data (without aspirin) with newer $P2Y_{12}$ antagonists plus oral anticoagulants. The ISAR-TRIPLE study [85] was an open-label randomized study in 614 patients receiving OAC therapy who underwent coronary stenting with DES. The study was designed to test whether shortening the duration of triple therapy from 6 months to 6 weeks affected net clinical outcomes. At 9 months, there was no significant difference between the two treatment arms in the composite primary endpoint (death, myocardial infarction, strike, definite stent thrombosis or TIMI major bleeding).

The most recent ESC NSTEACS guidelines [86] do not recommend using ticagrelor or prasugrel as part of a triple-therapy regimen, giving it a class III recommendation. A number of other studies, such as PIONEER-AF [87], REDUAL-PCI [88], GEMINI ACS 1 [89] and MANJUSRI [90], are continuing to explore this issue.

Future Directions

ISAR-REACT 5

On important ongoing ACS trial is ISAR-REACT 5 [91], a head-to-head, randomized trial comparing ticagrelor and prasugrel in approximately 4000 ACS patients (STEMI and NSTEACS). The primary endpoint is the composite of death, myocardial infarction or stroke at 12 months.

Monotherapy (Without Aspirin)

Two ongoing studies are examining ways to simplify post-procedure antiplatelet regimens, looking specifically at the issue of $P2Y_{12}$ monotherapy with a more potent agent. GLOBAL LEADERS is a 16,000 patient all-comers, open-label PCI trial (using a Biomatrix™ stent) that compares a standard 12-month DAPT regimen (aspirin plus clopidogrel in non-ACS patients and aspirin plus ticagrelor in ACS patients) followed by 12 months of aspirin alone to a novel modified regimen consisting of 1 month of ticagrelor plus aspirin, followed by 23 months of ticagrelor monotherapy [92]. The primary endpoint is death and Q-wave myocardial infarction at 2 years. TWILIGHT [93] is a blinded study looking at approximately 9000 high-risk PCI patients, who after 3 months of DAPT with aspirin plus ticagrelor are randomized to either continue dual therapy, or to switch to ticagrelor monotherapy, with a primary endpoint of Bleeding Academic Research Consortium bleeding (superiority) and as secondary outcome endpoint of MACE (non-inferiority).

Potential Reversal Strategies

One important clinical consideration in orally administered $P2Y_{12}$ inhibitors is how to reverse the effects if emergency surgery is necessary. While this is admittedly rare in the setting of an acute STEMI, work continues to explore how to improve the safety of surgery in these circumstances. Two particular areas of focus are the use of platelet transfusions and the potential for reversal agents, similar to those recently available for some of the newer oral anticoagulants. A number of studies have explored the use of platelet transfusions to reverse the effects of oral $P2Y_{12}$ inhibitors. Theoretically, this could be more effective in the setting of irreversibly bound thienopyridines as opposed to reversibly bound CPTPs (which might redistribute to transfused platelets if plasma levels were still high).

At the present time, the general view is that platelet transfusions may be somewhat useful with thienopyridines (if given after the active metabolite is gone), but are not effective very early after discontinuation of ticagrelor [94–98]. One provocative recent observation is that platelet-rich plasma, pooled platelets with human serum, and even human serum alone may be more effective than platelets alone in reversing the antiplatelet effects of ticagrelor, although this has only been demonstrated to date in preliminary ex-vivo studies [99].

An antigen-binding fragment (Fab) antidote for ticagrelor has been described [100] and is currently being considered for clinical development. The Fab has an extremely high (20 pM) affinity for ticagrelor and its active metabolite, more than two orders of magnitude greater than the affinity of ticagrelor and its metabolite for the $P2Y_{12}$ receptor. Because ticagrelor is reversibly bound to the receptor, the Fab can, by mass action, selectively remove it from the circulation. This mechanistic approach will not work with the thienopyridines because of their irreversible binding to $P2Y_{12}$. The Fab has been shown to be very specific for ticagrelor and its metabolite, and does not appear to bind to adenosine, ATP, ADP, or other structurally similar drugs. To date, it has only been tested in vitro in human prion protein and in vivo in mice.

Another novel reversal strategy that has shown encouraging preliminary data in ex-vivo systems is the use of styrene copolymer beads that can bind ticagrelor and remove it from blood that is passed through sorbent columns [101].

Summary

The standard of care for antiplatelet therapy in the setting of ACS and coronary intervention has evolved substantially over recent years. Clopidogrel, the previous gold standard, has been supplanted by two newer-generation options, the thienopyridine prasugrel and the CPTP ticagrelor, both having a faster onset of action, more potent platelet inhibition, and less genetic variability in response than clopidogrel. Large-scale clinical trial have consistently shown that clopidogrel cannot be viewed as the optimal foundation therapy. However, the potency and faster onset of prasugrel and ticagrelor does have to be balanced against a commensurate increase in major bleeding. Moreover, it has also become clear that longer-term antiplatelet therapy is also important in STEMI patients. We should not lose sight of the underlying disease that brought the patient to medical attention in the first place; oral antiplatelet therapy may be viewed as a key component of longer-term secondary prevention therapy in STEMI patients.

In the acute STEMI setting, there are potential problems with oral absorption of medications, especially with concomitant morphine use. Crushing ticagrelor tablets (and perhaps prasugrel and clopidogrel) may overcome some of this problem, and GP IIb/IIIa have been an option when more rapid onset of an antiplatelet effect is desired, but more recently cangrelor has also come forward as an alternative for rapidly achieving antiplatelet effects, with an equally fast offset of activity, although most of the benefits noted in the cangrelor clinical studies were in the setting of elective PCI, rather than the STEMI setting.

There are still major uncertainties remaining around how antiplatelet agents should be managed in STEMI patients who also have indications for oral anticoagulant therapy. Future studies will also help inform us on the longer-term use of newer agents as monotherapy, without aspirin, in an attempt to mitigate some of the potential bleeding risks that accompany aspirin, and on any potential clinical role of the PAR-1 antagonist vorapaxar in the setting of STEMI.

References

1 Libby P. Current concepts of the pathogenesis of the acute coronary syndromes. *Circulation*, 2001; 104: 365–372.
2 DeWood MA, Spores J, Notske R, et al. Prevalence of total coronary occlusion during the early hours of transmural myocardial infarction. *N Engl J Med*, 1980; 303: 897–902.
3 de Feyter PJ, van den Brand M, Serruys PW, et al. Early angiography after myocardial infarction: what have we learned? *Am Heart J*, 1985; 109: 194–199.
4 DeWood MA, Stifter WF, Simpson CS, et al. Coronary arteriographic findings soon after non-Q-wave myocardial infarction. *N Engl J Med*, 1986; 315: 417–423.
5 Kristensen SD, Ravn HB, Falk E. Insights into the pathophysiology of unstable coronary artery disease. *Am J Cardiol*, 1997; 80: 5E–9E.
6 Laskey MA, Deutsch E, Barnathan E, et al. Influence of heparin therapy on percutaneous transluminal coronary angioplasty outcome in unstable angina pectoris. *Am J Cardiol*, 1990; 65: 1425–1429.

7 Schafer AI. A practical guide to blood coagulation. In: Ferguson JJ, Chronos NA, Harrington RA Eds. *Antiplatelet Therapy in Clinical Practice*, pp. 3–14. London: Martin Dunitz. 2000.

8 Haynes LM, Bouchard BA, Tracy PB, et al. Prothrombin activation by platelet-associated prothrombinase proceeds through the prethrombin-2 pathway via a concerted mechanism. *J Biol Chem*, 2012; 287(46): 38647–38655.

9 Badimon L, Vilahur G. Neutophil extracellular traps: a new source of tissue factor in atherosclerosis. *Eur Heart J*, 2015; 36: 1364–1366.

10 Agbani EO, van den Bosch MJT, Brown E, et al. Coordinated membrane ballooning and procoagulant spreading in human platelets. *Circulation*, 2015; 132; 1414–1424.

11 Battinelli EM. Progoagulant platelets: Not just full of hot air. *Circulation*, 2015; 132; 1374–1376.

12 Patrono C, García Rodrígue LA, Landolfi R, et al. Low-dose aspirin for the prevention of atherothrombosis. *N Engl J Med*, 2005; 353: 2373–2383.

13 Schrör K. Ticlopidine and clopidogrel. In: Ferguson JJ, Chronos NAF, Harrington RA (eds.), *Antiplatelet Therapy in Clinical Practice*, pp. 93–111. London: Martin Dunitz; 2000.

14 Angiolillo DJ, Fernandez-Ortiz A, Bernardo E, et al. Variability in individual responsiveness to clopidogrel: Clinical implications, management, and future perspectives. *J Am Coll Cardiol*, 2007; 49: 1505–1516.

15 Sugidachi A, Ogawa T, Kurihara A, et al. The greater in vivo anti-platelet effects of prasugrel as compared to clopidogrel reflect more efficient generation of its active metabolite with similar anti-platelet activity to that of clopidogrel's active metabolite. *J Thromb Haemost*, 2007; 5: 1545–1551.

16 Wiviott SD, Antman EM, Winters KJ, et al. Randomized comparison of prasugrel (CS-747, LY640315), a novel thienopyridine P2Y$_{12}$ antagonist, with clopidogrel in percutaneous coronary intervention: results of the Joint Utilization of Medications to Block Platelets Optimally (JUMBO)-TIMI 26 trial. *Circulation*, 2005; 111: 3366–3373.

17 Hulot JS, Collet JP, Silvain J, et al. Cardiovascular risk in clopidogrel-treated patients according to cytochrome P450 2C19*2 loss-of-function allele or proton pump inhibitor co-administration. A systematic meta-analysis. *J Am Coll Cardiol*, 2010; 56: 134–143.

18 Storey RF, Oldroyd KG, Wilcox RG. Open multicentre study of the P2T receptor antagonist AR-C69931MX assessing safety, tolerability and activity in patients with acute coronary syndromes. *Thromb Haemost*, 2001; 85: 401–407.

19 Greenbaum AB, Grines CL, Bittl JA, et al. Initial experience with an intravenous P2Y$_{12}$ platelet receptor antagonist in patients undergoing percutaneous coronary intervention: results from a 2-part, phase II, multicenter, randomized, placebo- and active-controlled trial. *Am Heart J*, 2006; 151: 689 e1–689 e10.

20 Harrington RA, Stone GW, McNulty S, et al. Platelet inhibition with cangrelor in patients undergoing PCI. *N Engl J Med*, 2009; 361: 2318–2329.

21 Cannon, CP, Husted S, Harrington RA, et al. Safety, tolerability, and initial efficacy of AZD6140, the first reversible oral adenosine diphosphate receptor antagonist, compared with clopidogrel in patients with non-ST segment elevation acute coronary syndrome; Primary results of the DISPERSE-2 Trial. *J Am Coll Cardiol*, 2007; 50: 1844–1851.

22 Storey, RF, Husted S, Harrington, RA, et al. Inhibition of platelet aggregation by AZD6140, a reversible oral P2Y$_{12}$ receptor antagonist, compared with clopidogrel in patients with acute coronary syndromes. *J Am Coll Cardiol*, 2007; 50: 1852–1856.

23 Armstrong D, Summers C, Ewart L, et al. Characterization of the adenosine pharmacology of ticagrelor reveals therapeutically relevant inhibition of equilibrative nucleoside transporter 1. *J Cardiovasc Pharmacol Ther*, 2014; 19: 209–219.

24 Nylander S, Femia EA, Scavone M, et al. Ticagrelor inhibits human platelet aggregation via adenosine in addition to P2Y$_{12}$ antagonism. *J Thromb Haemost*, 2013; 11(10): 1867–1876.

25 Cattaneo M, Schulz R, Nylander S. Adenosine-mediated effects of ticagrelor: Evidence and potential clinical relevance. *J Am Coll Cardiol*, 2014; 63: 2503–2509.

26 Cattaneo M. The platelet P2Y$_{12}$ receptor for adenosine diphosphate: Congenital and drug-induced defects. *Blood*, 2011; 117(7): 2102–2012.

27 Björquist A, Di Buduo CA, Femia EA, et al. Studies of the interaction of ticagrelor with the P2Y$_{13}$ receptor and with the P2Y$_{13}$-dependent pro-platelet formation by human megakaryocytes. 2016; 116(6): 1079–1088.

28 Bonello L, Frere C, Cointe S, et al. Ticagrelor increases endothelial progenitor cell level compared to clopidogrel in acute coronary syndromes: A prospective, randomized study. *Int J Cardiol*, 2015; 187: 502–507.

29 Phillips DR, Scarborough RM. Clinical pharmacology of eptifibatide. *Am J Cardiol*, 1997; 80: 11B–20B.

30 Coughlin SR. Thrombin signaling and protease activated receptors. *Nature*, 2000; 407: 258–264.

31 Steinberg SF. The cardiovascular actions of protease-activated receptors. *Mol Pharmacol*, 2005; 67: 2–11.

32 Ossovskaya VS, Bunnett NW. Protease-activated receptors: Contribution to physiology and disease. *Physiol Rev*, 2004; 84: 579–621.

33 Merck, & Co., Inc. *Zontivity® (Vorapaxar) Prescribing Information*. Whitehouse Station, NJ: Merck; 2013. Available at http://www.accessdata.fda.gov/drugsatfda_docs/label/2014/204886s000lbl.pdf (accessed March 10, 2017).

34 Second International Study of Infarct Survival (ISIS-2) Collaborative Group. Randomized trial of intravenous streptokinase, oral aspirin, both, or neither among 17,187 cases of suspected acute myocardial infarction: ISIS-2. *Lancet*, 1988; 2; 349–360.

35 Roux S, Christeller S, Ludin E. Effects of aspirin on coronary reocclusion and recurrent ischemia after thrombolysis: a meta-analysis. *J Am Coll Cardiol*, 1992; 19: 671–677.

36 Bertrand ME, Rupprecht HJ, Urban P, et al. Double-blind study of the safety of clopidogrel with and without a loading dose in combination with aspirin compared with ticlopidine in combination with aspirin after coronary stenting: the clopidogrel aspirin stent international cooperative study (CLASSICS). *Circulation*, 2000; 102: 624–629.

37 Yusuf S, Zhao F, Mehta SR, et al., for the Clopidogrel in Unstable Angina to Prevent Recurrent Events Trial Investigators. Effects of clopidogrel in addition to aspirin in patients with acute coronary syndromes without ST-segment elevation. *N Engl J Med*, 2001; 345: 494–502.

38 Mehta SR, Yusuf S, Peters RJ, et al., for the Clopidogrel in Unstable Angina to Prevent Recurrent Events Trial (CURE) Investigators. Effects of pretreatment with clopidogrel and aspirin followed by long-term therapy in patients undergoing percutaneous coronary intervention: the PCI-CURE study. *Lancet*, 2001; 358: 527–533.

39 Steinhubl SR, Berger PB, Mann JT 3rd, et al., for the Clopidogrel for the Reduction of Events During Observation (CREDO) Investigators. Early and sustained dual oral anti-platelet therapy following percutaneous coronary intervention: a randomized controlled trial. *JAMA*, 2002; 288: 2411–2420.

40 The CURRENT-OASIS 7 Investigators. Dose comparisons of clopidogrel and aspirin in acute coronary syndromes. *N Engl J Med*, 2010; 363: 930–942.

41 Sabatine MS, Cannon CP, Gibson CM, et al., for the Clopidogrel as Adjunctive Reperfusion Therapy – Thrombolysis in Myocardial Infarction (CLARITY-TIMI) 28 Investigators. Addition of clopidogrel to aspirin and fibrinolytic therapy for myocardial infarction with ST-segment elevation. *N Engl J Med*, 2005; 352: 1179–1189.

42 Chen ZM, Jiang LX, Chen YP, et al., for the COMMIT (ClOpidogrel and Metoprolol in Myocardial Infarction Trial) collaborative group. Addition of clopidogrel to aspirin in 45,852 patients with acute myocardial infarction: randomised placebo-controlled trial. *Lancet*, 2005; 366: 1607–1621.

43 Wiviott SD, Braunwald E, McCabe CH, et al., for the Trial to Assess Improvement in Therapeutic Outcomes by optimizing platelet Inhibition with Prasugrel Thrombolysis In Myocardial Infarction 38 (TRITON-TIMI 38) investigators. Prasugrel versus clopidogrel in patients with acute coronary syndromes. *N Engl J Med*, 2007; 357: 2001–2015.

44 Montalescot G, Wiviott SD, Braunwald E, et al. for the TRITON-TIMI 38 investigators. Prasugrel compared with clopidogrel in patients undergoing percutaneous coronary intervention for ST-elevation myocardial infarction (TRITON-TIMI 38): double-blind, randomised controlled trial. *Lancet*, 2009; 373: 723–731.

45 Roe MT, Armstrong PW, Fox KAA, et al. Prasugrel versus clopidogrel for acute coronary syndromes without revascularization. *N Engl J Med*, 2012; 367: 1297–1309.

46 Montalescot G, Bolognese L, Dudek D, et al. Pretreatment with prasugrel in non-ST-segment-elevation acute coronary syndromes. *N Engl J Med*, 2013; 369: 999–1010.

47 Wallentin L, Becker RC, Budaj A, et al. Ticagrelor versus clopidogrel in patients with acute coronary syndromes. *N Engl J Med*, 2009; 361(11): 1045–1057.

48 Steg G, James S, Harrington R, et al. Ticagrelor versus clopidogrel in patients with ST-elevation acute coronary syndromes intended for reperfusion with primary percutaneous coronary intervention: A PLATO Trial subgroup analysis. *Circulation*, 2010; 122: 2131–2141.

49 Montalescot G, van't Hof AW, Lapostolle F, et al. Prehospital Ticagrelor in ST-segment elevation myocardial infarction. *N Engl J Med*, 2014; 371: 1016–1027.

50 Bonaca MP, Bhatt DL, Cohen M, et al. Long-term use of ticagrelor in patients prior myocardial infaction. *N Engl J Med*, 2015; 372: 1791–1800.

51 Harrington RA, Stone GW, McNulty S, et al. Platelet inhibition with cangrelor in patients undergoing PCI. *N Engl J Med*, 2009; 361(24): 2318–2329.

52 Bhatt DL, Lincoff AM, Gibson CM, et al. Intravenous platelet blockade with cangrelor during PCI. *N Engl J Med*. 2009; 361: 2330–2341.

53 Bhatt DL, Stone GW, Mahaffey KW, et al. Effect of platelet inhibition with cangrelor during PCI on ischemic events. *N Eng J Med*, 2013 368: 1303–1313.

54 European Medicines Agency. Kengrexal (cangrelor). Available at http://www.ema.europa.eu/ema/index.jsp?curl=pages/medicines/human/medicines/003773/human_med_001852.jsp&mid=WC0b01ac058001d124 (accessed March 10, 2017).

55 US Food and Drug Administration. Drug Trials Snapshots: Kengreal. Available at https://www.fda.gov/Drugs/InformationOnDrugs/ucm453966.htm (accessed March 10, 2017).

56 Steinhubl SR, Oh JJ, Oestreich JH, et al. Transitioning patients from cangrelor to clopidogrel: Pharmacodynamics evidence of a competitive effect. *Thromb Res*, 2008; 121: 527–534.

57 Dovlatova NL, Jakubowski JA, Sugidachi A, et al. The reversible P2Y antagonist cangrelor influences the ability of the active metabolites of clopidogrel and prasugrel to produce irreversible inhibition of platelet function. *J Thromb Haemost*, 2008; 6: 1153–1159.

58 Schneider DJ, Seecheran N, Raza SS, et al. Pharmacodynamic effects during the transition between cangrelor and prasugrel. *Coron Artery Dis*, 2015; 26: 42–48.

59 Schneider DJ, Agarwal Z, Seecheran N, et al. Pharmacodynamic effects during the transition between cangrelor and ticagrelor. *J Am Coll Cardiol Interv*, 2014; 7: 435–442.

60 Udell JA, Braunwald E, Antman EM, et al. Prasugrel versus clopidogrel in patients with ST-segment elevation myocardial infarction according to the timing of percutaneous coronary intervention. *J Am Coll Cardiol Interv*, 2014; 7: 604–612.

61 Heestermans A, van Werkum JW, Taubert D, et al. Impaired bioavailability of clopidogrel in patients with a ST-segment elevation myocardial infarction. *Thrombosis Res*, 2008; 122: 776–781.

62 Osmancik P, Jirmar R, Hulikova, et al. A comparison of VASP index between patients with hemodynamically complicated and uncomplicated myocardial infarction. *Cath Cardiov Interv*, 2010; 75: 158–166.

63 Nimmo WS, Heading RC, Wilson J, et al. Inhibition of gastric emptying and drug absorption by narcotic analgesics. *Br J Clin Pharmacol*, 1975; 2: 509–513.

64 Hobl EL, Stimpfl T, Ebner J, et al. Morphine decreases clopidogrel concentrations and effects: a randomized, double-blind, placebo-controlled trial. *J Am Coll Cardiol*, 2014; 63: 630–635.

65 Alexopoulos D, Xanthopoulou I, Gkizas V, et al. Randomized assessment of ticagrelor versus prasugrel antiplatelet effects in patients with ST-segment-elevation myocardial infaction. *Circ Cardiovasc Interv*, 2012; 5: 797–804.

66 Parodi G, Valenti R, Bellandi B, et al. Comparison of prasugrel and ticagrelor loading doses in ST-segment elevation myocardial infarction patients. *J Am Coll Cardiol*, 2013; 61: 1601–1606.

67 Morton AC, Hossain R, Ecob R, et al. Morphine delays the onset of action of prasugrel in patients with prior history of ST elevation myocardial infarction. *Circulation*, 2013; 128: A11449.

68 Parodi G, Bellandi B, Xanthopoulou I, et al. Morphine is associated with a delayed activity of oral antiplatelet agents in patients with ST-elevation acute myocardial infarction undergoing primary percutaneous coronary intervention. *Circulation*, 2015; 8(1): e001593.

69 Franchi F, Rollini F, Cho JR, et al. Impact of morphine on pharmacokinetic and pharmacodynamic profiles of ticagrelor in patients with ST-Segment elevation myocardial infarction undergoing primary percutaneous coronary intervention. *J Am Coll Cardiol*, 2015; 65(10S): A1751.

70 Franchi F, Rollini F, Cho JR, et al. Impact of escalating loading dose regimens of ticagrelor in patients with ST-segment elevation myocardial infarction undergoing primary percutaneous coronary intervention. *J Am Coll Cardiol Interv*, 2015; 8: 1457–1467.

71 Kubica JK, Adamski PA, Ostrowska M, et al. Morphine delays and attenuates ticagrelor exposure and action in patients with myocardial infarction: The randomized, double-blind, placebo-controlled IMPRESSION trial. *Eur Heart J*, 2015; 37(3): 245–252.

72 Zafar MU, Farkouh ME, Fuster V, et al. Crushed clopidogrel administered via nasogastric tube has faster and greater absorption than oral whole tablets. *J Interv Cardiol*, 2009; 22: 385–389.

73 Teng R, Carlson G, Hsia J. An open-label, randomized bioavailability study with alternative methods of administration of crushed Ticagrelor tablets in healthy volunteers. *Int J Clin Pharm and Therap* 2015; 53: 182–189.

74 Parodi G, Xanthopoulou I, Bellandi B, et al. Ticagrelor crushed tablet administration in STEMI patients. *J Am Coll Cardiol*, 2015; 65: 511–512.

75 Alexopoulos D, Barampoutis N, Gkizas V, et al. Crushed versus integral tablets of ticagrelor in ST-segment elevation myocardial infarction patients: A randomized pharmacokinetic/pharmacodynamics study. *Clin Pharmacokinet*, 2015; 55(3): 359–367.

76 Mauri L, Kereiakes DJ, Yeh RW, et al. Twelve or 30 months of dual antiplatelet therapy after drug-eluting stents. *N Engl J Med* 2014; 371: 2155–2166.

77 Yeh RW, Kereiakes DJ, Steg PG, et al. Benefits and risks of extended duration dual antiplatelet therapy after PCI in patients with and without myocardial infarction. *J Am Coll Cardiol*, 2015; 65: 2211–2221.

78 AstraZeneca LP. *Brilinta*. Wilmington, DE: AstraZeneca; 2015. Available at http://www.accessdata.fda.gov/drugsatfda_docs/label/2015/022433s017lbl.pdf (accessed March 10, 2017).

79 Giustino G, Baber U, Sartori S, et al. Duration of dual antiplatelet therapy after drug-eluting stent implantation. *J Am Coll Cardiol*, 2015; 65: 1298–1310.

80 Montalescot G, Brieger D, Dalby AJ, et al. Duration of dual antiplatelet therapy after coronary stenting: A review of the evidence. *J Am Coll Cardiol*, 2015; 66: 832–487.

81 Palmerini T, Benedetto U, Bacchi-Reggiani L et al. Mortality in patients treated with extended duration dual antiplatelet therapy after drug-eluting stent implantation: A pairwise and Bayesian network meta-analysis or randomized trials. *Lancet* 2015; 385: 2371–2382.

82 Udell JA, Bonaca MP, Collet J-P. Long-term dual antiplatelet therapy for secondary prevention of cardiovascular events in the subgroup of patients with previous myocardial infarction: A collaborative meta-analysis of randomized trials. *Eur Heart J*, 2015; 37(4): 390–399.

83 Dewilde WJM, Oirbans T, Verheugt FWA, et al. Use of clopidogrel with or without aspirin in patients taking oral anticoagulant therapy and undergoing percutaneous coronary intervention: an open-label, randomized, controlled trial. *Lancet*, 2013; 381: 1107–1115.

84 Sarafoff N, Martishnig A, Wealer J, et al. Triple therapy with aspirin, prasugrel, and vitamin k antagonists in patients with drug-eluting stent implantation and an indication for oral anticoagulation. *J Am Coll Cardiol*, 2013; 61: 2060–2066.

85 Fiedler KA, Maeng M, Mehilli J, et al. Duration of triple therapy in patients requiring oral anticoagulation after drug-eluting stent implantation: The ISAR-TRIPLE trial. *J Am Coll Cardiol* 2015; 65: 1619–1629.

86 Roffi M, Patrono C, Collet J-P, et al. 2015 ESC Guidelines for the management of acute coronary syndromes in patients presenting without persistent ST-segment elevation. *Eur Heart J*, 2015; 37(3): 267–315.

87 Gibson CM, Mehran R, Bode C, et al. An open-label, randomized, controlled, multicenter study exploring two treatment strategies of rivaroxaban and a dose-adjusted oral vitamin k antagonist treatment strategy in subjects with atrial fibrillation who undergo percutaneous coronary intervention (PIONEER AF-PCI). *Am Heart J*, 2015; 169: 472–478.

88 Evaluation of Dual Therapy With Dabigatran vs. Triple Therapy With Warfarin in Patients With AF That Undergo a PCI With Stenting (REDUAL-PCI). ClinicalTrials.gov. Available online at https://clinicaltrials.gov/ct2/show/NCT02164864 (accessed March 10, 2017).

89 A Study to Compare the Safety of Rivaroxaban versus Acetylsalicylic Acid in Addition to Either Clopidogrel or Ticagrelor Therapy in Participants with Acute Coronary Syndromes (GEMINI ACS 1). ClinicalTrials.gov. Available online at https://clinicaltrials.gov/ct2/show/NCT02293395 (accessed March 10, 2017).

90 Lu W, Chen L, Wang Y, et al. Rationale and design of MANJUSRI trial: A randomized, open-label, active controlled multicenter study to evaluate the safety of combined therapy with Ticagrelor and warfarin in AF subjects after PCI-eS. *Contemp Clin Trials*, 2015; 40: 166–171.

91 Schulz, Angiolillo DJ, Antoniucci D, et al. Randomized comparison of ticagrelor versus prasugrel in patients with acute coronary syndrome and planned invasive strategy – design and rationale of the Intracoronary Stenting and Antithrombitic Regimen: Rapid Early Action for Coronary Treatment (ISAR-REACT) 5 Trial. *J Cardiov Trans Res*, 2014; 7(1): 91–100.

92 GLOBAL LEADERS: A Clinical Study Comparing Two Forms of Anti-platelet Therapy After Stent Implantation. ClinicalTrials.gov. Available online at https://clinicaltrials.gov/ct2/show/NCT01813435 (accessed March 10, 2017).

93 Ticagrelor With Aspirin or Alone in High–Risk Patients After Coronary Intervention (TWILIGHT). ClinicalTrials.gov. Available online at https://clinicaltrials.gov/ct2/show/NCT02270242 (accessed March 10, 2017).

94 Martin AC, Berndt C, Calmette L, et al. The effectiveness of platelet supplementation for the reversal of Ticagrelor-induced inhibition of platelet aggregation: An in-vitro study. *Eur J Anaesthesiol*, 2016; 23(5): 361–367.

95 Vilahur G, Choi BG, Zafar MU, et al. Normalization of platelet reactivity in clopidogrel-treated subjects. *J Thromb Haemost* 2007; 5: 82–90.

96 Thiele T, Sümnig A, Hron G, et al. Platelet transfusion for reversal of dual antiplatelet therapy in patients requiring urgent surgery: A pilot study. *Thromb Haemost*, 2012; 10: 968–971.

97 Godier A, Taylor G, Gaussem P. Inefficacy of platelet transfusion to reverse ticagrelor. *N Engl J Med*, 2015; 372:196–197.

98 Scharbert G, Wetzel L, Schrottmaier WC, et al. Comparison of patient intake of ticagrelor, prasugrel or clopidogrel on restoring platelet function by donor platelets. *Transfusion* 2015; 55: 1320–1326.

99 Schoener L, Richter B, Pfluecke C, et al. A new strategy to reverse the platelet inhibitory effect of ticagrelor. *Eur Heart J*, 2015; 36(1 Supplement): 860.

100 Buchanan A, Newton P, Pehrsson S, et al. Structure and functional characterization of a specific antidote for ticagrelor. *Blood*, 2015; 125: 3484–3490.

101 Angheloiu GO, Gugiu BG, Pandey R, et al. Ticagrelor removal from human blood. *Circulation*, 2015; 132: A12904.

102 Bhatt DL, Fox KAA, Hacke W, et al. Clopidogrel and aspirin versus aspirin alone for the prevention of atherothrombotic events. *N Engl J Med*, 354: 1706–1717.

Part II

The STEMI Procedure

6

The Role of Acute Circulatory Support in STEMI

Yousef Bader MD, Navin K. Kapur MD

Introduction

A well-established therapeutic benchmark in the setting of ST-segment elevation myocardial infarction (STEMI) is a "door to balloon" time of less than 90 minutes, which is defined as the interval from the first electrocardiogram showing ST-segment elevation in the emergency department to mechanical reperfusion of the occluded coronary artery. However, despite timely reperfusion, nearly 10% of patients with acute myocardial infarction (AMI) die during their index hospitalization and 76% of survivors progress to develop chronic heart failure within the next 5 years [1–3]. These findings suggest that new approaches are needed to reduce the burden of myocardial injury in AMI.

Described best by Braunwald and Kloner in 1985, myocardial reperfusion is a "double-edged sword" owing to the fact that reperfusion of ischemic myocardium promotes cardiomyocyte death and microvascular damage through a process referred to as myocardial ischemia–reperfusion injury [4]. As an estimate of how much residual damage exists after successful, timely reperfusion therapy in an anterior STEMI, the CRISP-AMI trial demonstrated that up to 40% of the myocardium is injured, as measured by magnetic resonance imaging within 1 week of successful reperfusion therapy [5]. The percentage of these patients going on to develop systolic heart failure remains unknown.

Primary treatment objectives in the setting of STEMI and cardiogenic shock include: 1) early myocardial reperfusion; 2) maintenance of systemic perfusion pressure; and 3) a reduction in left ventricular stroke work. Objective one is met by coronary angioplasty. However, objectives two and three are nearly impossible to achieve without the use of an acute circulatory support pump. Since the 1990s, percutaneously delivered mechanical circulatory support (pMCS) devices have evolved to include pulsatile, axial flow, and centrifugal flow options that can be rapidly deployed in patients with STEMI and hemodynamic compromise. The overall goals of percutaneous circulatory support systems are: 1) to improve native cardiac output; 2) to augment coronary perfusion; 3) to reduce ventricular volume and filling pressures, thereby reducing wall stress, stroke work, and myocardial oxygen consumption; and 4) to maintain vital organ perfusion [6]. A 2014 analysis of the Nationwide Inpatient Sample from the Healthcare Cost and Utilization Project identified stable rates of intra-aortic balloon pump (IABP) implantation in the United States and increasing use of pMCS devices, including the Impella axial flow catheter, the TandemHeart® left atrial-to-femoral artery bypass system, and venoarterial extracorporeal membrane oxygenation (VA-ECMO) [7] (Figure 6.1). In this chapter, we discuss the hemodynamic impact of each pMCS device and clinical data surrounding their use in the setting of STEMI.

Manual of STEMI Interventions, First Edition. Edited by Sameer Mehta.

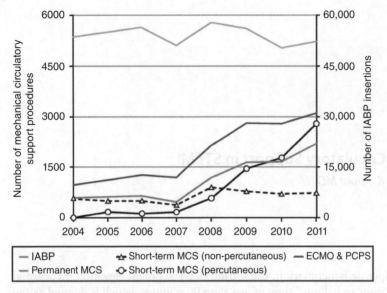

Figure 6.1 Number of mechanical circulatory support (MCS) and intra-aortic balloon counter pulsation (IABP) insertions. Use of short-term (acute) circulatory support pumps is increasing. Coincident with the growth in use of durable or permanent MCS, the use of short-term percutaneous MCS, extracorporeal membrane oxygenation (ECMO), and percutaneous cardiopulmonary support (PCPS) options have been steadily increasing since 2007 (reproduced with permission from *Journal of the American College of Cardiologists*, 2014; 64: 1407–1415).

Intra-Aortic Balloon Counterpulsation

The intra-aortic balloon pump (IABP) is a catheter-mounted balloon that augments pulsatile blood flow by inflating during diastole, which displaces blood volume in the descending aorta and increases mean aortic pressure, thereby potentially augmenting coronary perfusion (Figure 6.2a). Upon deflation, during systole, the IABP generates a pressure sink, which is filled by ejecting blood from the heart. As a result, an IABP reduces ventricular afterload, increases mean arterial pressure, and augments ventricular stroke volume. IABPs also augment myocardial perfusion in the setting of myocardial ischemia (Figure 6.3). The pioneering work of Kantrowitz, Weber, Janicki, Sarnoff, Schreuder, Kern, and many others has established that the hemodynamic impact of balloon counterpulsation is primarily determined by four factors: (1) the magnitude of diastolic pressure augmentation; (2) the magnitude of reduced systolic pressure; (3) the magnitude of volume displacement; and (4) the timing of balloon inflation and deflation. More recently, larger capacity IABPs, known as the MEGA® family (Maquet Inc.), have been introduced into clinical practice. Advantages of IABPs include the ease of insertion, global familiarity with the technology, and relative cost [8–15].

Registry data have historically supported the use of IABPs [16–19]. In the thrombolysis era, the Thrombolysis and Angioplasty in Myocardial Infarction trials assessed the use of IABP in patients after thrombolysis for STEMI. Of 810 patients, 85 received an IABP and were found to have less reocclusion of the culprit vessel (7% vs. 13%) at 1-week follow-up. In this nonrandomized study, there was, however, higher mortality among IABP recipients, which may reflect a selection bias toward sicker patients receiving IABP therapy. Despite this initial signal of potential benefit for IABP therapy in the setting of thrombolysis, data from primary percutaneous coronary intervention (PCI) cohorts have been less clear. Van't Hof and colleagues

(a)   (b)   (c)   (d)   (e)

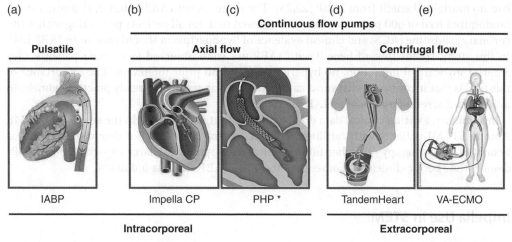

Continuous flow pumps

Pulsatile   **Axial flow**   **Centrifugal flow**

IABP   Impella CP   PHP *   TandemHeart   VA-ECMO

Intracorporeal   **Extracorporeal**

* Investigational

Figure 6.2 Classification of acute circulatory support devices. a) Intra-aortic balloon pump (IABP). b) Impella CP® axial flow catheter. c) Percutaneous heart pump (PHP) an investigational axial flow catheter. d) TandemHeart centrifugal flow pump. e) Venoarterial extracorporeal membrane oxygenation (VA-ECMO).

Figure 6.3 Intra-aortic balloon counter pulsation (IABP) augments myocardial perfusion during ischemia. During ischemia, dysregulation of microvascular autoregulation creates a hyperemic state that allows for a linear relationship between forward compression wave energy generated by an IABP (IABP-FCW) and coronary flow (average peak velocity; APV) (reproduced from *JACC Cardiovascular Interventions*, 2014; 7(6): 631–640, with permission).

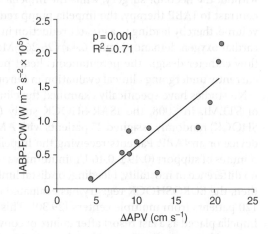

randomized 238 patients at high risk for myocardial infarction post-PCI to receive either IABP or usual care and found no difference in mortality, nonfatal myocardial infarction, stroke and ejection fraction. Similar findings were observed in the Primary Angioplasty in Myocardial Infarction-II trial, an international multicenter randomized trial in which patients presenting with STEMI were randomized to primary PCI and IABP versus IABP alone. No differences in death, reinfarction, infarct-related artery reocclusion, stroke, new heart failure, or ventricular arrhythmias were observed between groups [20,21].

Observational and randomized data do not support the routine use of IABP therapy among patients with AMI complicated by cardiogenic shock. Both the SHOCK (SHould we emergently revascularize Occluded Coronary arteries for cardiogenic shock) trial, as well as the National Registry of Myocardial Infarction-2 (NRMI-2) trial, showed no clear benefit for IABP use in the setting of AMI and shock. Consistent with prior data, NRMI-2 showed lower in-hospital mortality among patients who received thrombolysis for STEMI and had an IABP placed compared with those receiving thrombolysis alone. In the NRMI-2 trial, however, patients receiving PCI had no mortality benefit from IABP [22,23]. The more recent IABP-SHOCK II study, a large, randomized trial of 600 patients, effectively showed that not all patients presenting with acute coronary syndrome (ACS) and clinical evidence of hypoperfusion should receive an IABP [24]. In this study, trends toward benefit with IABP use were observed in younger patients with anterior myocardial infarction, no hypertension, and no prior infarction. The importance of this trial is that it confirms what most catheterization laboratories already practice, namely, to avoid non-discretionary use of an IABP in ACS.

In summary, existing clinical data do not support routine IABP use in the setting of STEMI. Among STEMI patients with cardiogenic shock, recent data have not demonstrated a clear benefit of IABP therapy. Whether future clinical trials employing large capacity, 50-cc IABPs demonstrate better clinical outcomes than the 40-cc IABP remains unknown.

Impella Use in STEMI

The Impella devices are catheter-mounted axial flow pumps that are placed into the left ventricle in retrograde fashion across the aortic valve. The pump transfers kinetic energy from a circulating impeller to the blood stream, which results in continuous blood flow from the left ventricle to ascending aorta (Figure 6.2b). The Impella 2.5 LP and CP devices can be deployed without the need for surgery, while the Impella 5.0 device requires surgical vascular access. In contrast to IABP therapy, the Impella pump reduces both native left ventricular pressure and volume, thereby leading to a greater reduction in left ventricular stroke work (LVSW) and myocardial oxygen demand (Figure 6.4a) [25,26]. More recently, preclinical data for another axial flow catheter design, the percutaneous heart pump (Thoratec Inc.) was reported [27] and is currently undergoing clinical evaluation in Europe (Figure 6.2c).

No studies have specifically examined the clinical utility of Impella unloading in the setting of STEMI. In 2008, the ISAR-SHOCK study (Impella LP 2.5 versus IABP in Cardiogenic SHOCK) randomly assigned 25 patients with AMI and cardiogenic shock to the Impella 2.5 LP device or an IABP. Patients receiving the Impella had a greater rise in cardiac index after 30 minutes of support (0.49 ± 0.46 l/minute/m^2 vs. $-.11 \pm 0.31$ l/minute/m^2). However, there was no difference in mortality, bleeding, or distal limb ischemia between the two groups [28]. Since then, the EUROSHOCK registry has evaluated the safety and efficacy of the Impella 25 LP in 120 patients from multiple centers [29,30]. This patient population had severe shock and had Impella placed as a last resort after failure of conventional therapy. Cardiopulmonary resuscitation prior to Impella implantation occurred in 41% of patients. The investigators found that, within 24 hours of support, there was a significant decrease in plasma lactate levels, suggesting improved organ perfusion. The mortality rate in this population was 64% at 30 days, reflecting a sick patient population with poor baseline hemodynamics and high risk of impending death.

Figure 6.4 Distinct hemodynamic effects of acute circulatory support devices percutaneous mechanical circulatory support systems. (a) The Impella axial flow catheters are deployed in retrograde fashion across the aortic valve and directly displace blood from the left ventricle (LV) into the proximal aorta. Immediate effects of the Impella activation include reduced LV pressure and volume as shown by pressure–volume (PV) loops. (b) The TandemHeart centrifugal flow pump displaces oxygenated blood from the left atrium (LA) to a femoral artery, thereby reducing LV preload. The net effect of immediate TandemHeart activation is a reduction in total LV volume and native LV stroke volume (width of the PV loop). (c) Venoarterial extracorporeal membrane oxygenation (VA-ECMO) displaces venous blood from the right atrium (RA) through an extracorporeal centrifugal pump and oxygenator, then returns oxygenated blood into the femoral artery. The immediate effect of VA-ECMO without an LV decompression mechanism is an increase in LV pressures and a reduction in LV stroke volume.

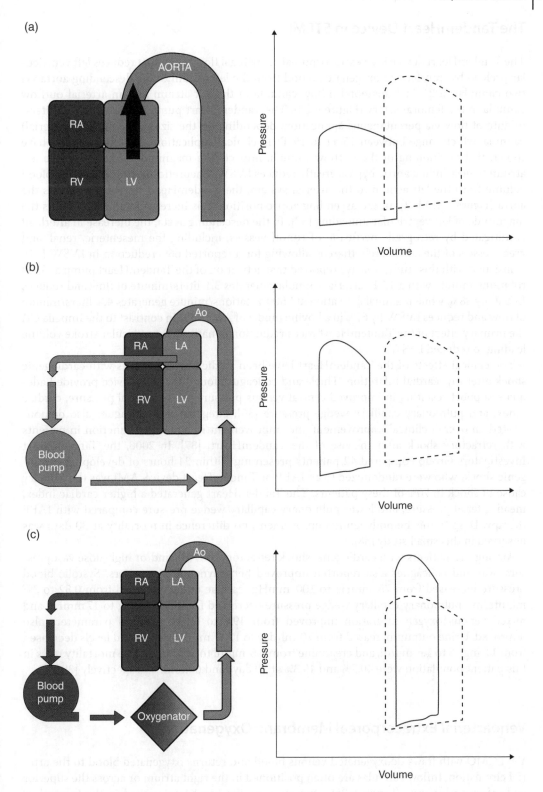

The TandemHeart Device in STEMI

The TandemHeart device is an extracorporeal centrifugal flow pump that reduces left ventricular preload by transferring oxygenated blood from the left atrium to the descending aorta via two cannulas: a 21 Fr transseptal inflow cannula in the left atrium and an arterial outflow cannula in the femoral artery (Figure 6.2d). The TandemHeart pump can provide 3–5 liters/minute of flow via percutaneous application, depending on the size of the outflow (arterial) cannula, which range between 15 Fr to 19 Fr in clinical application [31]. Prior reports have shown that positioning of the outflow cannula impacts the magnitude of LVSW, while left atrium to descending aortic bypass greatly reduces LVSW. Theoretically, by transferring blood volume from the left atrium to the arterial system, the TandemHeart device pressurizes the aorta (Figure 6.4b) [32]. In the ascending aortic position, this increase in afterload limits the magnitude of left ventricular unloading [33]. In the descending aorta, the increase in afterload is mitigated by retrograde perfusion of runoff vessels, including the mesenteric, renal, and great vessels of the aortic arch, thereby allowing for a reported 66% reduction in LVSW [34]. Consistent with this study, we have reported that activation of the TandemHeart pump at 5500 rotations/minute with a 17 Fr arterial cannula generates 3.1 liters/minute of flow and reduces LVSW by 38%, while maximal activation at 7500 rotations/minute generates 4.4 liters/minute of flow and reduces LVSW by 67% in a bovine model of AMI. [35] In contrast to the Impella CP, the primary effect of the TandemHeart was a reduction in native left ventricular stroke volume leading to reduced LVSW.

The clinical effects of the TandemHeart have been studied in 18 patients with cardiogenic shock after myocardial infarction. Thiele and colleagues found that the device provided adequate support resulting in improved central venous pressure, mean arterial pressure, cardiac index, and pulmonary capillary wedge pressure [36]. Gregoric and colleagues also demonstrated an overall clinical improvement and improvement in end-organ function in patients with refractory shock after the use of the TandemHeart. [37]. In 2006, the TandemHeart Investigators Group compared 42 patients presenting within 24 hours of developing cardiogenic shock, who were randomized to an IABP or TandemHeart device. AMI was the primary cause of shock in 70% of these patients. The TandemHeart generated a higher cardiac index, mean arterial pressure, and lower pulmonary capillary wedge pressure compared with IABP therapy. Despite this hemodynamic improvement, no difference in mortality at 30 days was observed in this small study [38].

Among 117 patients with cardiogenic shock refractory to IABP and/or high-dose vasopressors, Kar and colleagues also reported improved hemodynamic parameters. Systolic blood pressure increased from 75 mmHg to 100 mmHg, cardiac index increased from 0.52 to 3l/minute/m^2, pulmonary capillary wedge pressure decreased from 31 mmHg to 17 mmHg and mixed venous oxygen saturation improved from 49% to 69.3%. Clinical parameters also improved. Urine output increased from 70 ml/day to 1200 ml/day; lactic acid levels decreased from 11 mg/dl to 1.5 mg/dl; and creatinine from 1.5 mg/dl to 1.2 mg/dl. The mortality rates in this patient population were 40.2% and 45.3% at 30 days and 6 months, respectively [39].

Venoarterial Extracorporeal Membrane Oxygenation

VA-ECMO withdraws deoxygenated venous blood and returns oxygenated blood to the arterial circulation. Inflow cannulas are often positioned in the right atrium or across the superior and inferior vena cava (Figure 6.2e). Outflow cannulas can be positioned in the femoral or subclavian arteries. Since no venous reservoir is employed, VA-ECMO cannot be described as cardiopulmonary bypass. The primary hemodynamic effect of VA-ECMO is to displace blood volume from the venous to the arterial circulation. As a result, reduced right and left ventricular volumes can be observed with a concomitant increase in mean arterial pressure. Depending on the native left ventricular function and the presence or absence of aortic valve disease, VA-ECMO can be associated with increased left ventricular systolic and diastolic pressures (Figure 6.4c) [40].

The utility of VA-ECMO in AMI remains unknown. Several limitations preclude the use of VA-ECMO in AMI including: 1) the possibility for left ventricular distention and increased LVSW; 2) a potentially higher risk for bleeding complications due to the need for large bore cannulas in the setting of aggressive antithrombotic and antiplatelet therapy; and 3) the risk of other complications including vascular injury, limb ischemia and insufficient upper body oxygenation in cases of relatively preserved left ventricular systolic function. A 2015 single-center study reported a 67% survival to discharge rate among 18 patients with acute coronary syndromes complicated by cardiogenic shock. Bleeding complications were observed in 94% (17 of 18) patients in this study [41].

Right Ventricular Myocardial Infarction

Several studies have examined the clinical importance of right ventricular failure in the setting of an AMI. Right ventricular dysfunction, as defined by echocardiography, can be identified in up to 50% of patients presenting with an acute inferior wall myocardial infarction [42]. Of these patients, 15–25% will exhibit hemodynamic instability suggestive of right ventricular involvement, yet histologic infarction of the right ventricular free wall occurs in only 3–5% of patients with an acute inferior wall myocardial infarction. In a substudy of the SHOCK trial, right ventricular-dominant cardiogenic shock was associated with similar in-hospital mortality rates as left ventricular-dominant cardiogenic shock (53.1% vs. 60.8%, $P = 0.3$), despite a younger age, lower rate of anterior myocardial infarction, and higher likelihood of single-vessel disease among right ventricular-dominant shock patients [42]. Furthermore, a meta-analysis of several studies showed significantly higher in-hospital mortality and higher incidence of shock, ventricular arrhythmias, and advanced atrioventricular block if AMI involved the right ventricle [43].

Contemporary management of right ventricle failure includes reversal of the primary cause, volume resuscitation, inotropic support, and pulmonary vasodilation, which serves respectively to maintain preload, enhance contractility, and reduce afterload in the right ventricle. In refractory right ventricle failure, treatment options are limited to surgical right ventricle assist devices, ECMO, atrial septostomy, and cardiac transplantation. Percutaneously delivered circulatory support for right ventricle failure is an emerging field, with several device options available, including the IABP, the TandemHeart centrifugal flow pump, the axial flow Impella RP catheter, and VA-ECMO (Figure 6.5).

At present, minimal data exploring the clinical utility of percutaneous right ventricle support devices in right ventricular myocardial infarction exist. Several studies have shown the potential benefits of centrifugal flow pumps in right ventricle failure using surgical and hybridized surgical–percutaneous deployment with the Centrimag (Thoratec Inc.) [44], Rotaflow (Maquet Inc.) [45], and TandemHeart pumps [46,47]. Most recently, the Recover Right trial evaluated the Impella RP device in the setting of right ventricular myocardial infarction or post-cardiotomy right ventricle failure [48]. As experience with percutaneous right ventricle support devices grows, their role in the armamentarium of the mechanical therapies for right ventricular

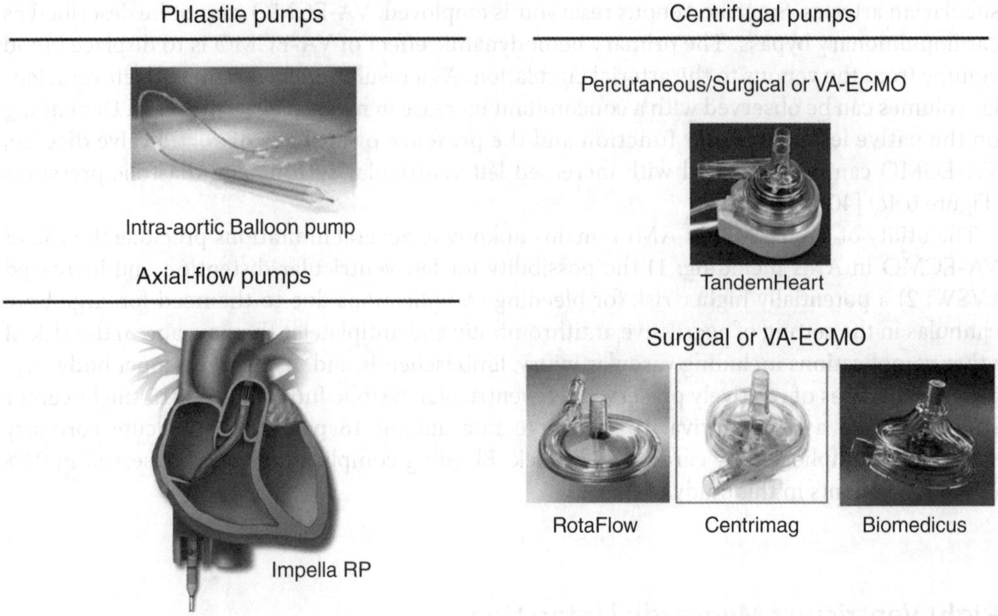

Pulastile pumps

Intra-aortic Balloon pump

Axial-flow pumps

Impella RP

Centrifugal pumps

Percutaneous/Surgical or VA-ECMO

TandemHeart

Surgical or VA-ECMO

RotaFlow   Centrimag   Biomedicus

Figure 6.5 Acute right ventricular support devices.

myocardial infarction will depend less on the technical ability to place the device, but rather on improved algorithms for patient selection, patient and device monitoring, and weaning protocols.

Time for a Paradigm Shift: From Primary Reperfusion to Primary Unloading in STEMI

In-hospital mortality due to cardiogenic shock in the setting of AMI remains prohibitively high, at between 30% and 50%. Furthermore, a recent analysis of nearly 8000 patients over the age of 65 years presenting with an AMI who underwent early revascularization confirmed that nearly 76% of patients who survive to discharge go on to develop heart failure within 5 years [2]. While coronary reperfusion to restore the myocardial oxygen supply is ultimately necessary, perhaps future approaches should focus on first reducing myocardial oxygen demand and supporting systemic hemodynamics before coronary reperfusion.

Historically, surgical implementation of cardiopulmonary bypass has been an effective method of reducing myocardial oxygen demand and has been associated with improved clinical outcomes and reduced infarct size in AMI complicated by cardiogenic shock [49,50]. Based on these early observations, activation of an IABP or catheter-mounted axial flow pump prior to coronary occlusion was found to reduce infarct size in preclinical models of AMI [51–53]. We previously reported that reducing left ventricle wall stress using the TandemHeart left atrial-to-femoral artery bypass pump and delaying coronary reperfusion by 30 minutes significantly decreased infarct size in a preclinical model of AMI [54]. This preclinical study led to the TandemHeart to Reduce Infarct Size trial, which commenced in 2015 in the United States [55]. We recently reported that mechanically conditioning the myocardium using a the Impella CP pump while delaying coronary reperfusion by 60 minutes reduces LV wall stress and activates

Figure 6.6 Future directions: Primary reperfusion versus primary unloading. a) Future studies are required to test the utility of preclinical observations showing that first unloading the left ventricle, then delaying reperfusion (primary unloading) reduces infarct size compared with primary reperfusion alone. b) Representative left ventricular sections after staining with triphenyltetrazolium chloride. Infarct zones are outlined in black.

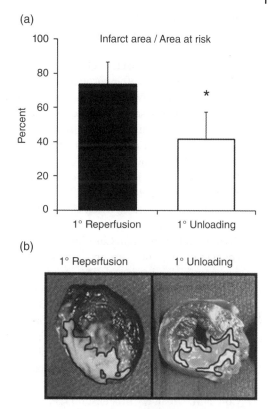

a myocardial protection program that upregulates expression of the cytokine stromal derived factor 1 alpha (SDF-1α), increases cardioprotective signaling, reduces apoptosis, and limits myocardial damage in AMI [56] (Figure 6.6). Future clinical studies are needed to examine the utility of primary unloading versus primary reperfusion in AMI.

References

1 Menees DS, Peterson ED, Wang Y, et al. Door-to-balloon time and mortality among patients undergoing primary PCI. *N Engl J Med*, 2013; 369: 901–909.
2 Ezekowitz JA, Kaul P, Bakal JA, et al. Declining in-hospital mortality and increasing heart failure incidence in elderly patients with first myocardial infarction. *J Am Coll Cardiol*, 2009; 53: 13–20.
3 Ezekowitz JA, Armstrong PW, Granger CB, et al. Predicting chronic left ventricular dysfunction 90 days after ST-segment elevation myocardial infarction: An Assessment of Pexelizumab in Acute Myocardial Infarction (APEX-AMI) Substudy. *Am Heart J*, 2010;160: 272–278.
4 Braunwald E, Kloner R. Myocardial Reperfusion: A Double-Edged Sword. *J Clin Invest*, 1985; 76(5): 1713–1719.
5 Patel M, Smalling R, Thiele H, et al. Intra-aortic Balloon Counterpulsation and Infarct Size in Patients With Acute Anterior Myocardial Infarction Without Shock The CRISP AMI Randomized Trial. *JAMA*, 2011; 306(12): 1329–1337.
6 Rihal C, Naidu S, Givertz M, et al. 2015 SCAI/ACC/HFSA/STS Clinical expert consensus statement on the use of percutaneous mechanical circulatory support devices in cardiovascular care. *J Am Coll Cardiol*, 2015; 65(19): e7–e26.

7 Stretch R, Sauer C, Bonde P. National trends in the utilization of short-term mechanical circulatory supportincidence, outcomes, and cost analysis. *J Am Coll Cardiol*, 2014; 64(14): 1407–1415.

8 Kern MJ, Aguirre F, Bach R, et al. Augmentation of coronary blood flow by intra-aortic balloon pumping in patients after coronary angioplasty. *Circulation*, 1993; 87(2): 500–511.

9 Kern MJ, Aguirre FV, Tatineni S, et al. Enhanced coronary blood flow velocity during intraaortic balloon counterpulsation in critically ill patients. *J Am Coll Cardiol*, 1993; 21(2): 359–368.

10 Schreuder JJ, Maisano F, Donelli A, et al. Beat-to-beat effects of intraaortic balloon pump timing on left ventricular performance in patients with low ejection fraction. *Ann Thorac Surg*, 2005; 79(3): 872–880.

11 De Silva K, Lumley M, Kailey B, et al. Coronary and microvascular physiology during intra-aortic balloon counterpulsation. *JACC Cardiovasc Interv*, 2014; 7(6): 631–640.

12 Sarnoff SJ, Braunwald E, Welch GH, et al. Hemodynamic determinants of oxygen consumption of the heart with special reference to the tension–time index. *Am J Physiol*, 1958; 192(1): 148–156.

13 Braunwald E, Sarnoff SJ, Case RB, et al. Hemodynamic determinants of coronary flow: effect of changes in aortic pressure and cardiac output on the relationship between myocardial oxygen consumption and coronary flow. *Am J Physiol*, 1958; 192(1): 157–163.

14 Weber KT, Janicki JS. Coronary collateral flow and intraaortic ballooncounterpulsation. *Trans Am Soc Artif Intern Organs*, 1973; 19: 395–401.

15 Weber KT, Janicki JS. Intraaortic balloon counterpulsation. A review of physiological principles, clinical results, and device safety. *Ann Thorac Surg*, 1974; 17(6): 602–636.

16 Stone GW, Ohman EM, Miller MF, et al. Contemporary utilization and outcomes of intraaortic balloon counterpulsation in acute myocardial infarction: the benchmark registry. *J Am Coll Cardiol*, 2003; 41(11): 1940–1945.

17 Cohen M, Urban P, Christenson JT, et al. Intra-aortic balloon counterpulsation in US and non-US centres: results of the Benchmark Registry. *Eur Heart J*, 2003; 24(19): 1763–1770.

18 Abdel-Wahab M, Saad M, Kynast J, et al. Comparison of hospital mortality with intraaortic balloon counterpulsation insertion before versus after primary percutaneous coronary intervention for cardiogenic shock complicating acute myocardial infarction. *Am J Cardiol*, 2010; 105(7): 967–971.

19 Curtis JP, Rathore SS, Wang Y, et al. Use and effectiveness of intra-aortic balloon pumps among patients undergoing high-risk percutaneous coronary intervention: insights from the National Cardiovascular Data Registry. *Circ Cardiovasc Qual Outcomes*, 2012; 5(1): 21–30.

20 Van't Hof A, Liem A de Boer M, et al. A randomized comparison of intra-aortic balloon pumping after primary coronary angioplasty in high risk patients with acute myocardial infarction. *Eur Heart J*, 1999; 20(9): 659–65.

21 Stone G, Marsalese D, Brodie B, et al. A prospective, randomized evaluation of prophylactic intraaortic balloon counterpulsation in high risk patients with acute myocardial infarction treated with primary angioplasty. *J Am Coll Cardiol*, 1997; 29: 1459–67.

22 Hochman J, Sleeper L, Webb J, et al. Early revascularization in acute myocardial infarction complicated by cardiogenic shock. *N Engl J Med*, 1999; 341: 625–634.

23 Barron HV, Every NR, Parsons LS, et al. The use of intra-aortic balloon counterpulsation in patients with cardiogenic shock complicating acute myocardial infarction: data from the National Registry of Myocardial Infarction 2. *Am Heart J*, 2001; 141: 933–939.

24 Thiele H, Zeymer U, Neumann F et al. Intraaortic balloon support for myocardial infarction with cardiogenic shock. *N Engl J Med*, 2012; 367:1287–1296.

25 Henriques JP, Remmelink M, Baan Jr J, et al. Safety and feasibility of elective high-risk percutaneous coronary intervention procedures with left ventricular support of the Impella Recover Lp 2.5. *Am J Cardiol*, 2006; 97: 990–992.

26 Sjauw KD, Remmelink M, Baan Jr J, et al. Left ventricular unloading in acute ST-segment elevation myocardial infarction patients is safe and feasible and provides acute and sustained left ventricular recovery. *J Am Coll Cardiol*, 2008; 51: 1044–1046.

27 Thoractec percutanous heart pump. *TCT Conference 2012*. www.tctconference.com (accessed 8 August 2015).

28 Seyfarth M, Sibbing D Bauer I, et al. A randomized clinical trial to evaluate the safety and efficacy of a percutaneous left ventricular assist device versus intra-aortic balloon pumping for treatment of cardiogenic shock caused by myocardial infarction. *J Am Coll Cardiol*, 2008; 52: 1584–1588.

29 Lauten A, Engstrom A, Jung C, et al. Percutaneous left-ventricular support with the Impella–2.5-assist device in acute cardiogenic shock results of the Impella-EUROSHOCK-Registry. *Circ Heart Fail*, 2013; 6: 23–30.

30 Acharya D, Loyaga-Rendon RY, Tallaj JA, et al. Circulatory support for shock complicating myocardial infarction. *J Invasive Cardiol*, 2014; 26(8): E109–114.

31 Kar B, Gregoric ID, Basra SS, et al. The percutaneous ventricular assist device in severe refractory cardiogenic shock. *J Am Coll Cardiol*, 2011; 57: 688–696.

32 Burkhoff D, Naidu SS. The science behind percutaneous hemodynamic support: a review and comparison of support strategies. *Catheter Cardiovasc Interv*, 2012; 80: 816–829.

33 Kono S, Nishimura K, Nishina T, et al. Autosynchronized systolic unloading during left ventricular assist with a centrifugal pump. *J Thorac Cardiovasc Surg*, 2003; 125: 353–360.

34 Goldstein AH, Pacella JJ, Clark RE. Predictable reduction in left ventricular stroke work and oxygen utilization with an implantable centrifugal pump. *Ann Thorac Surg*, 1994; 58: 1018–1024.

35 Sauren LD, Accord RE, Hamzeh K, et al. Combined Impella and intra-aortic balloon pump support to improve both ventricular unloading and coronary blood flow for myocardial recovery: an experimental study. *Artif Organs*, 2007; 31: 839–882.

36 Kapur N, Paruchuri V, Pham D, et al. Hemodynamic effects of left atrial or left ventricular cannulation for acute circulatory support in a bovine model of left heart injury. *ASAIO J*, 2015; 61(3): 301–306.

37 Thiele H, Lauer B, Hambrecht R, et al. Reversal of cardiogenic shock by percutaneous left atrial-to-femoral arterial bypass assistance. *Circulation*, 2001; 104: 2917–2922.

38 Bruckner BA, Jacob LP, Gregoric ID, et al. Clinical experience with the TandemHeart percutaneous ventricular assist device as a bridge to cardiac transplantation. *Tex Heart Inst J*, 2008; 35: 447–450.

39 Burkhoff D, Cohen H, Brunckhorst C, et al. TandemHeart Investigators Group. A randomized multicenter clinical study to evaluate the safety and efficacy of the TandemHeart percutaneous ventricular assist device versus conventional therapy with intraaortic balloon pumping for treatment of cardiogenic shock. *Am Heart J*, 2006; 152(3): 469.e.1–8.

40 Kar B, Gregoric ID, Basra SS, et al. The percutaneous ventricular assist device in severe refractory cardiogenic shock. *J Am Coll Cardiol*, 2011; 57(6): 688–696.

41 Aghili N, Kang S, Kapur NK. The fundamentals of extra-corporeal membrane oxygenation. *Minerva Cardioangiol*, 2015; 63(1): 75–85.

42 Esper SA, Bermudez C, Dueweke EJ, et al. Extracorporeal membrane oxygenation support in acute coronary syndromes complicated by cardiogenic shock. *Cathet Cardiovasc Interv*, 2015; 86 Suppl 1: S45–50.

43 Jacobs AK, Leopold JA, Bates E, et al. Cardiogenic shock caused by right ventricular infarction: a report from the SHOCK registry. *J Am Coll Cardiol*, 2003; 41: 1273–1279.

44 Mehta SR, Elkelboom JW, Natarajan MK, et al. Impact of right ventricular involvement on mortality and morbidity in patients with inferior myocardial infarction. *J Am Coll Cardiol*, 2001; 37(1): 37–43.

45 Takayama H, Naka Y, Kodali SK, et al. A novel approach to percutaneous right-ventricular mechanical support. *Eur J Cardiothorac Surg*, 2012; 41(2): 423–426.

46 Loor G, Khani-Hanjani A, Gonzalez–Stawinski GV. Use of RotaFlow (Maquet) for temporary right ventricular support during implantation of HeartMate II left ventricular assist device. *ASAIO J*, 2012; 58(3): 275–277.

47 Kapur NK, Paruchuri V, Korabathina R, et al. Effects of a percutaneous mechanical circulatory support device for medically refractory right ventricular failure. *J Heart Lung Transplant*, 2011; 30(12): 1360–1367.

48 Kapur NK, Paruchuri V, Jagannathan A, et al. Mechanical circulatory support for right ventricular failure: The TandemHeart in RIght VEntricular support (THRIVE) Registry. 32nd IHSLT 2012 Annual Meeting. *J Heart Lung Transplant*, 2012; 31(4 Suppl): S110.

49 Samuels L. The Recover Right™ trial: Use of the Impella RP percutaneous right ventricular assist device: An Hde study. *J Clin Exp Cardiolog*, 2015; 6: 4.

50 Kanter KR, Schaff HV, Gott VL, et al. Reduced oxygen consumption with effective left ventricular venting during postischemic reperfusion. *Circulation*, 1982; 66: 150–154.

51 Allen BS, Buckberg GD, Fontan FM, et al. Superiority of controlled surgical reperfusion versus percutaneous transluminal coronary angioplasty in acute coronary occlusion. *J Thorac Cardiovasc Surg*, 1993; 105: 864–879.

52 Smalling RW, Cassidy DB, Barrett R, et al. Improved regional myocardial blood flow, left ventricular unloading, and infarct salvage using an axial-flow, transvalvular left ventricular assist device. A comparison with intra-aortic balloon counterpulsation and reperfusion alone in a canine infarction model. *Circulation*, 1992; 85: 1152–1159.

53 Achour H, Boccalandro F, Felli P, et al. Mechanical left ventricular unloading prior to reperfusion reduces infarct size in a canine infarction model. *Catheter Cardiovasc Interv*, 2005; 64: 182–192.

54 Meyns B, Stolinski J, Leunens V, et al. Left ventricular support by catheter-mounted axial flow pump reduces infarct size. *J Am Coll Cardiol*, 2003; 41: 1087–1095.

55 Kapur NK, Paruchuri V, Urbano-Morales JA, et al. Mechanically unloading the left ventricle before coronary reperfusion reduces left ventricular wall stress and myocardial infarct size. *Circulation*, 2013; 128: 328–336.

56 Kapur NK, Qiao X, Paruchuri V, et al. Mechanical Preconditioning with Acute Circulatory Support Before Reperfusion Limits Infarct Size in Acute Myocardial Infarction. *JACC Heart Fail*, 2015; 3(11): 873–882.

7

Thrombus Management for STEMI Interventions

Sameer Mehta MD, Olga Reynbakh MD, Daniel Rodriguez MD, Tracy Zhang BS,
Michael Schweitzer MD, Maria Teresa Bedoya Reina MD, Miguel Vega Arango MD,
Juanita Gonzalez Arango MD, Maria Botero Urrea MD

Introduction

Thrombus is central to the pathophysiology of ST-elevated myocardial infarction (STEMI). Its identification and management constitute absolute essentials in optimal door-to-balloon STEMI interventions. Distal thrombus embolization during STEMI occurs frequently and is also associated with compromised long-term outcomes, not limited to larger enzymatic infarct size, increased major in-hospital complications, lower left ventricular ejection fraction at discharge, higher long-term mortality in STEMI, and increased incidence of emergency bypass surgery [1–4]. A high thrombus burden in STEMI has been associated with post-procedural epicardial and myocardial perfusion and higher no-reflow and distal embolization. Several mechanical adjunctive devices and pharmacologic options have shown diverse benefits in managing thrombus [5,6].

Pathophysiology of Thrombus

Atherosclerosis is a chronic inflammatory process that is fundamental to intimal plaque development in human vasculature, including the coronary vessels. Several risk factors, including advanced age, male sex, genetics, hyperlipidemia, hypertension, tobacco use, and diabetes mellitus predispose to endothelial injury. Atherogenesis, or plaque formation, involves a dynamic interplay between endothelial injury and inflammatory element recruitment (lipoproteins, macrophages, platelets, smooth muscle cells, collagen, etc.) and deposition [8].

In addition to locally produced mediators, products of blood coagulation and thrombosis are likely to contribute to atheroma evolution and complications. This involvement justifies the use of the term "atherothrombosis" to convey the inextricable links between atherosclerosis and thrombosis [8]. Plaque is subjected to a variety of intrinsic and extrinsic stressors that lead to an acute plaque change [9]. The rupture, fissuring, erosion, or ulceration of plaque initiates the thrombosis cascade in one of two pathways [8]. The first pathway involves exposed collagen of the vessel wall. The exposed collagen of disrupted endothelium interacts with platelet glycoproteins. Specifically, platelet glycoprotein VI binds with the collagen of the exposed vessel, while platelet glycoprotein Ib-V-IX interacts with the collagen-bound von Willebrand factor. This process not only secures the adherence of platelets to the vessel wall, but also initiates

Manual of STEMI Interventions, First Edition. Edited by Sameer Mehta.
© 2017 John Wiley & Sons Ltd. Published 2017 by John Wiley & Sons Ltd.

platelet activation and granule release, independent of thrombin [10]. Ultimately, this pathway leads to the formation of *white thrombus*, which consists of varying amounts of cellular debris, fibrin, and platelets, and a limited number of erythrocytes. Succeeding the white thrombus, the second pathway leads to formation of a *red thrombus*, which represents an erythrocyte- and thrombin-rich complex [11].

A membrane protein (tissue factor) mediates the second pathway. Among its functions, tissue factor initiates the extrinsic coagulation cascade. It binds to the activated factor VII, which then activates factor IX, ultimately leading to the cascade that generates thrombin. Thrombin then cleaves protease-activated receptor 4 on the platelet surface. This cleavage in turn activates platelets, causing the release of adenosine diphosphate (ADP), serotonin, and thromboxane A2, all of which are agonists in the activation of other platelets [10]. Depending on the initial size of plaque, both pathways can occlude the lumen of the coronary vessel, leading to a myocardial infarction [12–16]. The timing and intrinsic ability of the second pathway to stabilize, enlarge, and increase the density of the primary white thrombus [11] contributes to the complexity of management of thrombus, especially in the setting of door-to-balloon time constraints.

Thrombus and STEMI

In the very early stages of acute myocardial infarction, thrombus presents as a platelet-based white thrombus that progresses in the next few hours into a dense, organized red thrombus comprising red blood cells and fibrin strands. Figure 7.1 demonstrates the dynamic pathophysiology of thrombus and provides a framework for early and aggressive thrombus management.

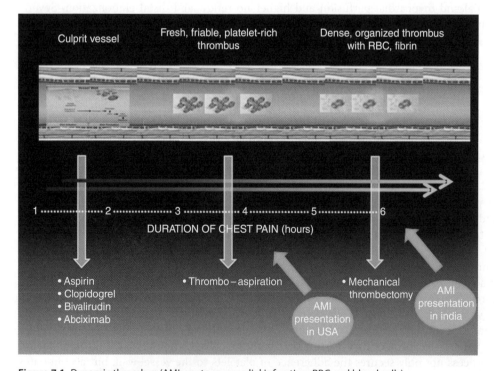

Figure 7.1 Dynamic thrombus (AMI, acute myocardial infarction; RBC, red blood cells).

Table 7.1 Thrombolysis in myocardial infarction (TIMI) thrombus grade.

Grade	Definition
0	No cine-angiographic characteristics of thrombus present.
1	Possible thrombus present. Angiography demonstrates characteristics such as reduced contrast density, haziness, irregular lesion contour or a smooth convex "meniscus" at the site of total occlusion suggestive but not diagnostic of thrombus.
2	Thrombus present; small size. Definite thrombus with greatest dimensions ≤ 0.5 vessel diameter.
3	Thrombus present; moderate size. Definite thrombus but with greatest linear dimension > 0.5 but < 2 vessel diameters.
4	Thrombus present; large size. As for grade 3 but with the largest dimension ≥ 2 vessel diameters.
5	Total occlusion.

Sources:
TIMI-IIIA Investigators. Early effects of tissue-type plasminogen activator added to conventional therapy on the culprit coronary lesion in patients presenting with ischemic cardiac pain at rest. *Circulation*, 1993; 87: 38–52.
van't Hof AW, Liem A, Suryapranata H, et al. Angiographic assessment of myocardial reperfusion in patients treated with primary angioplasty for acute myocardial infarction: myocardial blush grade. Zwolle Myocardial Infarction Study Group. *Circulation*, 1998; 97: 2302–2306.

Among the procedural variables, assessment of thrombus grade and applying a thrombus grade-based thrombectomy strategy are strongly advocated.

Thrombus burden has been shown to adversely affect clinical outcomes in both cerebrovascular accidents and acute coronary syndromes [25–28]. Barreto et al. [29] undertook a retrospective review of stroke patients and correlated the clinical outcomes to the angiographic thrombus burden, using the classification scheme outlined in Table 7.1. Compared with patients with thrombus grades 0–3, patients with thrombus grade 4 required longer treatment times, and experienced increased mechanical clot disruption, poor outcomes, and mortality [29]. Using the same classification scheme, Sianos et al. demonstrated in their landmark work the importance of thrombus burden in clinical outcomes in acute coronary syndromes [17]. Compared with a lower thrombus burden (grades 0–3), the study found that large intracoronary thrombus burden (grade 4) was an independent predictor of mortality and major adverse cardiovascular event (MACE). Evidently, clinical outcome is dependent upon thrombus burden.

Mehta Strategy

In our structured approach to door-to-balloon STEMI interventions that are particularly challenged by the constraints of a ticking clock, identification of the culprit lesion and compulsive management of thrombus remain the critical determinant of procedural success. Our methodology for thrombus management in STEMI interventions has been developed from our extensive work with the SINCERE (Single INdividual Community Experience Registry) database, which has included 1302 short door-to-balloon interventions. The Mehta Strategy for selective thrombus management was published in *Interventional Cardiology Clinics* [7] and we anticipate that the simplicity of our quantitatively based strategy will make it an attractive management option.

The thrombolysis in myocardial infarction (TIMI) thrombus grade classifies the thrombus based on angiography (Table 7.1) and is the basis for the Mehta Strategy for Thrombus Management (Table 7.2). The pioneering work by Sianos et al. [17] led to this classification, which has now been routinely put into practice in over 1145 short door-to-balloon STEMI interventions in the SINCERE database [18]. Table 7.3 formulates the stepwise technique for performing the entire STEMI procedure using this standardized algorithm.

Optimal angiographic visualization of thrombus is the first step; however, thrombus is very labile and its grading for the purpose of further management is better done after crossing the thrombotic STEMI lesion with the guide wire. Balloon catheters are not recommended, as they cause distal embolization and myocardial necrosis. We recommend using balloon catheters only for three rare situations:

1) Uncertainty, whether the guide wire is in the true lumen, after it has crossed a thrombotically occluded segment; in this situation, a small 2.0 mm balloon can be rapidly inflated.
2) For a patient with overwhelming ischemia and massive ST-segment elevation. The role of the balloon in this situation is to achieve some TIMI flow rapidly. However, this may result in thrombus migration and this strategy must be used with great discretion.
3) Unavailability of thrombectomy catheters and/or devices.

Often, there is no change in thrombus grade, but thrombus grade 5 most commonly is downsized after wire passage. If the extent of thrombus is small (thrombus grade 0–1), direct angioplasty and stenting may be sufficient (Figures 7.2–7.5). Moderate thrombus burden, grades 2–3, warrants pretreatment with an aspiration catheter. Several randomized controlled trials have demonstrated that aspiration catheters result in superior myocardial blush grade (MBG), ST-segment resolution, improved clinical outcome, TIMI 3 flow rates, and decreased angiographic evidence of distal embolization [18–20]. Figures 7.6–7.9 demonstrate aspiration pretreatment in a STEMI with moderate thrombus burden.

Mehta Strategy: Techniques and Results

Grade 0–1

With low thrombus grades, direct stenting is an acceptable strategy, and we advocate it over the use of pre-dilatation that carries its individual risk of distal embolization. We complement this strategy with the use of intracoronary vasodilators, as with all STEMI interventions. Although various pharmacological agents can be used for this purpose (adenosine, verapamil, diltiazem, nicardipine, clevidipine), our preferred agent as an intracoronary vasodilator is nitroprusside. Post- stenting, intracoronary vasodilators augment distal microvasculature flow and improve MBG.

Grade 2–3

Moderate thrombus burden management with aspiration catheters can be augmented with some practical techniques. Passes with the aspiration catheters should be made until there is no angiographic evidence of thrombus. Often, just two passes is sufficient. It is important to advance the catheter throughout the entire length of thrombus. Despite their ease of use and effectiveness, the aspiration catheters are not perfect monorail devices and attention should be paid to the tip of the guide wire as these catheters are advanced. Reducing the imaging magnification and monitoring the distal end of the guide wire as the aspiration catheter is advanced are practical techniques in preventing adverse results. Thrombus will often clog the aspiration holes of these catheters halting aspiration. Before abandoning them as unsuccessful, it is important to remove the catheter, flush it profusely, and reuse. Finally, in rare situations, the aspiration

Table 7.2 Strategy for the management of the STEMI lesion based on thrombus grade; Mehta Classification (source: Clinics of America, September 2009).

Grade	Thrombus Definition	Angiographic Examples	Mehta Classification	Technical Tips for Use	
				Aspiration catheter	AngioJet
0	No cine-angiographic characteristics of thrombus present			• Most effective with fresh clot; organized clot is more resistant to debulking.	• Can be used via the radial route. Although LAD and some LCX may not need TPM, I PLACE TPMS in all AngioJet procedures.
1	Possible thrombus present. Angiography demonstrates reduced contrast destiny, haziness, irregular lesion contour or a smooth convex "meniscus" at the site of total occlusion suggestive but not diagnostic of thrombus.		Direct stent ± predilation	• Have different profiles, different push-ability, tractability and aspiration rates. • All are 6 Fr compatible. It is useful to stock and be familiar with the use of at least one version. • Flush catheter lumen well before use, as this facilitates better tracking over the wire.	• Often, multiple passes will be required. Try to pause after every 2–3 passes to enable hemodynamics to be restored, to optimize guide wire and guiding catheter support, and to evaluate the results.
2	Thrombus present – small size. Definite thrombus with greatest dimensions ≤ half vessel diameter.			• Avoid kinking the catheter – advance slowly over the initial, softer portion of the catheter.	• Often, just the first passage will restore adequate flow. • Resistant and stubborn thrombi will require more distal advancement, which must be done more carefully.
3	Thrombus present – moderate size. Definite thrombus but with greatest linear dimension > half but < 2 vessel diameters.		Aspiration thrombectomy	• Monitor distal tip of the guide wire as the aspiration catheter is advanced – it is not uncommon for the guide wire to advance during the maneuver. • Advance the aspiration catheter through the entire length of occlusive disease.	• Avoid advancing in severe tortuosity and in vessels < 2 mm. • Since the AngioJet is used for large thrombus burden and high thrombus grade, consider abciximab as adjunctive therapy.

(Continued)

Table 7.2 (Continued)

			Technical Tips for Use	
			Aspiration catheter	AngioJet
Grade	Thrombus Definition	Angiographic Examples	Mehta Classification	
4	Thrombus present –large size. As for grade 3 but with the largest dimension ≥ 2 vessel diameters.		AngioJet	
5	Total occlusion.			

LAD, left anterior descending; LCX, left circumflex coronary artery; TPM, temporary pacemaker.

Table 7.3 Step by step technique for STEMI interventions.

Step	Technique	Comments
1	Obtain a clean, 6 Fr arterial access.	Routinely from the right femoral route (radial route for failed attempt with both groins, and for selected pharmaco-invasive, transfer patients).
2	Cine-angiography with 6 Fr diagnostic catheter of the non-infarct-related vessel.	Two orthogonal views for LCA and a single LAO projection for the RCA.
3	6 Fr guiding catheter for culprit vessel cannulation.	Obtain set-up shots that precisely define the occluded segment.
4	Hydrophilic 0.014-inch guide wire	Particularly useful for crossing thrombotic lesions.
5	Accurately assess thrombus grade using a selective thrombectomy strategy.	Direct stenting for low-grade thrombus, thrombo-aspiration for moderate thrombus and mechanical thrombectomy for large thrombus burden.
6	Abciximab for large thrombus burden.	Preferably via intracoronary use.
7	Stenting.	Drug-eluting stent for LAD, diabetic, long lesions and small vessels.
8	Liberal intracoronary nitroprusside.	After confirming satisfactory stent result and removing the guide wire.
9	Left ventriculography.	In RAO projection.
10	Sheath removal.	With closure device

Preferred rheolytic mechanical thrombectomy:

A	For thrombus grade 4 and 5
B	In large vessels with voluminous thrombus
C	SVG STEMI interventions
D	For treating dense, organized thrombus, in particular, in patients that present late
E	Failure to treat thrombotic lesions with aspiration thrombectomy

LAD, left anterior descending; LAO, left anterior oblique; LCA, left coronary artery; RAO, right anterior oblique; RCA, right coronary artery; STEMI, ST-elevation myocardial infarction; SVG, saphenous vein graft.

(a)   (b)   (c)

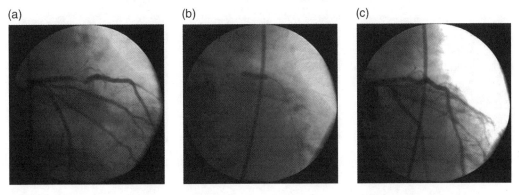

Figure 7.2 Primary percutaneous coronary intervention for STEMI with low thrombus burden. Lesions with low-grade thrombus can be treated safely without the need for more complex catheters or procedures. Angiograms from a patient who presented with an acute anterior wall STEMI. The initial angiogram demonstrated a critical mid left anterior descending culprit lesion with a low-grade 0–1 thrombus burden (a). The lesion was direct stented with a 3.5-mm drug-eluting stent (b), with a door-to-balloon time of 56 minutes. The final angiography demonstrates TIMI 3 flow (c).

(a) (b) (c)

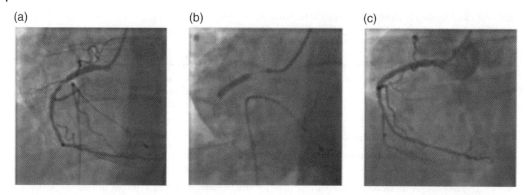

Figure 7.3 Direct stenting for low grade thrombus. a) Grade 1 thrombus. b) Direct stenting with 4-mm bare-metal stent. c) Post stenting.

(a) (b) (c)

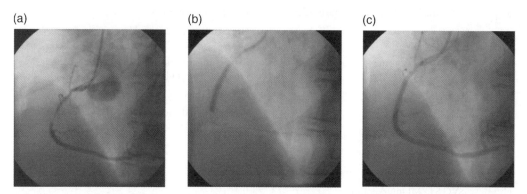

Figure 7.4 Direct stenting for low-grade thrombus. a) Grade 1 thrombus. b) Direct stenting with 4-mm bare-metal stent. c) Post stenting.

(a) (b) (c)

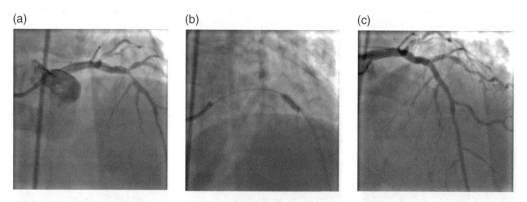

Figure 7.5 Direct stenting for low-grade thrombus. a) Grade 1 thrombus. b) Direct stenting with 4-mm bare-metal stent. c) Post stenting.

catheter will drag the tail of a long thread thrombus that may get dislodged. In one clinical case documented in the SINCERE database, a thrombus was dragged from the obtuse marginal branch and lodged at the bifurcation of the left circumflex – this was managed by suctioning with the AngioJet® peripheral thrombectomy system. The newer aspiration catheters are very

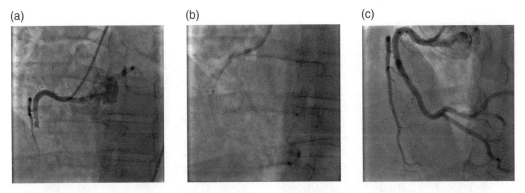

Figure 7.6 Primary percutaneous coronary intervention for STEMI with moderate thrombus burden. Lesions with moderate grade thrombus are best treated with aspiration thrombectomy devices, prior to definitive treatment and stenting. The angiograms show a moderate thrombus (grade 3) in a patient with ST-elevation in leads DII-III. The first angiogram demonstrates a discerning mid right coronary artery culprit lesion with a moderate grade thrombus (a). The lesion was treated then with an aspiration catheter (b) followed by angioplasty and stenting with a 4-mm bare-metal stent with a door-to-balloon time of 61 minutes, with good results (c).

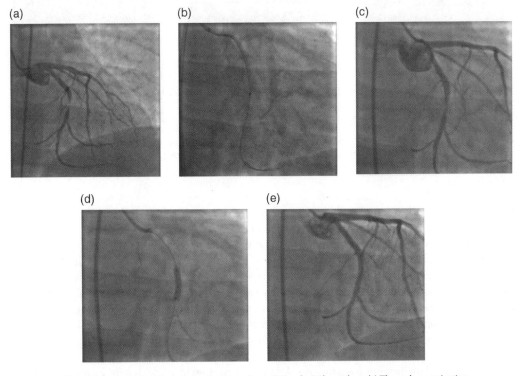

Figure 7.7 Thrombo-aspiration for moderate thrombus. a) Grade 2 thrombus. b) Thrombo-aspiration performed by Export Catheter. c) Post thrombectomy. d) 3.5-mm bare-metal stent. e) Post stenting.

easy to use and their use has now become the default strategy for managing thrombus for most lesions, except for those with very large thrombus burden, where mechanical thrombectomy is beneficial.

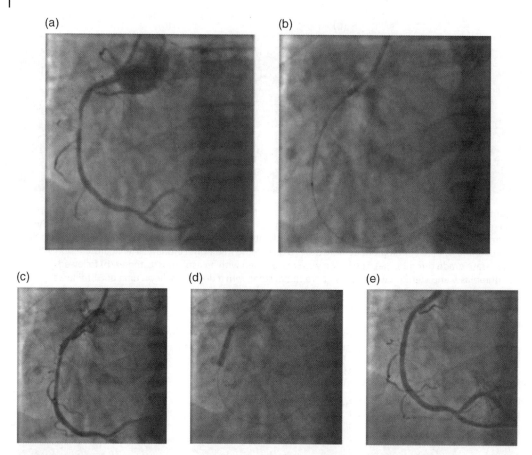

Figure 7.8 Thrombo-aspiration for moderate thrombus. a) Grade 1–2 thrombus. b) Thrombo-aspiration performed by Export Catheter. c) Post thrombectomy. d) 3.5-mm bare-metal stent. e) Post stenting.

Grade 4–5

Larger thrombus burden (grades 4–5) presents more challenges. As demonstrated in Figures 7.10–7.13, aspiration may be insufficient in cases with grade 4–5 thrombus. In such cases, thrombectomy may be justified. The AngioJet catheter is an effective device for debulking such voluminous thrombi. The thrombus is aspirated and extracted after high-velocity water jets have created a vacuum in this catheter-based system [21]. Compared with stenting alone, trials have found the AngioJet to be very successful in improving epicardial flow, frame count, MBG, and infarct size [20,22]. The Vein Graft AngioJet Study 2 trial found that the AngioJet catheter system was superior to intracoronary urokinase administration in improving device and procedural success, with lower major adverse effects, bleeding, and vascular complications [23].

Some practical techniques for using the AngioJet thrombectomy device may improve clinical outcomes. The new Spiroflex® AngioJet device is very quick to set up; the speed of set-up is vital to maintain the goals of achieving short door-to-balloon times. The new catheters, including the 4F thrombectomy catheter, track well. Thrombectomy should be performed through the entire length of the thrombus; in fact, the most frequent errors with this device are an inadequate number of passes, and not ablating through the complete length of the thrombotic segment. In addition to being a critical device for removing large and bulky thrombus, the AngioJet

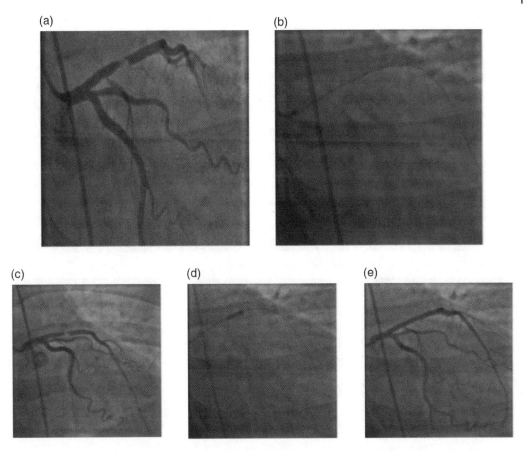

Figure 7.9 Thrombo-aspiration for moderate thrombus. a) Grade 2–3 thrombus. b) Thrombo-aspiration performed by Export Catheter. c) Post thrombectomy. d) 3.5-mm drug-eluting stent. e) Post stenting.

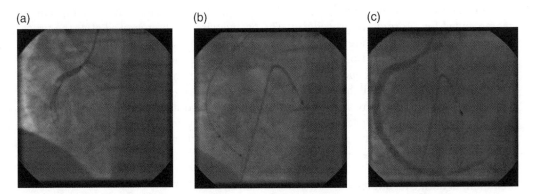

Figure 7.10 Primary percutaneous coronary intervention for STEMI with large thrombus burden. Lesions with high-grade thrombus may require some thrombectomy prior to definitive treatment and stenting. The initial angiogram on this patient, who presented with an acute inferior wall STEMI, demonstrated a large amount of thrombus (grade 3–4) (a). An AngioJet catheter (b) was initially used for rheolytic thrombectomy and after angioplasty and stenting, the final angiographic result was excellent (c).

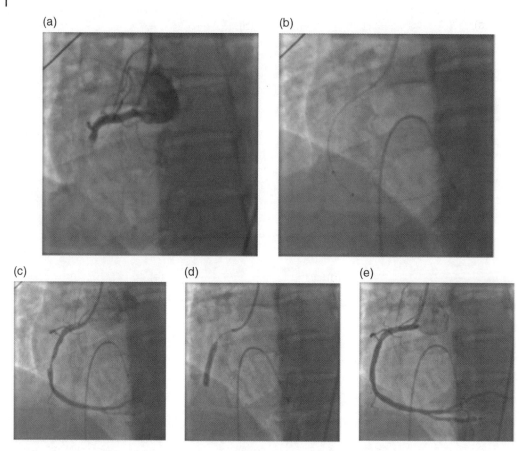

Figure 7.11 Rheolytic thrombectomy for large thrombus. a) Grade 5 thrombus. b) Rheolytic thrombectomy performed with AngioJet. c) Post thrombectomy. d) 4-mm bare-metal stent. e) Post stenting.

is invaluable in managing organized thrombus in late-presenting patients. The SINCERE database includes several successful AngioJet procedures where aspiration thrombectomy catheters were unsuccessful in aspirating such dense, organized thrombi. Temporary pacing is recommended for all AngioJet procedures. The pacing wire can be removed after the procedure, even though pacing is rare.

We offer another valuable tip for using both the aspiration and mechanical catheters when thrombectomy is deemed adequate. To reach this point of optimal thrombectomy, we advocate making successive passes until the last pass makes no further progress in debulking. Sometimes, it can be difficult to assess by angiography, but this broad strategy provides a philosophical approach to these thrombotic lesions with thrombectomy devices. For unsuitable anatomy or where rheolytic thrombectomy is not available, a strategy using intracoronary abciximab via the Clearway™ (Atrium) catheter is an acceptable option.

Limitations of the Mehta Strategy

1) Several catheterization laboratories are not equipped with mechanical thrombectomy devices (AngioJet, X-sizer®, and ThromCat®), or operators are not familiar with their use or their use causes door-to-balloon delays. In these situations, we feel that drug delivery of abciximab via the Clearway catheter provides a good alternative.

(a) (b)

(c) (d)

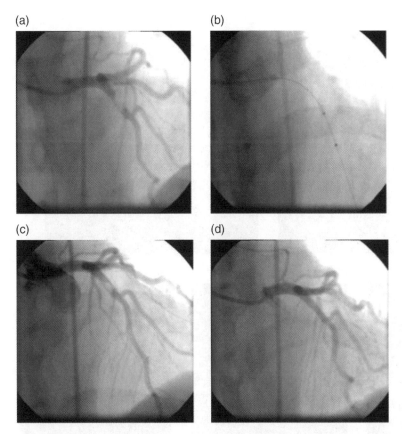

Figure 7.12 Rheolytic thrombectomy for large thrombus. a) Large, bulky thrombus in mid left anterior descending coronary artery. b) Rheolytic thrombectomy performed with AngioJet. c) Post thrombectomy. d) Post stenting, final result.

2) The same limitations as in #1 exist with unfavorable anatomy for the AngioJet (our preferred mechanical thrombectomy device), although the newer 4F catheters have narrowed our relative contraindications for their use in STEMI interventions (< 2.5 mm vessel size and severe tortuosity).

3) Although we recommend mechanical thrombectomy for large thrombus grade, in numerous cases, thrombo-aspiration works extremely well in large-grade thrombi. We have presented numerous examples of these situations (Figures 7.14–7.19). The thrombus grade is high (4–5), yet excellent debulking is observed with the simple aspiration catheters. We suspect that this happens in patients who present very early, with a fresh, red, soft, thrombus that is easily and completely aspirated with these catheters. This observation is contrary to our proposed hypothesis; however, this powerful observation is shared for its tremendous practical benefit. We have observed this finding most often in thrombotic occlusions where it was logical to advance a small aspiration catheter rather than a more bulky mechanical device. Incidentally, this is a rare situation, where we will use a low-profile balloon to verify that the guide wire is in the true lumen. Based upon an increasing number of similar cases (Figures 7.14–7.19), we are currently postulating thrombo-aspiration as a default strategy. The rationale for this is simple: The aspiration catheters are user friendly, relatively inexpensive, and take no more than a balloon catheter to prepare and

(a)   (b)

(c)   (d)   (e)

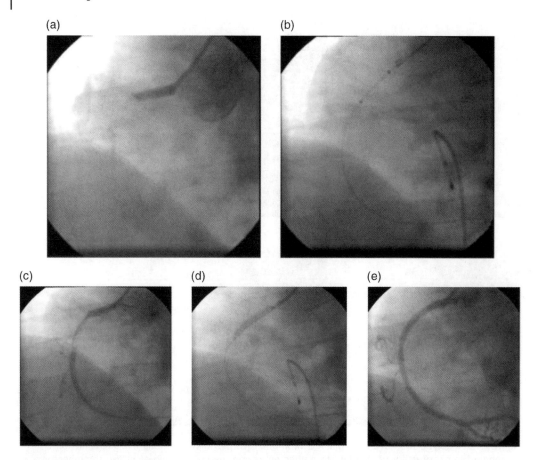

Figure 7.13 Rheolytic thrombectomy for large thrombus. a) Grade 5 thrombus. b) Rheolytic thrombectomy performed with AngioJet. c) Post thrombectomy. d) 4.5-mm bare-metal stent. e) Post stenting.

deploy. With this methodology, we grade thrombus, then quickly make a pass with the aspiration catheter, and either persist with more thrombo-aspiration or advance to using mechanical thrombectomy.

4) Similarly, we have also experienced numerous cases, even with a moderate thrombus burden, where the dense, organized, thrombus cannot be debulked with thrombo-aspiration. In these situations, the default strategy gives a way to using mechanical thrombectomy, consistent with the Mehta Strategy.

5) Although several newer trials appear to validate our strategy with the appropriate presently available device, greater scientific validity is needed. Founded on extensive experience, we feel confident in our strategy for effective thrombus management for STEMI interventions. Nevertheless, this strategy needs endorsement by clinical trials. A single individual experience, irrespective of its expertise, cannot substitute for data from large, randomized, clinical trials and/or established guidelines.

6) We have also explored possibilities of using a time to presentation-based strategy for applying a thrombectomy device. This idea is akin to the use of pre-hospital lysis, as in the CAPTIM (Comparison of Angioplasty and Pre-hospital Thrombolysis in Acute Myocardial Infarction) trial, where the cohorts of patients presenting with very early acute myocardial infarction (AMI) benefit from very early lysis [24]. This probably results from effective lysis

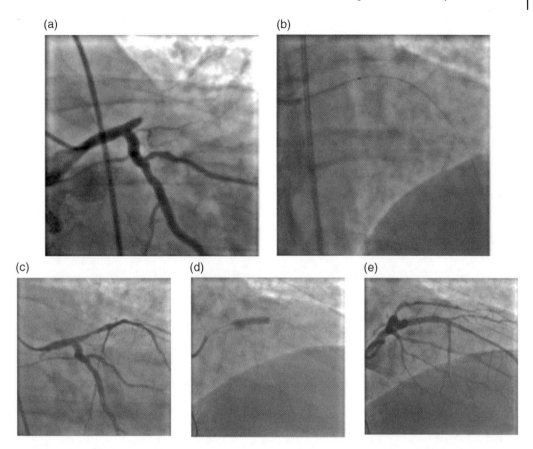

(a) (b) (c) (d) (e)

Figure 7.14 Thrombo-aspiration as default strategy. a) Grade 5 thrombus. b) Thrombo-aspiration performed by Export Catheter. c) Post thrombectomy. d) 3.5-mm Xience drug-eluting stent. e) Post stenting.

of a fresh clot. The same principles as very early lysis may be extended to the use of a thrombectomy device during STEMI with thrombo-aspiration working as very effective therapy for early presenters (less than 3 hours) and mechanical thrombectomy for late presenters (over 3 hours). Of course, calculating the time to presentation is not without its challenges. We also recognize the numerous variables that affect thrombus presentation in STEMI and the heterogeneity of thrombus and of its over simplification. Yet, this topic deserves further attention as the interventional management of a soft, white, early, thrombus is quite different from that of dense, organized thrombus.

Global Strategies of Thrombectomy and Recent Trials

Figure 7.20 presents a flow chart describing interventional options based on the thrombus dynamic in different STEMI systems. With early patient presentation, early hospital triage, intelligent ambulance systems and pre-hospital management, a STEMI procedure involves managing a white thrombus that is relatively easy to treat. The gray zone shows the approach in these efficient STEMI systems. It is usual to have maximal benefit from simple thrombectomy devices in this group. As is depicted in the figure, several of these early-presenting patients,

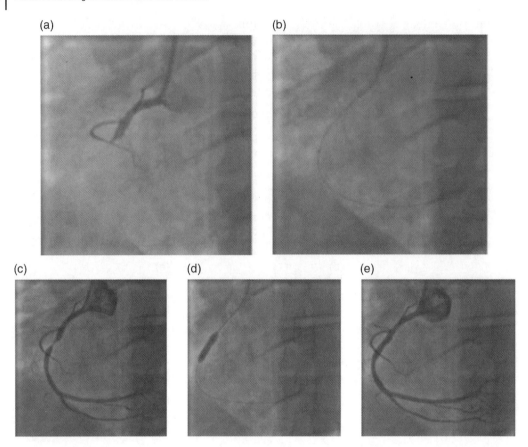

Figure 7.15 Thrombo-aspiration as default strategy. a) Grade 5 thrombus. b) Thrombo-aspiration performed by Export Catheter. c) Post thrombectomy. d) 4-mm bare-metal stent. e) Post stenting.

in particular those who have been treated with effective antiplatelet and anticoagulants, will demonstrate TIMI 3 flow and thrombus removal with simple thrombectomy techniques. This differentiation demonstrates how an efficient STEMI process contributes to an easier and better STEMI procedure.

The red section in Figure 7.20 describes the approach to the thrombus management when operators confront dense, organized thrombus that is formed due to a thrombus dynamics proceeding over time into a red thrombus with erythrocytes and fibrin strands. This type of late STEMI presentation is often seen in developing countries with less-structured STEMI management responses and delayed treatment. For such dense, organized thrombi, as advocated in our thrombus strategy, more complex thrombectomy techniques, including mechanical thrombectomy may be required.

Management of this type of thrombus is completely different to that of the soft, friable thrombus. Mechanical thrombectomy devices are of particular benefit in treating such thrombotic lesions provided that the anatomy is suitable – large vessels without excessive tortuosity. Although it is not commonly used in this particular situation, laser angioplasty is also an attractive modality for ablating thrombus in dense, organized, late-presenting lesions. In particular, the MGuard™ stent may be very useful in such situations [8]. If large, randomized clinical trials can demonstrate that it does not increase target-vessel revascularization, this device could become a front-line management for treating STEMI lesions.

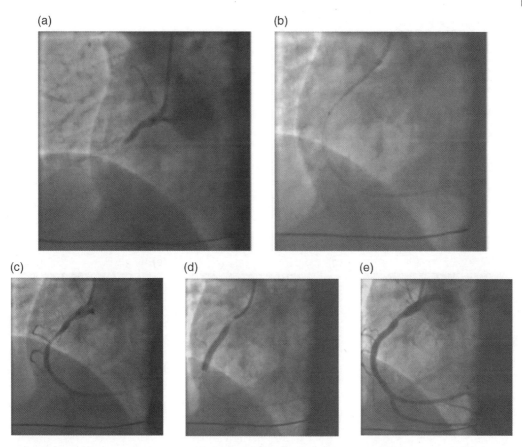

Figure 7.16 Thrombo-aspiration as default strategy. a) Grade 5 thrombus. b) Thrombo-aspiration performed by Export Catheter. c) Post thrombectomy. d) 4-mm bare-metal stent. e) Post stenting.

Improvements in the STEMI process and short door-to-balloon times therefore directly help the STEMI procedure, as the operators engage the easier to treat white thrombus. Unless the fresh thrombus in the early-presenting patient is voluminous (MBG 4 or 5), using the AngioJet in these cases is unnecessary, and is associated with higher complications. This observation should explain why several AngioJet trials demonstrated higher MACE events [4,5].

Figure 7.20 also presents a flow chart for interventional options when there is residual thrombus and less than TIMI 3 flow. An essential component of this strategy is to avoid stenting in the presence of residual thrombus. The most common scenario, in particular, in late-presenting lesions with dense thrombus, is where these devices are either unavailable or do not work. In such cases that demonstrate residual thrombus and inadequate flow, we strongly recommend not to stent, to use ample antiplatelets and anticoagulants, and return the patient to the catheterization laboratory for a staged and definitive management of thrombus and the STEMI lesion.

Thrombus removal prior to STEMI intervention in comparison with standard percutaneous coronary intervention (PCI) alone has been investigated in many randomized controlled trials and retrospective studies. Based on the results from these trials, it is apparent that prior meta-analyses from both single and multicenter trials, such as TAPAS [19], JETSTENT (AngioJET Thrombectomy and STENTing for Treatment of Acute Myocardial Infarction) [20], MUSTELA (MUltidevice thrombectomy in acute ST-Segment ELevation Acute myocardial infarction)

(a) (b)

(c) (d) (e)

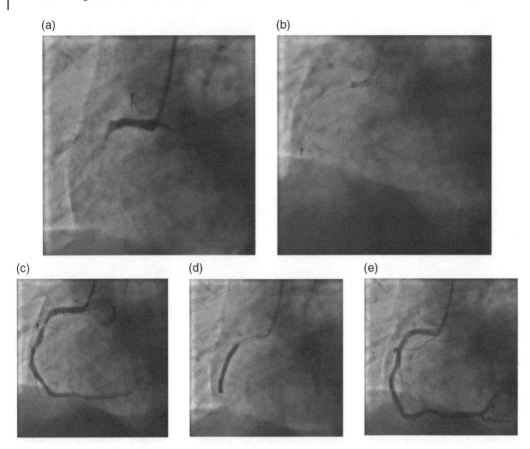

Figure 7.17 Thrombo-aspiration as default strategy. a) Grade 5 thrombus. b) Thrombo-aspiration performed by Export Catheter. c) Post thrombectomy. d) 4-mm bare-metal stent. e) Post stenting.

[30], INFUSE-AMI[31] and SMART-AMI [32], showed both positive and negative results with a wide variety of primary endpoints. Lack of consistent primary endpoints across studies also makes interpreting and comparing studies challenging if not impossible.

Despite the mixed clinical outcomes of these trials, we strongly believe that these studies are constrained by having a single strategy for all-comers without volumetric adjustments for thrombus burden. Although, philosophically, we remain in complete agreement with the intent to aspirate thrombus, as is clearly demonstrable in the TAPAS trial [19], we believe that this sole aspiration strategy does not suffice for all thrombus grades, and it particularly fails to effectively treat dense, organized thrombus that is commonly seen in delayed presentations. Dense, organized thrombus in late-presenting AMI is the most common presentation in developing countries that lack well-organized ambulance systems and efficient STEMI systems of care. In such situations, it is infrequent that the physician encounters a white thrombus that is easy to treat with aspiration thrombectomy, as was demonstrable in the TAPAS trial. Dense, organized thrombus that are often present in STEMI cases are too complex to manage with aspiration catheters. Based upon our work, we strongly consider that such lesions are better managed by mechanical devices, such as the AngioJet, provided that the anatomy is favorable (avoiding severe tortuosity and vessels less than 2.5 mm). So far as clinical support for our selective thrombus management strategy, the drawback of using a single aspiration thrombectomy

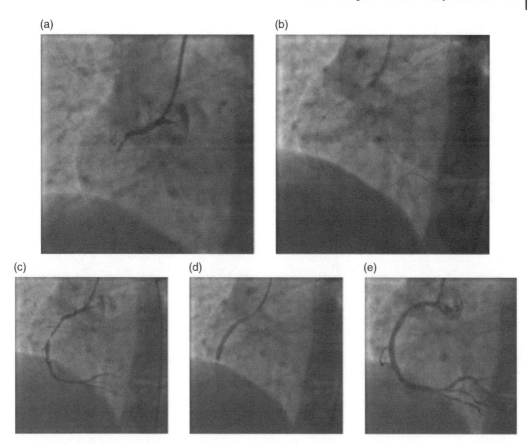

Figure 7.18 Thrombo-aspiration as default strategy. a) Grade 5 thrombus. b) Thrombo-aspiration performed by Export Catheter. c) Post thrombectomy. d) 4-mm bare-metal stent. e) Post stenting.

strategy has been partially corrected in the JETSTENT trial, which uses angiography to grade the thrombus burden prior to thrombus aspiration and subsequent PCI intervention [20].

We recognize the scientific observations of the large TASTE [33] trial, which raised doubts over thrombectomy. The Swedish group has performed an exceptional long-term evaluation of thrombectomy in STEMI. The TASTE trial is a multicenter, prospective, open-label, randomized, controlled clinical trial. This study presented long-term follow-up data on 7244 patients with STEMI, which increases the strength of the trial. The results showed that routine thrombus aspiration before PCI as compared with PCI alone did not reduce 30-day mortality among patients with STEMI. These comparisons remained non-significant when the data were analyzed for the longer-term follow-up (up to 1 year), although the 30-day mortality was observed to be lower than expected (2.9%) in the study cohort. Overall, 78.4% of patients had a high thrombus burden (TIMI thrombus grade 4 or 5). The rate of crossover was 4.6% from thrombectomy to PCI alone and 1.4% from PCI alone to thrombectomy. In addition, bailout thrombectomy was used in 7.1% of the control group. Investigators also acknowledge some limitations of the trial, including the fact that interventionalists performing the procedures were not blinded to treatment assignment, the inclusion of some patients with low thrombus burden, and the inability to rule out a benefit of selective rather than routine use of thrombectomy.

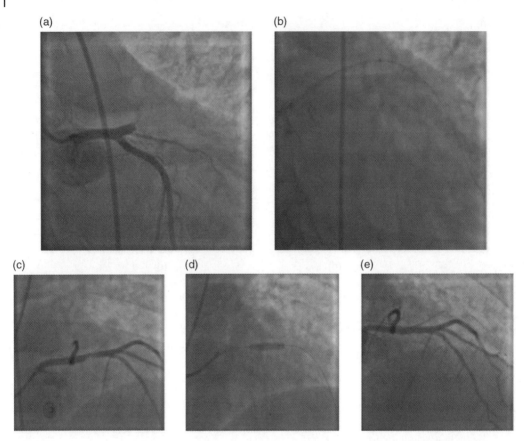

Figure 7.19 Thrombo-aspiration as default strategy. a) Grade 5 thrombus. b) Thrombo-aspiration performed by Export Catheter. c) Post thrombectomy. d) 4-mm Xience V drug-eluting stent. e) Post stenting.

Based on the meta-analyses, aspiration thrombectomy is a class IIa recommendation with level of evidence B in the 2013 American College of Cardiology/American Heart Association STEMI guidelines. However, it is still our firm believe that thrombectomy is most effective when it is directed in a selective fashion and when selection is based on thrombosis grade. Therefore, not discounting the robust findings, we state our viewpoint or a strategy that has been successfully employed in the SINCERE database for more than a decade. For almost the same reasons of lacking a selective strategy, we have some reluctance in accepting the results of the INFUSE-AMI, MUSTELA and TOTAL [34] trials.

The most recent and the largest randomized trial to date to redefine the guidelines for the thrombectomy is the TOTAL trial (Randomized Trial of Primary PCI with or without Routine Manual Thrombectomy), an international, multicenter, prospective, randomized trial that included 10,066 patients [35]. The primary efficacy outcome was death from cardiovascular causes, recurrent myocardial infarction, cardiogenic shock, or new or worsening New York Heart Association class IV heart failure within 180 days. This study showed that there were no substantial differences between the groups with routine manual thrombectomy or direct stenting in cardiovascular death, recurrent myocardial infarction, cardiogenic shock or heart failure within 6 months. The investigators also reported higher stroke rates in patients who had undergone routine thrombectomy than in those who underwent PCI alone. This finding should be further investigated, since the study was not powered to detect a difference in stroke, the number

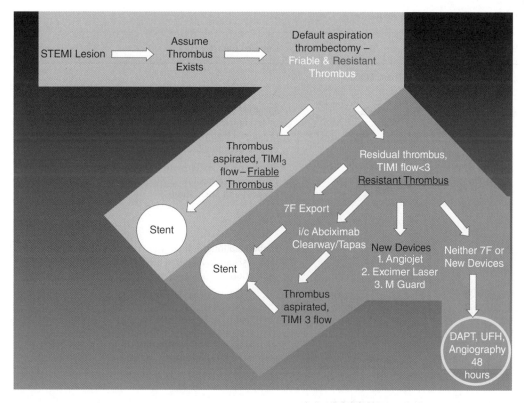

Figure 7.20 Thrombus management strategy (DAPT, dual antiplatelet therapy; i/c, intracoronary; TIMI, thrombolysis in myocardial infarction; UFH, unfractionated heparin).

of events was small, and the stroke risk was not in connection with the periprocedural period, thus raising doubts that the procedure was the cause. This study did not investigate selective thrombectomy and the authors agree that when ballooning does not open the artery, bailout aspiration thrombectomy is a reasonable strategy. In these 300–400 patients, no strokes in the post-procedure period were noted.

Since thrombus burden or grade can be quickly assessed angiographically, a thrombus grade approach is practical. This is the major advantage of the Mehta Strategy (Table 7.2), as it provides a selective strategy for thrombus management, based upon the thrombus grade. This methodology contradicts the notion that thrombus can be managed by a single modality, as proposed by the TAPAS [33], TASTE [37] and TOTAL [34,39] trials, which used thrombo-aspiration as an effective strategy, irrespective of the thrombus grade. In this chapter, we have presented numerous cases that support our rationale for a selective, thrombus grade-based strategy. Specifically, we cite numerous procedures where a dense, organized thrombus could not be effectively managed by thrombo-aspiration, instead requiring a change to mechanical thrombectomy. Table 7.4 outlines various thrombectomy devices for STEMI and PCI. In fact, some of the most memorable successes in the SINCERE database employed these tenets. The situation with an organized, dense thrombus in late-presenting STEMI patients is the most noteworthy of these cases. These can be extremely difficult cases and their management, from crossing the impenetrable lesions to debulking them, requires considerable skills, and often, mechanical thrombectomy.

Table 7.4 Thrombectomy devices.

Device	Unique Characteristics
ASPIRATION THROMBECTOMY	
Diver CE	Available in 2 versions: Aspiration lumen with side holes (for fresh thrombus removal, 2–6 hours post symptom onset) and aspiration lumen without side holes (for organized thrombus removal, 6–24 hours post symptom onset). Ultraflexible shaft from increased trackability.
Export	Distal end is flexible with high-density variable braiding. Proximal end has low-density variable braiding for support and push-ability.
Pronto	Embedded longitudinal wire enhances deliverability and kink resistance. Patented Silva distal tip provides vessel protection.
QuickCat	6 Fr aspiration catheter with a low profile. Moderate suction ability, kinks easily and could perform better with more tensile strength of catheter.
Fetch	Rapid exchange and 6 Fr compatible. Braided shaft with hydrophilic coating and convex tip.
Hunter	Rapid exchange with dual lumen and 6 F compatible.
Thrombuster	Low frictional resistance, kink resistance and deliverability enhanced with a metal braided shaft. Large aspiration lumen and hydrophilic coating.
F.A.S.T. Funnel Catheter	Delivered over guide wire proximal to the occlusion, funnel occluder stops blood from flowing through, preventing distal flow of debris. A standard syringe allows removal of thrombus and stagnant blood flow. 7 Fr compatible.

Table 7.4 (Continued)

Device		Unique Characteristics
Xtract	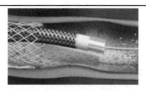	Large single lumen with a free floating guide wire. Circular right-angled tip to allow catheter placement immediately adjacent to lesion. Curved, directional tip with excellent torque response to enable full sweep of the vessel.
5Max reperfusion catheter		5 Fr and 6 Fr compatible. Short tip design. Large aspiration port allows higher rate of aspiration and great volume.
Fetch2		Coiled shaft for kink resistance. Low pitch distal shaft for flexibility with high pitch proximal shaft for pushability. Distal radiopaque band for visability.
Eliminate		Preloaded stylet, fully braided shaft and 6 Fr compatible.

MECHANICAL THROMBECTOMY

Angiojet	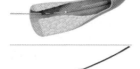	Rheolytic thrombectomy system that uses high-velocity saline jets at the distal catheter tip. The jets creates a negative pressure to collect the thrombus. Only thrombectomy device indicated for native coronary arteries and synthetic grafts.
X-Sizer		The Archimedes screw is designed to grab thrombus on contact – quickly drawing it in, shearing and removing it.
Rinspirator	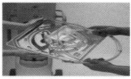	3 lumens; first allows passage of standard guidewire, second allows aspiration, third allows simultaneous saline infusion through exit points proximal to the aspiration lumen, yielding turbulence that may improve the efficiency of thrombus removal. Infusion holes at distal end direct rising spray and central lumen aspirate thrombi.
Rescue	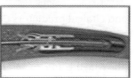	No active thrombus fragmentation, but connected to a vacuum motor unit. 4.5 Fr for monorail polyethylene catheter with a guidewire exit hole 30 cm from the distal tip, compatible with a 0.014-inch or smaller guide wire. Platinum marker band at the distal tip for visibility.
TVAC	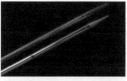	Effective length 1350 mm, radiopaque marker with 250 mm effective coating and 7 Fr compatible. Single lumen catheter with a beak-shaped distal tip. The catheter is attached to an aspiration pump for vacuum and removal of thrombotic material.

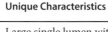
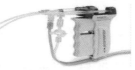
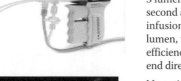

Conclusions

The management of thrombus in STEMI interventions is of paramount importance. To accomplish this complex task successfully, a systematic approach is necessary. Owing to the dynamic nature of thrombus formation, an interventional approach must incorporate a thrombus grading system, which also integrates mechanical adjunct devices. The limitations of equivocal clinical results from multiple trials fail to endorse the true potential of mechanical adjunct devices for STEMI intervention.

The Mehta Strategy successfully tackles this problem. Ultimately, the Mehta Strategy is offered as: a selective thrombus management strategy in STEMI interventions based upon the thrombus grade, with direct stenting recommended for low-grade thrombus, thrombo-aspiration for moderate thrombus, and rheolytic thrombectomy for high-grade thrombus (depending upon suitable anatomy). We propose simple aspiration thrombectomy as the initial therapy, as it is inexpensive, globally available and extremely easy to use. In addition, as the time course of STEMI is mostly unknown (and difficult to predict), selecting aspiration or mechanical thrombectomy on the basis of duration of chest pain is less certain. One may lean on the electrocardiogram for this approximation, using ST-segment elevation as a surrogate for white thrombus and early Q waves with residual ST-segment elevation as a proxy for red thrombus [7]. The vast majority of white thrombus will be aspirated with proper aspiration techniques. In fact, it has become a norm for us to make a reverse conclusion – if the thrombus aspirates, the lesion is often, although not always, white thrombus.

The algorithm has produced a thrombus-graded adjunct device approach to managing thrombus burden, which has produced excellent clinical results, as demonstrated in the SINCERE database.

References

1 Ellis SG, Roubin GS, King SB, 3rd, et al. Angiographic and clinical predictors of acute closure after native vessel coronary angioplasty. *Circulation*, 1988; 77(2): 372–379.
2 Singh M, Berger PB, Ting HH, et al. Influence of coronary thrombus on outcome of percutaneous coronary angioplasty in the current era (the Mayo Clinic experience). *Am J Cardiol*, 2001; 88(10): 1091–1096.
3 Mabin TA, Holmes DR, Jr., Smith HC, et al. Intracoronary thrombus: role in coronary occlusion complicating percutaneous transluminal coronary angioplasty. *J Am Coll Cardiol*, 1985; 5(2 Pt 1): 198–202.
4 White CJ, Ramee SR, Collins TJ, et al. Coronary thrombi increase PTCA risk. Angioscopy as a clinical tool. *Circulation*, 1996; 93(2): 253–258.
5 Tamhane UU, Chetcuti S, Hameed I, et al. Safety and efficacy of thrombectomy in patients undergoing primary percutaneous coronary intervention for acute ST elevation MI: a meta-analysis of randomized controlled trials. *BMC Cardiovasc Disord*, 2010; 10: 10.
6 Mongeon FP, Belisle P, Joseph L, et al. Adjunctive thrombectomy for acute myocardial infarction: A bayesian meta-analysis. *Circ Cardiovasc Interv*, 2010; 3(1): 6–16.
7 Mehta S, Kostela JC, Oliveros E, et al. Compulsive thrombus management in STEMI interventions. *Interv Cardiol Clin*, 2012; 1(4): 485–505.
8 Kumar V AA, Fausto N, Robbins SL, et al. *Robbins and Cotran Pathologic Basis of Disease.* 7th ed. Philadelphia: Elsevier Saunders; 2005.
9 Falk E, Shah PK, Fuster V. Coronary plaque disruption. *Circulation*, 1995; 92(3): 657–671.

10 Furie B, Furie BC. Mechanisms of thrombus formation. *N Engl J Med*, 2008; 359(9): 938–949.

11 Friedman M, Van den Bovenkamp GJ. The pathogenesis of a coronary thrombus. *Am J Pathol*, 1966; 48(1): 19–44.

12 DeWood MA, Spores J, Notske R, et al. Prevalence of total coronary occlusion during the early hours of transmural myocardial infarction. *N Engl J Med*, 1980; 303(16): 897–902.

13 Davies MJ, Thomas A. Thrombosis and acute coronary-artery lesions in sudden cardiac ischemic death. *N Engl J Med*, 1984; 310(18): 1137–1140.

14 Davies MJ, Thomas AC. Plaque fissuring: The cause of acute myocardial infarction, sudden ischaemic death, and crescendo angina. *Br Heart J*, 1985; 53(4): 363–373.

15 Horie T, Sekiguchi M, Hirosawa K. Coronary thrombosis in pathogenesis of acute myocardial infarction. Histopathological study of coronary arteries in 108 necropsied cases using serial section. *Br Heart J*, 1978; 40(2): 153–161.

16 Grines CL, Browne KF, Marco J, et al. A comparison of immediate angioplasty with thrombolytic therapy for acute myocardial infarction. The Primary Angioplasty in Myocardial Infarction Study Group. *N Engl J Med*, 1993; 328(10): 673–679.

17 Sianos G, Papafaklis MI, Daemen J, et al. Angiographic stent thrombosis after routine use of drug-eluting stents in ST-segment elevation myocardial infarction: the importance of thrombus burden. *J Am Coll Cardiol*, 2007; 50(7): 573–583.

18 Mehta S, Alfonso C, Oliveros E, et al. Lesson from the Single INdividual Community Experience REgistry for Primary PCI (SINCERE) Database. In: Kappur R, ed. *Textbook of STEMI Interventions*, 2nd ed. pp. 131–148. Malvern, UK: HMP Communications; 2010.

19 Svilaas T, Vlaar PJ, van der Horst IC, et al. Thrombus aspiration during primary percutaneous coronary intervention. *N Engl J Med*, 2008; 358(6): 557–567.

20 Antoniucci D, Valenti R, Migliorini A, et al. Comparison of rheolytic thrombectomy before direct infarct artery stenting versus direct stenting alone in patients undergoing percutaneous coronary intervention for acute myocardial infarction. *Am J Cardiol*, 2004; 93(8): 1033–1035.

21 Whisenant BK, Baim DS, Kuntz RE, et al. Rheolytic thrombectomy with the Possis AngioJet: technical considerations and initial clinical experience. *J Invasive Cardiol*, 1999; 11(7): 421–426.

22 Margheri M, Falai M, Vittori G, et al. Safety and efficacy of the AngioJet in patients with acute myocardial infarction: results from the Florence Appraisal Study of Rheolytic Thrombectomy (FAST). *J Invas Cardiol*, 2006; 18(10): 481–486.

23 Kuntz RE, Baim DS, Cohen DJ, et al. A trial comparing rheolytic thrombectomy with intracoronary urokinase for coronary and vein graft thrombus (the Vein Graft AngioJet Study, VeGAS 2). *Am J Cardiol*, 2002; 89(3): 326–330.

24 Szerlip M, Grines CL. The current role of AngioJet rheolytic thrombectomy in acute myocardial infarction. *J Invas Cardiol*, 2010; 22(10B): 21B–22B.

25 Stone GW, Abizaid A, Silber S, et al. Prospective, Randomized, Multicenter Evaluation of a Polyethylene Terephthalate Micronet Mesh-Covered Stent (MGuard) in ST-Segment Elevation Myocardial Infarction: The MASTER Trial. *J Am Coll Cardiol*, 2012; 60(19): 1975–1984.

26 Migliorini A, Stabile A, Rodriguez AE, et al. Comparison of AngioJet rheolytic thrombectomy before direct infarct artery stenting with direct stenting alone in patients with acute myocardial infarction. The JETSTENT trial. *J Am Coll Cardiol*, 2010; 56(16): 1298–1306.

27 Fukuda D, Tanaka A, Shimada K, et al. Predicting angiographic distal embolization following percutaneous coronary intervention in patients with acute myocardial infarction. *Am J Cardiol*, 2003; 91(4): 403–407.

28 Tanaka A, Kawarabayashi T, Nishibori Y, et al. No-reflow phenomenon and lesion morphology in patients with acute myocardial infarction. *Circulation*, 2002; 105(18): 2148–2152.

29 Barreto AD, Albright KC, Hallevi H, et al. Thrombus burden is associated with clinical outcome after intra-arterial therapy for acute ischemic stroke. *Stroke*, 2008; 39(12): 3231–3235.

30 De Carlo M, Aquaro GD, Palmieri C, et al. A prospective randomized trial of thrombectomy versus no thrombectomy in patients with ST-segment elevation myocardial infarction and thrombus-rich lesions: MUSTELA (MUltidevice Thrombectomy in Acute ST-Segment ELevation Acute Myocardial Infarction) trial. *JACC Cardiovasc Interv*, 2012; 5(12): 1223–1230.

31 The INFUSE-Anterior Myocardial Infarction (AMI) Study. ClinicalTrials.gov. Available at http://clinicaltrials.gov/ct2/show/NCT00976521 (accessed March 20, 2017).

32 G. Parodi, Valenti R, Migliorini A, et al. Comparison of manual thrombus aspiration with rheolytic thrombectomy in acute myocardial infarction. *Circ Cardiovasc Interv*, 2013; 6: 224–230.

33 Fröbert O, Lagerqvist B, Olivecrona GK, et al. Thrombus aspiration during ST-segment elevation myocardial infarction. *N Engl J Med*, 2013; 369(17): 1587–1597.

34 Jolly S. TOTAL trial: A Trial of Routine Aspiration Thrombectomy With Percutaneous Coronary Intervention (PCI) Versus PCI Alone in Patients With ST-Segment Elevation Myocardial Infarction (STEMI) Undergoing Primary PCI. ClinicalTrials.gov. Available at http://www.clinicaltrials.gov/ct2/show/NCT01149044 (accessed March 20, 2017).

35 Valente S, Lazzeri C, Mattesini A, et al. Thrombus aspiration in elderly STEMI patients: A single center experience. *Int J Cardiol*, 2013; 168(3): 3097–3099.

36 Steg PG, Bonnefoy E, Chabaud S, et al. Impact of time to treatment on mortality after prehospital fibrinolysis or primary angioplasty: data from the CAPTIM randomized clinical trial. *Circulation*, 2003; 108(23): 2851–2856.

37 Rezkalla SH, Kloner RA. No-reflow phenomenon. *Circulation*, 2002; 105(5): 656–662.

38 Okamura A, Ito H, Iwakura K, et al. Detection of embolic particles with the Doppler guide wire during coronary intervention in patients with acute myocardial infarction: efficacy of distal protection device. *J Am Coll Cardiol*, 2005; 45(2): 212–215.

39 Jolly S, Cairns J, Yusuf S, et al. Randomized trial of primary PCI with or without routine manual thrombectomy. *N Engl J Med*, 2015; 372:1389–1398.

8

Transradial Techniques to Improve STEMI Outcomes

Tejas Patel MD DM FACC FESC FSCAI, Sanjay Shah MD DM,
Samir Pancholy MD FACC FSCAI

Introduction and Historical Perspective

In 1989, Lucien Campeau described the first use of the radial route for coronary angiograms [1]. Subsequently, in 1993, Kiemeneij described the use of this route for percutaneous coronary intervention (PCI) using 6 Fr guide catheters, at a time when most interventional procedures were performed with larger 8 Fr guide catheters [2]. Since then, the transradial approach for PCI has evolved as an alternative to the transfemoral approach for most subsets of PCI, including multivessel lesions, left main coronary artery (LMCA) lesions, bifurcation lesions, chronic total occlusions, calcified lesions and acute coronary syndrome (ACS) [3–9]. Ochiai published the first observational pilot study of the transradial approach for acute myocardial infarction (AMI) interventions [10]. Since then, several randomized studies have been published comparing the transradial approach for AMI interventions with the transfemoral approach [4,10–19].

The Transradial Approach and STEMI Interventions

What is the Body of Evidence?

Keeley et al., in their quantitative review of 23 randomized trials, demonstrated that earlier treatment of STEMI with primary PCI (PPCI) improved outcomes compared with thrombolysis [11]. Ochiai et al. were the first to perform an observational pilot study to determine whether risk-stratified AMI patients could experience reduced bleeding complications and earlier mobilization with transradial coronary intervention and primary stenting [10]. Fifty-six patients with Killip class I or II had a transradial approach for AMI interventions, with 100% success in stent deployment and 97% success in normalization of distal coronary blood flow. No major vascular complications occurred in this experience. Philippe et al. also published similar results in their series of 119 consecutive patients with AMI having PPCI via the radial (64 patients) or femoral (55 patients) approach with adjunctive abciximab therapy [12]. The length of hospital stay was longer in the transfemoral group (5.9 days) compared with the transradial group (4.5 days; $P = 0.05$). There were no vascular complications in the transradial group, compared with three (5.5%) in the transfemoral group ($P = 0.04$), although longer radiation exposure times were observed in the transradial cohort.

Cruden and associates published observations of rescue PCI in 287 patients with unsuccessful thrombolysis for AMI [13]. In this retrospective analysis, procedural success was similar for

Manual of STEMI Interventions, First Edition. Edited by Sameer Mehta.
© 2017 John Wiley & Sons Ltd. Published 2017 by John Wiley & Sons Ltd.

transradial and transfemoral interventions (98% vs. 93%, $P = 0.3$). However, the rate of vascular complications (0% vs. 13%, $P < 0.01$) and length of stay (7.0 vs. 7.9 days, $P < 0.005$) favored the transradial over the transfemoral approach.

Cantor et al. in the RADIAL-AMI pilot study, randomized 50 patients having primary or rescue PCI to the transradial or transfemoral approach [14]. No major bleeding occurred and no transfusions were required in either group. Procedural time slightly favored the transfemoral over the transradial group. Final thrombolysis in myocardial infarction flow, contrast and fluoroscopy time were similar for both transradial and transfemoral interventions.

Saito et al., in the TEMPURA clinical study, randomized 149 patients with AMI less than 12 hours from onset to a transradial ($n = 77$) or transfemoral ($n = 72$) intervention [15]. Procedural success (radial 96.1% vs. femoral 97.1%, $P = $ NS) and adverse cardiac events (transradial 5.2% vs. transfemoral 8.3%, $P = $ NS) were similar in each group. Severe bleeding was seen in 3% of patients who underwent a transfemoral intervention and none who in the transradial group. Procedural time was slightly shorter with the transradial approach as compared with the transfemoral approach in this series.

Yan et al. compared the transradial with the transfemoral approach in elderly (aged over 65 years) Chinese patients undergoing AMI interventions [16]. There was no significant statistical difference between the two groups for success rate, puncture time, cannulation time, reperfusion time, and total procedural time. However, hospital stay was longer with the transfemoral approach (10.1 + 4.6 days) than with the transradial (7.2 + 2.6 days; $P < 0.01$), and vascular access site-related complications were higher in the transfemoral group (13.1% vs. 1.8%, $P < 0.05$).

De Carlo et al. published results of a prospective registry enrolling patients presenting with an ACS, either STEMI or high-risk non-ST-elevation ACS treated with either abciximab or tirofiban in addition to standard medical therapy, who underwent urgent or emergency PCI through the transradial route in a 2-year span [17]. All possible high-risk subsets, including patients above 80 years, patients undergoing rescue PCI after failed thrombolysis, and patients with cardiogenic shock were enrolled. The results of this study demonstrated that the transradial approach allows for near-abolition of vascular access bleeding and blood transfusions with no negative impact on procedural success rate, procedural duration, or 1-year clinical outcome.

Pancholy et al. compared door-to-balloon times for PPCI for the transradial and transfemoral approaches [18]; 313 consecutive patients with STEMI undergoing PPCI were divided in two groups: group 1 ($n = 204$) underwent PCI via the transfemoral route and group 2 ($n = 109$) via the transradial route. Door-to-balloon time was 72 ± 14 minutes for group 1 compared with 70 ± 17 minutes for group 2, although the difference was not statistically significant (P 0.27). Group 2 patients had significantly fewer access-site complications compared with group 1 ($P < 0.05$). Demographics, pre-discharge adverse events, and major adverse cardiac events at 1 year follow-up were comparable between the two groups.

Weaver et al. compared the transradial and transfemoral approaches for time to intervention for patients presenting with AMI [19]. Of the 240 patients in the study, 205 underwent successful PCI (124 in the transradial group, 116 in the transfemoral group). No significant difference was observed in pre-cardiac catheter laboratory times. Mean case start times were significantly longer in the transradial group (12.5 + 5.4 minutes) compared with the transfemoral group (10.5 + 5.7 minutes; $P = 0.005$) as patient preparation took more time. Once arterial access was obtained, balloon inflation occurred faster in the transradial group, (18.3 vs. 24.1 minutes, $P < 0.001$). Total time from patient arrival to catheter laboratory to PCI was reduced in the transradial group as compared with the transfemoral group (28.4 vs. 32.7 minutes, $P = 0.01$). There was a small, but statistically significant, difference in door-to-balloon time (76.4 minutes for transradial vs. 86.5 minutes for transfemoral, $P < 0.008$). The transradial group also had shorter fluoroscopy times as compared with the transfemoral group (12.5 + 7.9 minutes vs. 15.2 + 10.1 minutes, $P = 0.02$).

Siudak et al. gathered and analyzed consecutive data on 1650 STEMI patients transferred for PPCI in-hospital STEMI networks between November 2005 and January 2007 from seven countries in Europe (EUROTRANSFER registry) [20]. Abciximab was administered in 1086 patients (66%); 169 patients were assigned to the transradial approach and 917 to the trans-femoral route. Puncture site hematomas were more frequent in transradial group (1.2 vs. 9.4% $P < 0.001$). Major bleeding requiring blood transfusion occurred similarly in both the groups.

Vin et al. examined the feasibility of routinely using the transradial approach in PPCI for STEMI in 2209 procedures done between January 2001 and December 2008 in a single high-volume center [21]. In 84 patients (3.8%), access-site crossover was needed. Crossover rates decreased from 5.9% in 2001–02 to 1.5% in 2007–08 ($P = 0.001$). The procedural success rate was 94.1%, which remained stable over the years. Despite an increased complexity of PPCI, total procedural duration decreased from 38 minutes (interquartile range, IQR, 28–50) in 2001–02 to 24 minutes (IQR 18–33) in 2007–08 ($P < 0.001$). The study demonstrated that systematic use of the transradial route in PPCI yields low access-site crossover, high procedural success rates and excellent procedural performances. Hence, the transradial approach can represent the primary access site in the vast majority of STEMI patients.

The HORIZONS-AMI study investigators analyzed the outcomes for 3345 patients who underwent PPCI for STEMI [22]. They compared the transradial group ($n = 200$) and the trans-femoral group ($n = 3145$) with respect to endpoints including the 30-day, 1-year and 3-year rates of major adverse cardiovascular events (death, reinfarction, stroke, or target-vessel revas-cularization) and mortality. At 3-year follow-up, patients with in-hospital major bleeding had higher mortality (24.6% vs. 5.4%, $P < 0.0001$) and major adverse cardiovascular events (40.3% vs. 20%, $P < 0.0001$). The deleterious effect of major bleeding was observed within 1 month, between 1 month and 1 year, and between 1 and 3 years. A major bleed in hospital was an independent predictor of mortality (hazard ratio 2.80, 95% confidence interval, CI, 1.89 to 4.16, $P < 0.0001$) at 3-year follow-up. The study concluded that patients with a major bleed after PPCI have significantly increased morbidity and mortality rates up to 3 years.

The RIVAL study investigators enrolled 7021 patients with acute coronary syndrome from 158 hospitals in 32 countries; 3507 patients were randomly assigned to a transradial group and 3514 to a transfemoral group [23]. The study concluded that both approaches are safe and effective for PCI. The local vascular complication rate was significantly lower in the transradial group ($n = 42$) than the transfemoral group ($n = 106$; $P < 0.001$). Investigators also observed a statistically significant (40%) relative reduction in the risk of death, myocardial infarction, stroke or non-coronary artery bypass grafting-related major bleeding and a significant (61%) relative reduction in the risk of death among STEMI patients treated via radial route. They also reported a significant reduction in the risk of the primary outcome (51%) among PCI centers that performed the highest volume of radial procedures.

The RIFLE STEACS study was a prospective randomized parallel group multicenter trial to evaluate transradial versus transfemoral routes for PPCI [24]; 1001 patients were randomized between these two groups. The primary endpoint of 30-day net adverse cardiac events occurred in 68 patients (13.6%) in the radial arm and 105 patients (21.0%) in the femoral arm ($P = 0.003$). In particular, compared with the femoral route, radial access was associated with significantly lower rates of cardiac mortality (5.2% vs. 9.2%, $P = 0.02$), bleeding (7.8% vs. 12.5%, $P = 0.026$), and shorter hospital stay (5 days first to third quartile; range 4–7 days vs. 6 days; range 5–8 days; $P = 0.03$). The study concluded that the transradial route in patients with STEMI was associated with significant clinical benefits in terms of both lower morbidity and cardiac mortality.

Bernat et al., in the STEMI-RADIAL trial, compared the transradial and transfemoral approaches in patients undergoing PPCI by high-volume operators experienced in both access sites [51]. The primary endpoint (cumulative incidence of major bleeding and vascular access-site complications at 30 days) occurred in 1.4% of the radial group (n = 348) and 7.2% of the femoral group (n = 359; P = 0.0001). The net rate of adverse cardiac events was 4.6% in the radial group and 11.0% in the femoral group (P = 0.0028). Crossover from the radial to the femoral approach was 3.7%. Intensive care stay (2.5 + 1.7 days vs. 3.0 + 2.9 days, P = 0.0038), and contrast utilization (170 + 71 ml vs. 182 + 60 ml, P = 0.01) were significantly reduced in the radial group. Mortality was 2.3% in the radial group and 3.1% in the femoral group (P = 0.64) at 30 days, and 2.3% in the radial group compared with 3.6% in the femoral group (P = 0.31) at 6 months. The study concluded that in patients with STEMI undergoing PPCI by operators experienced in both access sites, the radial was associated with a significantly lower incidence of major bleeding, access sites complications and gave a superior net clinical benefit.

The literature clearly reflects that the transradial approach for AMI is safe, effective, reproducible and has fewer vascular access-related complications than the transfemoral route, particularly in the hands of experienced operators and support staff.

Rationale for Using the Transradial Route for STEMI Interventions

Sound reasons are necessary for a surgeon to learn and switch from a well-established time-tested technique to a different technique. It took almost two decades for the transradial approach to gain universal acceptance. The approach has proven its superiority over the trans-femoral route in different issues, including a reduction in local vascular complication rates (minor and major), increase in the comfort levels of patients and support staff, and a reduction in hospital management costs [29,30,32,33,47]. These benefits have been achieved in regular interventions, as well as in difficult and demanding subsets such as complex and calcified lesions, LMCA lesions, and bifurcation lesions [3–9].

An Important Bleeding Avoidance Strategy for Primary PCI

Studies have consistently shown that bleeding events associated with PCI are independent predictors of major adverse cardiac events and death [26–31]. The National Heart, Lung, and Blood Institute Dynamic Registry evaluated the relationship between access-site hematomas requiring blood transfusions and in-hospital and 1-year mortality [25]. This study included data on 6656 patients and captured 120 hematomas requiring transfusion, with an incidence of 1.8%; 97% of patients with hematomas had femoral artery access. In-hospital mortality was about nine times higher in those with hematomas requiring blood transfusions than in those without hematomas (9.9% vs. 1.2%). Similarly, at 1 year, mortality among those who developed hematoma requiring transfusion was approximately 4.5 times higher than those who did not require transfusion (18.8% vs. 9.9%).

The ACUITY trial analyzed the impact of major bleeding on mortality and clinical outcomes 30 days after surgery. Those patients with major bleeding had a higher 30-day mortality (7.3% vs. 1.2%, P < 0.0001) than patients without major bleeding [26]. In addition, at 30 days, those with major bleeding had higher rates of composite ischemia, defined as death, myocardial infarction, or unplanned revascularization for ischemia (23.1% vs. 6.8%, P < 0.0001), as well as stent thrombosis (3.4% vs. 0.6%, P < 0.0001).

The MORTAL study reported on reductions in mortality, likely mediated through reduced transfusions after PCI performed transradially or transfemorally [27]. The study evaluated 38,872 PCI procedures in 32,822 patients in British Columbia, Canada. The transfemoral approach was used in 79.5% and the transradial approach in 20.5% of PCI. In the femoral group, 2.8% of procedures were complicated by the need for periprocedural transfusions, while only 1.4% of the procedures were associated with a transfusion in the radial group. Thus, the transfusion rate was 50% lower in the radial group. The reduced transfusion rate was associated with a significant reduction in mortality at 30 days and 1 year. The death rates at 30 days of the transfused group versus the non-transfused group were 12.6% and 1.3%, respectively. At 1 year, the death rates were 22.9% and 3.2%, respectively.

Rao et al. retrospectively analyzed data from 5,93,094 procedures in the National Cardiovascular Data Registry (606 sites, 2004–2007) [28]. They evaluated trends in use and outcomes of the transradial approach to PCI. Transradial intervention was associated with procedural success rates similar to the femoral approach and with significantly lower rates of bleeding and vascular complications, even among high-risk groups such as elderly patients, women and patients with ACS.

A meta-analysis comparing radial and femoral approaches for PCI identified 12 studies that meet the criteria for inclusion [29]. The primary outcomes evaluated were major adverse cardiac events, access-site complications, including bleeding, and procedural success. The major adverse cardiac event rate in was not significantly different between the groups, at 2.4% and 2.1%, respectively. However, there were significantly fewer access-site complications in the radial group (0.3%) compared with the femoral group (2.8%).

Jolly and colleagues evaluated 23 randomized trials comparing both approaches and analyzed their impact on major bleeding and ischemic events [30]. There was a 73% reduction in major bleeding in the radial group (0.05% vs. 2.3%). Also noted was a non-statistically significant reduction in the rates of death, myocardial infarction, and stroke.

Eikelboom et al. evaluated the impact of bleeding on prognosis in 34,146 patients with ACS by combining patient data from the OASIS Registry, the OASIS-2 trial and the CURE trial [31]; 667 (2%) patients developed major bleeding. Those with major bleeding were five times more likely to die within the first 30 days (12.8% vs. 2.5%; $P < 0.0001$) and 1.5 times more likely to die between 30 days and 6 months (4.6% vs. 2.9%; $P < 0.002$).

Kwok et al. published a meta-analysis in 2015 which defined the prevalence and prognostic impact of blood transfusions in contemporary PCI practice [39]. Nineteen studies that included 2,258,711 patients with more than 54,000 transfusion events were identified (prevalence of blood transfusion 2.3%). Crude mortality rate was 6,435 of 50,979 (12.6%, eight studies) in patients who received a blood transfusion and 27,061 of 2,266,111 (1.2%, eight studies) in the remaining patients. Crude major adverse cardiac events rates were 17.4% (8,439 of 48,518) in patients who had a blood transfusion and 3.1% (68,062 of 2,212,730) in the remaining cohort. Meta-analysis demonstrated that blood transfusion was independently associated with an increase in mortality (odds ratio, OR, 3.02, 95% CI 2.16 to 4.21, $I^2 = 91\%$) and major adverse cardiac events (OR 3.15, 95% CI 2.59 to 3.82, $I^2 = 81\%$). Similar observations were recorded in studies that adjusted for baseline hematocrit, anemia, and bleeding. The study concluded that blood transfusion is independently associated with increased risk of mortality and major adverse cardiac events. Clinicians should minimize the risk for periprocedural transfusion by using available bleeding avoidance strategies and limiting liberal transfusion practices.

In summary, in-hospital major bleeding after PCI remains a significant complication which constitutes an adverse impact on short- and long-term outcomes. It is also noteworthy that patients with AMI are at the highest risk for bleeding for multiple reasons, but particularly related to their anticoagulation, antiplatelet, thrombolytic status, and the emergent nature of their procedures. Bleeding complications in this patient subset are more likely to be associated with repeated ischemia as well as short- and long-term adverse cardiac events, including mortality. If bleeding complications are associated with an increased risk for mortality (regardless of the mechanisms involved), then reduced bleeding risk should be associated with reduced mortality. Specifically, since the rate of bleeding is higher among STEMI patients undergoing

PPCI, and because the proportion of access-site bleeding is relatively higher in this population compared with the other subsets of PCI, the transradial route should lead to significantly lower rates of bleeding when compared with the transfemoral approach among patients undergoing PPCI. Thus, avoidance of major bleeding becomes a clinical priority in contemporary PPCI practice.

Economic Benefits and Quality of Life

Early ambulation provides a potential cost reduction through expedited room turnover, increased throughput (both through the catheter laboratory and the same-day or recovery unit), decreased intensity of care required by nursing and support staff, shorter length of stay, enhanced ability to perform same-day PCI, and a more rapid return to productivity for working patients [47].

AMI intervention is prone to higher bleeding and access site-related complications, particularly through the femoral route [27–30]. Large groin hematomas and retroperitoneal hematomas may necessitate several additional investigations (femoral vascular ultrasound, computed tomography of the abdomen/pelvis, laboratory investigations), blood transfusions and longer hospital stay [47]. This additional cost of treating the complications and prolonged hospital stay can be minimized or eliminated using the radial route for AMI interventions.

Cooper et al. studied and compared quality of life parameters of patients undergoing transfemoral and transradial interventions [32]. Among patients who have had both approaches, 80% had strong preference for the radial approach, 18% were undecided and only 2% had strong preference for the femoral route. Preference for the radial approach was related to more favorable rankings of back and body pain, social functioning, mental health, the ability to use the bathroom and to ambulate.

Amoroso et al. quantified the workload for both catheter laboratory and recovery area nurses following 260 consecutive radial ($n = 208$) and femoral ($n = 52$) procedures. The workload was significantly reduced for radial procedures (86 minutes) compared with femoral (174 minutes, $P < 0.001$) and for recovery time (radial, 386 minutes vs. femoral, 720 minutes) [33]. The workload and time savings were related to less time spent on sheath removal, early patient mobility, shorter recovery time, and shorter time to ambulation. The benefits of the radial approach should be profound in the complex and more demanding situations of AMI interventions.

Early ambulation and a secure access site may allow for an earlier return to productivity. It is also rational to expect that those patients experiencing access-site complications, significantly more frequent with the femoral route, would be delayed in returning to work by an extended recovery. Although early ambulation is possible with use of femoral vascular closure devices, there is no reduction in bleeding or vascular complication rates, and these devices involve approximately five times the closure cost of a radial hemostasis device [32,33]. Thus, improved quality of life for the patients, relatively shorter and more relaxed periprocedural care for the nursing and support staff, and significant cost savings for the hospital management are good reasons to use the transradial approach for AMI interventions.

Developing a Transradial Acute Myocardial Infarction Program

Currently, no formalized guidelines exist regarding development of transradial AMI (TR-AMI) program. However, it is reasonable to assume that this should be an important off-shoot of a standard elective transradial program. Based on the available literature combined with our own long experience in this area, we set out the following recommendations for the establishment of a new TR-AMI program.

Recommendation 1

The operator and support staff should have experience of managing well-selected, stable, and non-complex lesions in the elective setting to develop skill and experience with this approach. This elective experience should be gradually expanded to more complex areas, including bifurcations, LMCA lesions, calcified and/or tortuous segments, radial loops and subclavian loops. This will allow the operator to become more accustomed to the technique modification and device choices that are suited for these situations in a more controlled environment before encountering these circumstances in patients who are less stable and when time to perfusion is critical. Although it is not a routine practice in regular cases, we strongly recommend injecting contrast through the puncture cannula to define the vascular anatomy before introducing the sheath. If anatomy is unfavorable or very difficult, immediate switch-over to femoral access will save crucial time. With increasing experience of the operator, the number of crossovers will decrease remarkably. Figure 8.1a shows an example of a complex radiobrachial loop. Experienced operators should be able to work through this loop without wasting time Figure 8.1b,c. Although they are uncommon, beginners should switch to a contralateral radial or femoral approach. Figure 8.2 shows an example of working through the arteria lusoria to address left circumflex artery stenosis in an acute inferoposterior wall myocardial infarction. Figure 8.3a,b shows an example of balloon-assisted tracking of a catheter through a difficult radial anatomy. Figure 8.4a,b,c,d shows an example of a modified sheathless technique for atraumatic tracking of a 7 Fr guide catheter through the right atrium for addressing LMCA bifurcation lesions in acute anterior wall myocardial infarction.

(a) (b) (c)

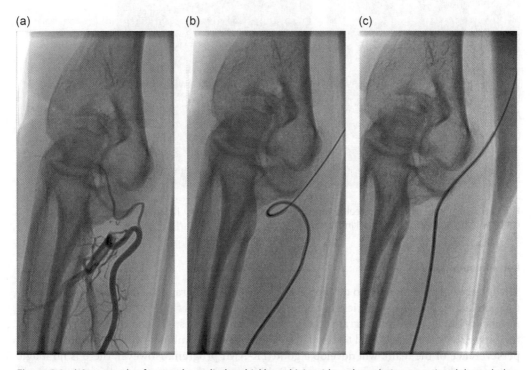

Figure 8.1 a) An example of a complex radio-brachial loop. b) A guide catheter being negotiated through the loop. c) The catheter is traversing beyond the loop.

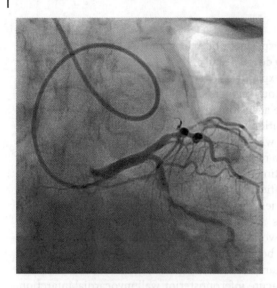

Figure 8.2 An example of left circumflex artery stenting in acute myocardial infarction through the arteria lusoria.

(a) (b)

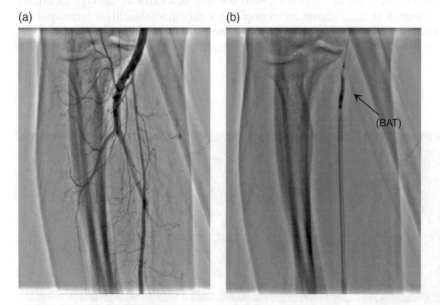

(BAT)

Figure 8.3 a) Contrast injection revealed very small caliber of radial artery. b) Smooth passage of a 6 Fr guide catheter using balloon-assisted tracking (arrow).

Recommendation 2

The number of cases needed to develop a stable TR-AMI program will depend on various factors, including operator experience, operator skills, number of operators in a group, overall number of procedures in a program, and number of supportive staff (including catheter laboratory, intensive care nurses, and technicians). These factors, combined with determination and perseverance of the team, will develop a good TR-AMI program. However, there is no magic number at which one suddenly becomes a TR-AMI expert; the more you do, the better you will get [34]. We recommend performing at least 250 coronary angiograms and 75 transradial PCI

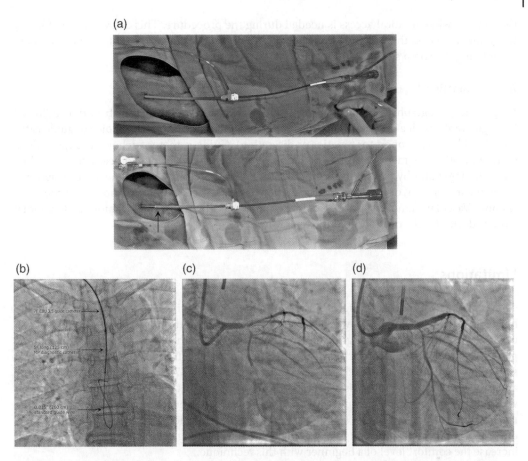

Figure 8.4 a) In vitro demonstration of modified sheathless technique (arrow). b) A 7 Fr extra backup (EBU) guide catheter is tracked over a long (125-cm) 5 Fr multipurpose (MP) diagnostic catheter and a standard 0.035-inch (260-cm) guide wire (arrow). c) Left main coronary artery bifurcation lesion is profiled. d) Optimal end result is obtained.

in stable cases before entering into a TR-AMI program. These numbers will enable an operator to handle an adequate number of anatomical variations in the radiobrachial and subclavian regions and will increase operator comfort levels while performing AMI interventions [35–38]. It is important to select at least 25 hemodynamically stable AMI cases in the initial stage of a TR-AMI program, to overcome the learning curve with no delay in reperfusion.

Recommendation 3

Catheter laboratory preparation and patient set-up are important for a TR-AMI program. The arm board for site access should be placed close to the femoral position, to mimic the transfemoral approach [39]. Many operators shift a standard femoral window drape so that the right femoral window is over the right radial artery (for right radial approach) and the left femoral window is overlying the right femoral artery (for femoral crossover or intra-aortic balloon pump (IABP)/hemodynamic support device placement). This method works well for patients who are not obese. An alternative method is to use towel drapes for the desired radial access site and standard femoral window drapes for the legs. Although the preparation time is slightly prolonged to prepare provisional femoral access, it is typically justified to minimize this activity when femoral access is needed during the procedure. This delay may be offset by the ability to access the radial without needing fluoroscopic guidance (that is, while staff are completing the room set up) [40].

Recommendation 4

Diagnostic angiography should be performed in the non-infarct vascular distribution, followed by angiography with a guide catheter for infarct-related distribution (the choice of guide catheter should be as per operator practice or discretion). Guide-catheter anchoring support, deep seating or other augmentation may be employed as needed. A 5 Fr guide catheter should be used sparingly and by an experienced operator. Thrombectomy, percutaneous transluminal coronary angioplasty, or direct stenting can then be performed, and PCI completed in the usual fashion. Vascular hemostasis can be achieved in a typically transradial fashion using a radial closure device (at the discretion of the operator).

Limitations

The transradial approach for STEMI interventions, despite having certain definite advantages, has been adopted relatively slowly because of certain procedure-related issues. The learning curve for a new procedure is slightly more difficult because of the unstable cardiac status of the patient and the mental pressure on the operator for early reperfusion. However, after achieving some experience in this approach, these issues are minimized [37,40]. Prolonged puncture time and procedural time are other issues [14–19], although Saito et al. [15] and Weaver et al. [19] showed shorter timings. The puncture and procedural times become shorter with increasing experience. Selecting relatively stable AMI cases for intervention and defining vascular anatomy by injecting contrast through a cannula before introducing the sheath in initial cases, will increase the comfort level of a beginner with this technique.

Comfortable use of bulky devices, including a thrombectomy device, distal protection device, or kissing balloons is possible with the transradial approach because most devices are 6 Fr guide catheter-compatible and most radials can accommodate 7 Fr guide catheters. There is an argument against using the radial route in AMI intervention when IABP support is required. However, puncturing one groin for IABP insertion and PCI through the radial approach for AMI intervention will spare the other groin. So, logically, groin-related vascular complications should be reduced by half.

Certain studies have shown increased radiation exposure and fluoroscopy time with the radial compared with femoral approach [12,41,42,48,49]. This is believed to be because of the relatively longer procedural time and the proximity of the operator to the x-ray tube during the procedure [34]. Keeping the arm board for the access site parallel and close to the femoral position, rather than perpendicular, should resolve this issue to a great extent. Increasing experience, smart application of procedure-related techniques and miniaturization of hardware should help an operator overcoming the perceived limitations.

Conclusions

A growing body of evidence now supports the use of the transradial approach as the preferred access site for STEMI interventions. Historically, this route has been avoided in the STEMI population, because of concerns over the longer procedural time, longer door-to-device time, higher crossover rates, increased radiation exposure and greater experience level required compared with the femoral route [48,49]. However, in recent years, recognition of the impact of periprocedural bleeding on mortality in patients with acute coronary syndromes has garnered great interest in the utility of the radial approach as an established method to reduce bleeding [25–31]. Registry data, meta-analyses and randomized control trials all similarly demonstrate that the radial route is associated with reduced periprocedural bleeding and lower mortality compared with the femoral route in the STEMI population [41–46]. Additional benefits include enhanced patient comfort, reduced hospital stay and reduced cost [33,47].

The 2012 European Society of Cardiology guidelines state that, "if performed by an experienced operator, radial access should be preferred over femoral access for PPCI". A class IIa indication with a level of evidence of B has been assigned. This is the first time that a guideline has specifically specified the transradial approach for PPCI.

References

1 Campeau L. Percutaneous radial artery approach for coronary angiography. *Cathet Cardiovasc Diagn*, 1989; 16 (1): 3–7.

2 Kiemeneij F, Laarman GJ. Percutaneous transradial artery approach for coronary stent implantation. *Cathet Cardiovasc Diagn*, 1993; 30 (2): 173–178.

3 Cheng CI, Wu CJ, Fang CY, et al. Feasibility and safety of transradial stenting for unprotected left main coronary artery stenosis. *Circ J*, 2007; 71: 855–861.

4 Ranjan A, Patel TM, Shah SC, et al. Transradial primary angioplasty and stenting in Indian patients with acute myocardial infarction: Acute results and 6-month follow-up. *Indian Heart J*, 2005; 57: 681–687.

5 Yip HK, Chung SY, Chai HT, et al. Safety and efficacy of transradial vs transfemoral arterial primary coronary angioplasty for acute myocardial infarction: Single-Center Experience. *Circ J*, 2009; 73: 2050–2055.

6 Rathore S, Hakeem A, Pauriah M, et al. A comparison of the transradial and the transfemoral approach in chronic total occlusion percutaneous coronary intervention. *Catheter Cardiovasc Interv*, 2009; 73: 883–887.

7 Yang YJ, Xu B, Chen JL, et al. Comparison of immediate and follow-up results between transradial and transfemoral approach for percutaneous coronary intervention in true bifurcational lesions. *Chin Med J (Engl)*, 2007; 120: 539–544.

8 Ziakas A, Klinke P, Mildenberger R, et al. A comparison of the radial and the femoral approach in vein graft PCI. A retrospective study. *Int J Cardiovasc Intervent*, 2005; 7: 93–96.

9 Ziakas A, Klinke P, Mildenberger R, et al. Comparison of the radial and femoral approaches in left main PCI: A retrospective study. *J Invasive Cardiol*, 2004; 16: 129–132.

10 Ochiai M, Isshiki T, Toyoizumi H, et al. Efficacy of transradial primary stenting in patients with acute myocardial infarction. *Am J Cardiol*, 1999; 83: 966–968.

11 Kelley EC, Boura JA, Grines CL. Primary angioplasty versus intravenous thrombolytic therapy for acute myocardial infarction: A quantitative review of 23 randomised trials. *Lancet*, 2003; 361: 13–20.

12 Philippe F, Larrazer F, Meziane T, et al. Comparison of transradial vs transfemoral approach in the treatment of acute myocardial infarction with primary angioplasty and abciximab. *Catheter Cardiovasc Interv*, 2004; 61: 67–73.

13 Cruden NL, The CH, Starkey IR, et al. Reduced vascular complications and length of stay with transradial rescue angioplasty for acute myocardial infarction. *Catheter Cardiovasc Interv*, 2007; 70: 670–675.

14 Cantor WJ, Puley G, Natarajan MK, et al. Radial versus femoral access for emergent percutaneous coronary intervention with adjunct glycoprotein IIb/IIIa inhibition in acute myocardial infarction – the RADIAL-AMI pilot randomized trial. *Am Heart J*, 2005; 1560: 543–549.

15 Saito S, Tanaka S, Hiroe Y, et al. Comparative study on transradial approach vs. transfemoral approach in primary stent implantation for patients with acute myocardial infarction: Results of the test for myocardial infarction by prospective unicenter randomization for access sites (TEMPURA) trial. *Caheter Cardiovasc Interv*, 2003; 59: 26–33.

16 Yan Z, Zhou Y, Zhao Y, et al. Safety and feasibility of transradial approach for primary percutaneous coronary intervention in elderly patients with acute myocardial infarction. *Chin Med J*, 2008; 121 (19): 782–786.

17 De Carlo M, Borelli G, Gistri R, et al. Effectiveness of the transradial approach to reduce bleedings in patients undergoing urgent coronary angioplasty with GP IIb/IIIa inhibitors for acute coronary syndromes. *Catheter Cardiovasc Interv*, 2009; 74: 408–415.

18 Pancholy S, Patel T, Sanghvi K et al. Comparison of door-to-balloon times for primary PCI using transradial versus transfemoral approach. *Catheter Cardiovasc Interv*, 2010; 75(7): 991–5.

19 Weaver AN, Henderson RA, Gilchrist IC, et al. Arterial access and door-to-balloon times for primary percutaneous coronary intervention in patients presenting with acute ST-elevation myocardial infarction. *Catheter Cardiovasc Interv*, 2010; 75: 695–699.

20 Siudak Z, Zawislak B, Dziewierz A, et al. Transradial approach in patients with ST-elevation myocardial infarction treated with abciximab results in fewer bleeding complications: data from EUROTRANSFER registry. *Coron Artery Dis*, 2010; 21(5): 292–297.

21 Vin MA, Amoroso G, Dirksen MT, et al. Routine use of the transradial approach in primary percutaneous coronary intervention: procedural aspects and outcomes in 2209 patients treated in a single high-volume centre. *Heart*, 2011; 97(23): 1938–1942.

22 Suh JW, Mehran R, Stone GW, et al. Impact of In-Hospital Major Bleeding on Late Clinical Outcomes After Primary Percutaneous Coronary Intervention in Acute Myocardial Infarction: the HORIZONS-AMI trial. *J Am Coll Cardiol*, 2011; 17: 1750–1756.

23 Jolly SS, Yusuf S, Cairns J, et al. Radial versus femoral access for coronary angiography and intervention in patients with acute coronary syndromes (RIVAL): a randomized, parallel group, multicentre trial. *Lancet*, 2011; 377: 1409–1420.

24 Romagnoli E, Biondi-Zoccai G, Sciahbasi A, et al. Radial versus femoral randomized investigation in ST elevation acute coronary syndrome: the RIFLE STEACS study. *J Am Coll Cardiol*, 2012; 60(24): 2481–2489.

25 Yatskar L, Selzer F, Feit F, et al. Access site hematoma requiring blood transfusion predicts mortality in patients undergoing percutaneous coronary intervention: Data from the National Heart, Lung and Blood Institute Dynamic Registry. *Catheter Cardiovasc Interv*, 2007; 69: 961–966.

26 Manoukian, SV, Feit F, Mehran R, et al. Impact of major bleeding on 30-day mortality and clinical outcomes in patients with acute coronary syndromes, an analysis from the ACUITY Trial. *J Am Coll Cardiol*, 2007; 49: 1362–1368.

27 Chase AJ, Fretz EB, Warbutton WP, et al. Association of the arterial access site at angioplasty with transfusion and mortality, the M.O.R.T.A.L. study (Mortality benefit Of Reduced Transfusion after percutaneous coronary intervention via the Arm or Leg). *Heart*, 2008; 94: 1019–1025.

28 Rao SV, Ou FS, Wang TY, et al. Trends in the prevalence and outcomes of radial and femoral approaches to percutaneous coronary intervention: A report from the National Cardiovascular Data Registry. *JACC Cardiovasc Interv*, 2008; 1: 379–386.

29 Agostoni P, Biondi-Zoccai GG, de Benedictis ML, et al. Radial versus femoral approach for percutaneous coronary diagnostic and interventional procedures; systematic overview and meta-analysis of randomized trials. *J Am Coll Cardiol*, 2004; 44: 349–356.

30 Jolly SS, Amlani S, Hamon M, et al. Radial versus femoral access for coronary angiography or intervention and the impact on major bleeding and ischemic events: a systematic review and meta-analysis of randomized trials. *Am Heart J*, 2009; 157 (1): 132–140.

31 Eikelboom JW, Mehta SR, Anand SS, et al. Adverse impact of bleeding on prognosis in patients with acute coronary syndromes. *Circulation*, 2006; 114: 774–782.

32 Cooper CJ, El-Shiekh RA, Cohen DJ, et al. Effect of transradial access on quality-of-life and cost of cardiac catheterization: A randomized comparison. *Am Heart J*, 1999; 138 (3 Pt 1): 430–436.

33 Amoroso G, Sarti M, Bellucci R, et al. Clinical and procedural predictors of nurse workload during and after invasive coronary procedures: The potential benefit of a systematic radial access. *Eur Cardiovasc Nurs*, 2005; 4: 234–241.

34 Trammel J. Launching a successful transradial program. *J Inv Cardiol*, 2009; 21(Suppl A): 3A–8A.

35 Patel T, Shah S, Pancholy S. *Patel's Atlas of Transradial Intervention: The Basics and Beyond.* pp. 37–106. Malvern, PA: HMP Communications; 2012.

36 Louvard Y, Lefèvre T. Loops and transradial approach in coronary diagnosis and intervention. *Cathet Cardiovasc Interv*, 2000; 51: 250–252.

37 Gilchrist IC. Transradial technical tips. *Cathet Cardiovasc Interv*, 2000; 49(3): 353–354.

38 Barbeau GR. Radial loop and extreme vessel tortuosity in the transradial approach: Advantage of hydrophilic-coated guidewires and catheters. *Cathet Cardiovasc Interv*, 2003; 59(4): 442–450.

39 Kwok CS, Sherwood MW, Mamas MA, et al. Blood transfusion after percutaneous coronary intervention and risk of subsequent adverse outcomes. a systematic review and meta-analysis. *JACC Cardiovasc Interv*, 2015; 8(3): 436–446.

40 Thompson CA. Transradial approach for percutaneous intervention in acute myocardial infarction. *J Inv Cardiol*, 2009; 21(Suppl A): 25A–27A.

41 Steg PG, James SK, Atar D, et al. ESC Guidelines for the management of acute myocardial infarction in patients presenting with ST-segment elevation. *Eur Heart J*, 2012; 33(20): 2569–2619.

42 Mehta SR, Bassand JP, Chrolavicius S, et al. Design and rationale of CURRENT-OASIS 7: A randomized, 2 x 2 factorial trial evaluating optimal dosing strategies for clopidogrel and aspirin in patients with ST and non-ST-elevation acute coronary syndromes managed with an early invasive strategy. *Am Heart J*, 2008; 156: 1080–1088.

43 Feit F, Voeltz MD, Attubato MJ, et al. Predictors and impact of major hemorrhage on mortality following percutaneous coronary intervention from the REPLACE-2 Trial. *Am J Cardiol*, 2007; 100: 1364–1369.

44 Singh M, Rihal CS, Gersh BJ, et al. Twenty-five-year trends in in-hospital and long-term outcome after percutaneous coronary intervention: A single-institution experience. *Circulation* 2007; 115: 2835–2841.

45 Fox KA, Steg PG, Eagle KA, et al. Decline in rates of death and heart failure in acute coronary syndromes, 1999–2006. *JAMA*, 2007; 297: 1892–1900.

46 Rao SV, Eikelboom JA, Granger CB, et al. Bleeding and blood transfusion issues in patients with non-ST-segment elevation acute coronary syndromes. *Eur Heart J*, 2007; 28: 1193–1204.

47 Doyle BJ, Rihal CS, Gastineau DA, et al. Bleeding, blood transfusion, and increased mortality after percutaneous coronary intervention: Implications for contemporary practice. *J Am Coll Cardiol*, 2009; 53: 2019–2027.

48 Caputo R. Transradial arterial access: Economical considerations. *J Inv Cardiol*, 2009; 21(Suppl A): 18A–20A.

49 Lange HW, von Boetticher H. Randomized comparison of operator radiation exposure during coronary angiography and intervention by radial or femoral approach. *Cathet Cardiovasc Interv*, 2006; 67: 12–16.

9

Management of Cardiogenic Shock

Holger Thiele MD, Suzanne de Waha MD

Diagnosis and Pathophysiology

Cardiogenic shock is defined as a state of critical end-organ hypoperfusion due to reduced cardiac output. Notably, it forms a spectrum that ranges from mild hypoperfusion to profound shock. Established criteria for the diagnosis of cardiogenic shock are outlined in Box 9.1. The diagnosis can usually be made on the basis of these easy-to-assess clinical criteria without additional advanced hemodynamic monitoring. However, assessment of cardiac index and pulmonary capillary wedge pressure may be helpful [1].

In the setting of acute myocardial infarction (AMI), ventricular dysfunction is the most frequent cause of cardiogenic shock, accounting for approximately 80% of cases. Mechanical complications such as ventricular septal defect (VSD, 4%) or free wall rupture (2%), and acute severe mitral regurgitation (7%) are less frequent causes after AMI [2]. The pathophysiology of cardiogenic shock is complex (Figure 9.1). In brief, ischemia induces profound depression of myocardial contractility, which initiates a vicious spiral of reduced cardiac index and low blood pressure which, in combination, impair cardiac power index and further promote coronary ischemia. The reduction in cardiac index causes severe tissue hypoperfusion, which is most sensitively measured by serum lactate and may finally lead to death if the circle is not successfully interrupted by adequate treatment measures. It has been recognized that cardiogenic shock cannot only be attributed to the loss of left ventricular function but is rather the result of derangements in the entire circulatory system. Initial compensatory vasoconstriction is subsequently counteracted by pathological vasodilation. Among others, development of systemic inflammation with capillary leakage, impairment of microcirculation, and vasodilation contribute to the vicious circle of cardiogenic shock. Bleeding and transfusion further contribute to inflammatory derangements in the shock spiral.

Incidence and Prognosis

Cardiogenic shock complicating AMI occurs in 5–15% of patients every year [3–5]. This translates to approximately 40,000–50,000 patients per year in the United States and approximately 60,000–70,000 in Europe [6]. Despite advances in treatment, mainly by early revascularization with subsequent mortality reduction, cardiogenic shock remains the leading cause of death in hospitalized patients with AMI, with mortality rates still approaching 40–50% according to registries and randomized trials [3–5,7].

Manual of STEMI Interventions, First Edition. Edited by Sameer Mehta.
© 2017 John Wiley & Sons Ltd. Published 2017 by John Wiley & Sons Ltd.

Box 9.1   Criteria for the Diagnosis of Cardiogenic Shock

1) Systolic blood pressure < 90 mmHg for > 30 minutes
   or
   Vasopressors required to achieve a blood pressure ≥ 90 mmHg
2) Pulmonary congestion
   or
   Elevated left ventricular filling pressures
3) Signs of impaired organ perfusion with at least one of the following criteria:
   a) Altered mental status
   b) Cold clammy skin
   c) Oliguria
   d) Increased serum lactate

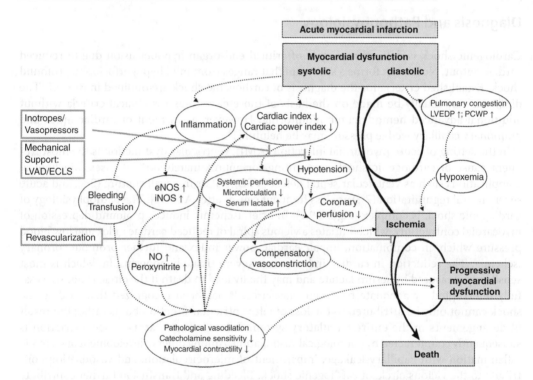

Figure 9.1 Current concept of CS pathophysiology. The classic shock spiral (black) and the parameters influencing the spiral by inflammation and bleeding/transfusion (blue) are shown. Treatment options such as: 1) revascularization; 2) mechanical support by left ventricular assist devices (LVAD) or extracorporeal life support systems (ECLS); and 3) inotropes or vasopressors to reverse the shock spiral are shown in green (LVEDP, left ventricular end-diastolic pressure; PCWP, pulmonary capillary wedge pressure).

According to multivariable modeling from the major cardiogenic shock trials (TRIUMPH [8], SHOCK [9], IABP-SHOCK II [10]), typical factors associated with higher mortality include older age, anoxic brain damage, lower left ventricular ejection fraction, lower cardiac power index, lower systolic blood pressure, need for vasopressor support, worse renal function, and higher serum lactate [8–10]. Multiple other biomarkers, which focus mainly on the degree of inflammation, as well as imaging methods such as sidestream darkfield imaging (which allows measurement of microcirculatory impairment) have been shown to be associated with mortality [11].

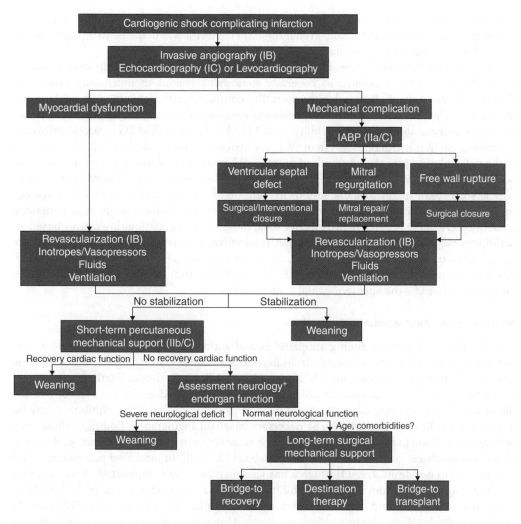

Figure 9.2 Treatment algorithm for patients with cardiogenic shock complicating acute myocardial infarction. Class of recommendation and level of evidence according to American College of Cardiology/ American Heart Association guidelines is provided if available (IABP, intra-aortic balloon pump) [12].

Interventional Management

Summarizing current evidence and American College of Cardiology/American Heart Association, as well as European Society of Cardiology guideline recommendations for cardiogenic shock management [12], a treatment algorithm reflecting clinical practice is shown in Figure 9.2.

Revascularization

Early revascularization by percutaneous coronary intervention (PCI) or coronary artery bypass grafting (CABG) is the most important treatment in cardiogenic shock complicating AMI [13]. This has first been demonstrated in the Should we emergently revascularize Occluded Coronaries for cardiogenic shocK (SHOCK) trial [9]. Although the trial failed to meet the primary endpoint (superiority of early revascularization over medical therapy on 30-day mortality) there was a significant mortality reduction at longer follow-up of 6 months, 1 year, and 6 years [13,14].

The primary therapeutic goal in cardiogenic shock complicated by AMI is therefore to perform revascularization in a timely fashion, even if the associated risk is anticipated to be high, such as in the elderly or following resuscitation.

Approximately 70–80% of patients with cardiogenic shock present with multivessel coronary artery disease, which is defined as coronary stenosis/occlusions in more than one vessel [7,13,15]. These patients have a higher mortality compared with patients with single-vessel disease [16]. Current guidelines recommend early revascularization by PCI or CABG, depending on coronary anatomy and amenability to PCI [12,17]. However, CABG is rarely performed in cardiogenic shock with rates less than 5% in registries and randomized trials [5,7]. Thus, PCI of the culprit lesion is accepted standard practice, whereas optimal management of additional non-culprit lesions is unclear. Current European guidelines encourage multivessel PCI of all critical stenoses or highly unstable lesions in addition to the culprit lesion (class IIa B recommendation) in cardiogenic shock, whereas no clear recommendation is given in American guidelines. Owing to the lack of prospective data, these recommendations are mainly based on pathophysiological considerations. Since non-randomized observational studies and registries are prone to treatment and selection bias, there is an urgent need for randomized data. The prospective, randomized, multicenter CULPRIT-SHOCK trial began enrolling patients in Europe in 2016 to fill the apparent gap of evidence [18].

Antiplatelet and Antithrombotic Medication

Antithrombotic therapy, including antiplatelets and anticoagulation, is a cornerstone procedure during PCI. There are no specific trials for oral antiplatelets in cardiogenic shock, but it is well known that enteral resorption is impaired in cardiogenic shock. Further, mechanical ventilation with inability to swallow prasugrel/ticagrelor or clopidogrel plays a major role for the bioavailability of these drugs. In general, administration of oral $P2Y_{12}$-inhibitors may be deferred, as CABG may immediately be necessary based on angiographic findings. All patients undergoing PCI are indicated aspirin in addition to prasugrel/ticagrelor or clopidogrel in case of contraindications for the newer oral antiplatelets [12,17,19]. In intubated patients, crushed tablets need to be administered through a nasogastric tube. This is supported by the fact that crushed ticagrelor can improve platelet inhibition in comparison with non-crushed tablets [20].

Because of the late and impaired onset of oral antiplatelets glycoprotein (GP) IIb/IIIa inhibitors may be beneficial in cardiogenic shock. However, routine upstream abciximab is not superior in comparison with standard treatment with optional abciximab use [21]. Therefore, current considerations and experience suggest a liberal use of GP IIb/IIIa inhibitors in patients with high thrombus burden and slow flow after PCI, in particular for the patient with cardiogenic shock.

During PCI, adjunctive anticoagulation including unfractionated heparin, low molecular weight heparin, or direct thrombin inhibitors should be co-administered with antiplatelets [12,17,19]. With a lack of specific randomized trials in cardiogenic shock, the same recommendations apply as for other types of acute coronary syndrome.

Treatment of Mechanical Complications

Early diagnosis of mechanical complications in AMI is of critical importance to optimize the otherwise often poor prognosis. Thus, repeated clinical evaluation and transthoracic echocardiography should be performed in all patients with AMI. In complicated cases, transesophageal echocardiography and use of pulmonary artery catheters to assess oxygen saturations or pulmonary capillary wedge pressure can further help to rule out or confirm the diagnosis. Surgical consultation should be obtained when a mechanical defect is suspected; intra-aortic balloon pumping (IABP) may provide temporary circulatory support [12].

Ventricular Septal Defect

The incidence of infarct-related VSD without reperfusion ranges from 1–2% [22,23], with a decrease to 0.2% in the era of reperfusion [24]. Without surgical repair of post-infarction VSD, 90% of patients die within 2 months [25]. However, even after surgical post-infarction VSD closure, mortality remains as high as 50% [26,27]. In patients with VSD and cardiogenic shock, the reported mortality rates are even higher, ranging from 81% to 100% in two prospective registries [24,28]. Thus, current guidelines recommend immediate surgical VSD closure independently of the patient's hemodynamic status [12,19]. As a result of the high mortality and suboptimal surgical results with a postoperative residual shunt, found in up to 20% of the treated patients [24,27,29], the technique of percutaneous VSD device closure has been developed [29]. Current data for post-infarction VSD interventional closure are limited. The largest single-center experience in 29 patients reported a survival rate at 30 days of 35%, with a much higher mortality in cardiogenic shock as opposed to non-shock patients (88% vs. 38%, $P < 0.001$) [30]. Procedure-related complications are frequent, which further demonstrates the requirement of technical improvement.

Free Wall Rupture

Since many patients with free wall rupture present with sudden profound cardiogenic shock (often rapidly leading to pulseless electrical activity caused by pericardial tamponade) there are limited treatment options. However, there may also be subacute presentations in case of a covered rupture. Immediate pericardiocentesis, in addition to echocardiography, can confirm the diagnosis. This is the cornerstone of diagnostic work-up. If available, pericardiocentesis relieves pericardial tamponade, at least momentarily, for immediate surgical repair. In a less acute clinical course, this allows for potentially life-saving therapeutic interventions. In the SHOCK trial registry, 28 patients presented with pericardial rupture or tamponade. The overall in-hospital mortality for this specific cohort (of which 75% underwent surgery) was as low as 39% [31]. However, this was a selected patient group with not all patients having overt clinical free wall rupture.

Acute Ischemic Mitral Regurgitation

In acute ischemic mitral regurgitation only papillary muscle rupture needs immediate repair. Other causes, such as left ventricular global or regional remodeling and ischemic papillary muscle dysfunction, may resolve after revascularization and recovery of left ventricular function. Accordingly, only 46% of the patients in the SHOCK trial registry underwent mitral valve surgery [32]. In contrast to VSD repair, surgery of papillary muscle rupture does not involve necrotic myocardium in suture lines. Therefore, mortality associated with this repair is lower [32]. The unpredictability of rapid deterioration and death with papillary muscle rupture makes early surgery necessary.

Right Ventricular Failure

In the treatment of cardiogenic shock from right ventricular failure it is of paramount importance to establish early reperfusion to reverse right ventricular ischemia. In addition to early revascularization, maintenance of adequate right ventricular preload with volume loading and preservation of synchronizing dual-chamber temporary pacing or even biventricular pacing, as well as reducing right ventricular afterload by IABP and inotropes, are of utmost importance. Traditionally, treatment of patients with right ventricular dysfunction with cardiogenic shock focused on ensuring adequate right-sided filling pressures in order to maintain cardiac output and adequate left ventricular preload. Nevertheless, patients with cardiogenic shock due to right ventricular dysfunction regularly have relatively high end-diastolic pressure, often exceeding 20 mmHg. This may result in shifting of the interventricular septum toward the left ventricle, impairing left ventricular filling and systolic function [33]. The common practice of aggressive fluid resuscitation for right ventricular dysfunction in cardiogenic shock can therefore be misleading and should be monitored via a pulmonary artery catheter. Inotropic therapy may thus be indicated for right ventricular failure when cardiogenic shock persists after preload optimization. In extreme cases, both pericardectomy and creation of atrial septal defects can be performed [34]. Cardiogenic shock due to isolated right ventricular dysfunction carries nearly the same mortality risk as left sided cardiogenic shock and the benefits of revascularization are similar, as shown in the SHOCK trial registry [35].

Intensive Care Unit Treatment

Vasopressors and Inotropes

Catecholamines increase myocardial oxygen consumption and vasoconstrictors may impair microcirculation and tissue perfusion. As a consequence, their use should be restricted to the shortest possible duration and the lowest possible dose. In analogy to septic shock, the target mean blood pressure should be titrated to 65–70 mmHg as a higher blood pressure is not associated with a beneficial outcome [36].

Although catecholamines are administered in approximately 90% of patients with cardiogenic shock [7], there is only limited evidence from randomized trials comparing catecholamines for cardiogenic shock. In a randomized comparison of 1679 patients with shock, including 280 patients treated with dopamine in comparison with norepinephrine, dopamine was associated with significantly more arrhythmic events for the overall study cohort and had no significant reduction in mortality. A predefined subgroup of patients with cardiogenic shock (the percentage of cardiogenic shock due to AMI is not reported) had lower mortality with norepinephrine [37]. When blood pressure is low, norepinephrine should therefore be considered as the first choice of vasopressor.

As inotropic agent, dobutamine may be given simultaneously to norepinephrine in an attempt to improve cardiac contractility, which is often performed in clinical practice [7]. Other inotropes such as levosimendan or phosphodiesterase-inhibitors are of interest in cardiogenic shock based on their improvement of myocardial contractility without increasing oxygen requirements and potential for vasodilation. However, the current evidence for inotropes and vasodilators in cardiogenic shock is limited [38].

Supportive Therapy

Optimal treatment to prevent or reverse multi-organ dysfunction syndrome in the intensive care unit is essential for the treatment of patients with cardiogenic shock and has a major impact on prognosis. Although not specifically investigated in cardiogenic shock, multiple measures are generally recommended [39]. Basic treatment measures include volume expansion to obtain euvolemia. Fluid administration in cardiogenic shock is mainly based on pathophysiological considerations. As the hemodynamic management depends on optimal filling pressures, pulmonary artery catheters, Pulse Contour Cardiac Output (PiCCO®) or other systems may be used in all complicated courses [39], although no specific randomized trial has been performed with these monitoring systems in cases of cardiogenic shock.

If invasive ventilation is required, lung-protective ventilation should be performed to prevent pulmonary injury. Urinary production should be measured, and continuous renal replacement therapy must be initiated in case of acute renal failure with clinical signs of uremia, hydropic decompensation, metabolic acidosis, and/or refractory hyperkalemia. Moreover, optimal nutrition and glycemic control to less than11 mmol/l for avoiding hypoglycemia, as well as thromboembolism and stress ulcer prophylaxis should be provided [39].

Further, moderate to severe bleeding is common in patients with cardiogenic shock, ranging from 20% to 90%, depending on the definition used. The degree of bleeding is also influenced by concomitant use of mechanical support devices [7,13,40,41]. Formerly, it was generally believed that raising hemoglobin levels via transfusion would increase oxygen delivery and lead to a beneficial effect. However, blood transfusions in acute coronary syndromes increase mortality [42]. Alterations in erythrocyte nitric oxide biology in stored blood may provide a partial explanation, leading to initial vasoconstriction, platelet aggregation, and ineffective oxygen delivery. In addition, bleeding, as well as transfusions, contribute to inflammation [42]. Trials in patients without cardiogenic shock who are bleeding demonstrate that a restrictive transfusion regimen can improve outcome. General accepted intensive care strategies include to avoiding the correction of laboratory anomalies unless there is a clinically relevant bleeding problem [43,44].

Mechanical Support

To improve hemodynamics and overcome the limitations of inotropes and vasopressors, mechanical circulatory support appears to be appealing. Figure 9.3 shows schematic drawings of the different devices and Table 9.1 provides an updated overview of technical features and left ventricular unloading properties [45].

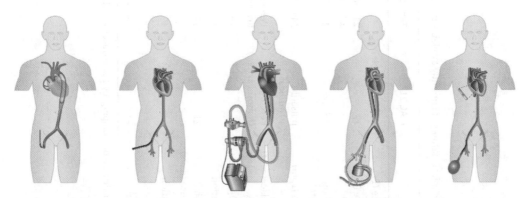

Figure 9.3 Current percutaneous mechanical support devices for cardiogenic shock: (left to right) intra-aortic balloon pump (IABP); Impella® 2.5, 3.5 or 5.0; TandemHeart™; extracorporeal life support system (ECMO) extracorporeal membrane oxygenation (ECMO); iVAC 2 L®.

Table 9.1 Technical features of currently available percutaneous support devices.

	iVAC 2 L®	TandemHeart™	Impella® 5.0	Impella® 2.5	Impella® CP	ECLS (multiple systems)
Catheter size (Fr)	11 (expandable)	–	9	9	9	–
Cannula size (Fr)	17	21 venous 12–19 arterial	21	12	–	17–21 venous 16–19 arterial
Maximum flow (liters/minute)	2.8	4	5	2.5	3.7–4	7
Pump speed (rpm)	pulsatile, 40 ml/beat	Max. 7,500	Max. 33,000	Max. 51,000	Max. 51,000	Max. 5,000
Insertion (placement)	Percutaneous (femoral artery)	Percutaneous (femoral artery + vein for left atrium)	Peripheral surgical (femoral artery)	Percutaneous (femoral artery)	Percutaneous (femoral artery)	Percutaneous (femoral artery + vein)
LV unloading	+	++	++	+	+	–
Anticoagulation	+	+	+	+	+	+
Recommended duration of use (days)	21	14	10	10	10	7
CE-certification	+	+	+	+	+	+
FDA	–	+	+	+	+	+
Relative costs	++	++++	++++	+++	++++	+(+)

IABP, intra-aortic balloon pumping; ECLS, extracorporeal life support system; LV, left ventricular; CE, European conformity; FDA, Food and Drug Administration; rpm, revolutions per minute.

Intra-aortic Balloon Pumping

IABP is the most widely used device for mechanical support [46]. IABP improves the diastolic and lowers the end-systolic pressure without affecting the mean blood pressure. In the largest randomized, multicenter trial in cardiogenic shock (IABP-SHOCK II trial), 600 patients with cardiogenic shock complicating AMI who were undergoing early revascularization were randomized to either IABP or conventional treatment. In the primary endpoint of 30-day mortality (39.7% versus 41.3%; $P = 0.69$) no significant difference could be observed between the two treatment groups [7]. There were also no differences in any of the secondary endpoints, such as serum lactate, renal function, catecholamine doses, or length of intensive care unit treatment. In addition, no subgroups could be identified with a potential advantage for IABP support [7]. The 12-month follow-up analysis confirmed these negative findings [10].

Since IABP support has been in place for nearly five decades, the negative results of IABP-SHOCK II triggered some discussion. The sample size calculation was based on the assumption of a higher mortality in the control group. However, the mortality was lower than anticipated and marginally lower in comparison to other previous trials in cardiogenic shock despite similar baseline characteristics [13,47]. Furthermore, as in all negative trials, a type II error cannot be definitely excluded. A certain crossover rate might also have influenced the results. However, the lack of benefit for any of the investigated secondary study endpoints, the neutral results in all subgroup analyses, and the lack of benefit at 12-month follow-up and in the as-treated analysis argue against any clinically meaningful IABP effect [10]. It has been criticized that timing of IABP insertion was left to the discretion of the operator resulting in IABP insertion pre-PCI in only 13.4% [7]. However, data on timing of IABP insertion derived from small registries in cardiogenic shock are limited and conflicting, with more data even showing harm than benefit by IABP insertion before PCI [48,49].

Percutaneous Left Ventricular Assist Devices

Active percutaneous left ventricular assist devices and extracorporeal life support systems are used in patients not responding to standard treatment. Despite an increasing number of different devices that include mechanical extracorporeal life support in cardiogenic shock, data derived from randomized clinical trials on their effectiveness and safety, differential indications for different devices, and optimal timing are limited. Despite these uncertainties, current European and American guidelines recommend considering the use of a mechanical assist device for circulatory support in refractory cardiogenic shock without any preference for device selection (evidence level IIa/C recommendation) [12,17,19].

Multiple open issues remain in mechanical device therapy, such as optimal timing of insertion. A potential benefit of an early use at onset of cardiogenic shock could be prevention of multi-organ dysfunction syndrome. However, early use might lead to complications associated with invasive mechanical support devices, and adverse clinical outcome in patients who still had noninvasive therapeutic options. Appropriate patient selection is also important, and is currently often based on subjective criteria. Approximately 60% of patients with cardiogenic shock will survive without any active device [7]. There may also be situations where even the best device available will not be able to change clinical outcome. Timing and appropriate patient selection is thus influenced by the balance between efficacy of any device and its device-related complications. Devices with low complication rates may be chosen more liberally in the early stage of cardiogenic shock, whereas more aggressive devices with higher flow rates may be reserved for more severe cases. Further, complication rates may be lowered by greater experience with respect to percutaneous implantation and patient management following the implantation.

Summary

Cardiogenic shock remains the most common cause of death in hospitalized patients with AMI. Following a rapid diagnosis, early revascularization is the therapeutic cornerstone in patients with cardiogenic shock and AMI. Repeated clinical examinations and transthoracic echocardiography should be performed to assess for mechanical complications. Optimal intensive care treatment and potentially implantation of mechanical support devices can further help to improve the prognosis for patients. However, there are multiple open questions over treatment for cardiogenic shock, as prospective clinical studies are difficult to perform and only few randomized clinical trials powered to detect differences in clinical outcome have achieved completion of the required patient numbers.

References

1 Reynolds HR, Hochman JS. Cardiogenic shock. Current concepts and improving outcomes. *Circulation*, 2008; 117: 686–697.

2 Hochman JS, Buller CE, Sleeper LA, et al. Cardiogenic shock complicating acute myocardial infarction: Etiologies, management and outcome. A report from the SHOCK Trial Registry. *J Am Coll Cardiol*, 2000; 36(3, Suppl 1): 1063–1070.

3 Aissaoui N, Puymirat E, Tabone X, et al. Improved outcome of cardiogenic shock at the acute stage of myocardial infarction: A report from the USIK 1995, USIC 2000, and FAST-MI French Nationwide Registries. *Eur Heart J* 2012; 33(20):2535–2543.

4 Goldberg RJ, Spencer FA, Gore JM, et al. Thirty-year trends (1975 to 2005) in the magnitude of, management of, and hospital death rates associated with cardiogenic shock in patients with acute myocardial infarction: a population-based perspective. *Circulation*, 2009; 119(9): 1211–1219.

5 Jeger RV, Radovanovic D, Hunziker PR, et al. Ten-year incidence and treatment of cardiogenic shock. *Ann Intern Med*, 2008; 149: 618–626.

6 Thiele H, Allam B, Chatellier G, et al. Shock in acute myocardial infarction: The Cape Horn for trials? *Eur Heart J*, 2010; 31: 1828–1835.

7 Thiele H, Zeymer U, Neumann F-J, et al. Intraaortic balloon support for myocardial infarction with cardiogenic shock. *N Engl J Med*, 2012; 367(14): 1287–1296.

8 Katz JN, Stebbins AL, Alexander JH, et al. Predictors of 30-day mortality in patients with refractory cardiogenic shock following acute myocardial infarction despite a patent infarct artery. *Am Heart J*, 2009; 158(4): 680–687.

9 Sleeper LA, Reynolds HR, White HD, et al. A severity scoring system for risk assessment of patients with cardiogenic shock: A report from the SHOCK Trial and Registry. *Am Heart J*, 2010; 160(3): 443–450.

10 Thiele H, Zeymer U, Neumann F-J, et al. Intraaortic balloon counterpulsation in acute myocardial infarction complicated by cardiogenic shock. Final 12-month results of the randomised IntraAortic Balloon Pump in cardiogenic shock II (IABP-SHOCK II) Trial. *Lancet*, 2013; 382: 1638–1645.

11 Prondzinsky R, Unverzagt S, Lemm H, et al. Interleukin-6, -7, -8 and -10 predict outcome in acute myocardial infarction complicated by cardiogenic shock. *Clin Res Cardiol*, 2012; 101: 375–384.

12 O'Gara PT, Kushner FG, Ascheim DD, et al. 2013 ACCF/AHA guideline for the management of ST-elevation myocardial infarction: a report of the American College of Cardiology Foundation/American Heart Association Task Force on Practice Guidelines. *J Am Coll Cardiol*, 2013; 61(4): e78–e140.

13 Hochman JS, Sleeper LA, Webb JG, et al. Early revascularization in acute myocardial infarction complicated by cardiogenic shock. SHOCK Investigators. Should We Emergently Revascularize Occluded Coronaries for Cardiogenic Shock. *N Engl J Med*, 1999; 341(9): 625–634.

14 Hochman JS, Sleeper LA, Webb JG, et al. Early revascularization and long-term survival in cardiogenic shock complicating acute myocardial infarction. *JAMA*, 2006; 295: 2511–2515.

15 Webb JG, Lowe AM, Sanborn TA, et al. Percutaneous coronary intervention for cardiogenic shock in the SHOCK trial. *J Am Coll Cardiol*, 2003; 42(8): 1380–1386.

16 Sanborn TA, Sleeper LA, Webb JG, et al. Correlates of one-year survival in patients with cardiogenic shock complicating acute myocardial infarction: angiographic findings from the SHOCK trial. *J Am Coll Cardiol*, 2003; 42: 1373–1379.

17 Windecker S, Kolh P, Alfonso F, et al. 2014 ESC/EACTS Guidelines on myocardial revascularization: The Task Force on Myocardial Revascularization of the European Society of Cardiology (ESC) and the European Association for Cardio-Thoracic Surgery (EACTS) Developed with the special contribution of the European Association of Percutaneous Cardiovascular Interventions (EAPCI). *Eur Heart J*, 2014; 35(37): 2541–2619.

18 Culprit Lesion Only PCI Versus Multivessel PCI in Cardiogenic Shock (CULPRIT-SHOCK). Clinicaltrials.gov: NCT01927549. Available at https://clinicaltrials.gov/ct2/show/NCT01927549 (accessed March 11, 2017).

19 Steg PG, James SK, Atar D, et al. ESC Guidelines for the management of acute myocardial infarction in patients presenting with ST-segment elevation. *Eur Heart J*, 2012; 33: 2569–2619.

20 Parodi G, Xanthopoulou I, Bellandi B, et al. Ticagrelor crushed tablets administration in STEMI patients: The Mashed Or Just Integral Tablets of ticagrelOr (MOJITO) study. *Eur Heart J* 2014; 35 (Abstract Supplement): 1030.

21 Tousek P, Rokyta R, Tesarova J, et al. Routine upfront abciximab versus standard periprocedural therapy in patients undergoing primary percutaneous coronary intervention for cardiogenic shock: The PRAGUE-7 Study. An open randomized multicentre study. *Acute Card Care*, 2011; 13(3): 116–122.

22 Heitmiller R, Jacobs ML, Daggett WM. Surgical management of postinfarction ventricular septal rupture. *Ann Thorac Surg*, 1986; 41(6): 683–691.

23 Topaz O, Taylor AL. Interventricular septal rupture complicating acute myocardial infarction: from pathophysiologic features to the role of invasive and noninvasive diagnostic modalities in current management. *Am J Med*, 1992; 93: 683–688.

24 Crenshaw BS, Granger CB, Birnbaum Y, et al. Risk factors, angiographic patterns, and outcomes in patients with ventricular septal defect complicating acute myocardial infarction. GUSTO-I (Global Utilization of Streptokinase and TPA for Occluded Coronary Arteries) Trial Investigators. *Circulation*, 2000; 101(1): 27–32.

25 Lee WY, Cardon L, Slodki SJ. Perforation of infarcted interventricular septum. Report of a case with prolonged survival and review of the literature. *Arch Intern Med*, 1962; 109: 731–735.

26 Bouchart F, Bessou JP, Tabley A, et al. Urgent surgical repair of postinfarction ventricular septal rupture: Early and late outcome. *J Card Surg*, 1998; 13:104–112.

27 Deja MA, Szostek J, Widenka K, et al. Post infarction ventricular septal defect: Can we do better? *Eur J Cardiothorac Surg*, 2000; 18(2): 194–201.

28 Menon V, Webb JG, Hillis LD, et al. Outcome and profile of ventricular septal rupture with cardiogenic shock after myocardial infarction: a report from the SHOCK Trial Registry. SHould we emergently revascularize Occluded Coronaries in cardiogenic shocK? *J Am Coll Cardiol*, 2000; 36(3 Suppl A): 1110–1116.

29 Caputo M, Wilde P, Angelini GD. Management of postinfarction ventricular septal defect. *Br J Hosp Med*, 1995; 54(11): 562–566.

30 Thiele H, Kaulfersch C, Daehnert I, Schoenauer M, Eitel I, Borger M, Schuler G. Immediate primary transcatheter closure of postinfarction ventricular septal defects. *Eur Heart J* 2009; 30:81–88.

31 Slater J, Brown RJ, Antonelli TA, et al. Cardiogenic shock due to cardiac free-wall rupture or tamponade after acute myocardial infarction: a report from the SHOCK Trial Registry. *J Am Coll Cardiol*, 2000; 36(3, Suppl 1): 1117–1122.

32 Thompson CR, Buller CE, Sleeper LA, et al. Cardiogenic shock due to acute severe mitral regurgitation complicating acute myocardial infarction: A report from the SHOCK Trial Registry. *J Am Coll Cardiol*, 2000; 36(3, Suppl 1): 1104–1109.

33 Brookes C, Ravn H, White P, et al. Acute right ventricular dilatation in response to ischemia significantly impairs left ventricular systolic performance. *Circulation*, 1999; 100(7): 761–767.

34 Goldstein JA. Pathophysiology and managment of right heart ischemia. *J Am Coll Cardiol*, 2002; 40: 841–853.

35 Jacobs AK, Leopold JA, Bates E, et al. Cardiogenic shock caused by right ventricular infarction: A report from the SHOCK registry. *J Am Coll Cardiol*, 2003; 41(8): 1273–1279.

36 Asfar P, Meziani F, Hamel J-F, et al. High versus low blood-pressure target in patients with septic shock. *N Engl J Med*, 2014; 370(17): 1583–1593.

37 De Backer D, Biston P, Devriendt J, et al. Comparison of dopamine and norepinephrine in the treatment of shock. *N Engl J Med*, 2010; 362(9): 779–789.

38 Unverzagt S, Wachsmuth L, Hirsch K, et al. Inotropic agents and vasodilator strategies for acute myocardial infarction complicated by cardiogenic shock or low cardiac output syndrome. *Cochrane Database Syst Rev*, 2014; (1): CD009669. doi: 10.1002/14651858.CD009669.pub2.

39 Werdan K, Ruß M, Buerke M, et al. Cardiogenic shock due to myocardial infarction: diagnosis, monitoring and treatment: A German–Austrian S3 Guideline. *Dtsch Arztebl Int*, 2012; 109(18): 343–351.

40 Cheng JM, den Uil CA, Hoeks SE, et al. Percutaneous left ventricular assist devices vs. intra-aortic balloon pump counterpulsation for treatment of cardiogenic shock: a meta-analysis of controlled trials. *Eur Heart J*, 2009; 30(17): 2102–2108.

41 Cheng R, Hachamovitch R, Kittleson M, et al. Complications of extracorporeal membrane oxygenation for treatment of cardiogenic shock and cardiac arrest: A meta-analysis of 1,866 adult patients. *Ann Thorac Surg*, 2014; 97(2): 610–616.

42 Rao SV, Jollis JG, Harrington RA, et al. Relationship of blood transfusion and clinical outcomes in patients with acute coronary syndromes. *JAMA*, 2004; 292: 1555–1562.

43 Hunt BJ. Bleeding and coagulopathies in critical care. *N Engl J Med*, 2014; 370(9): 847–859.

44 Villanueva C, Colomo A, Bosch A, et al. Transfusion strategies for acute upper gastrointestinal bleeding. *N Engl J Med*, 2013; 368(1): 11–21.

45 Thiele H, Ohman EM, Desch S, et al. Management of cardiogenic shock. *Eur Heart J*, 2015; 36(20): 1223–1230.

46 Stretch R, Sauer CM, Yuh DD, et al. National trends in the utilization of short-term mechanical circulatory support: Incidence, outcomes, and cost analysis. *J Am Coll Cardiol*, 2014; 64(14): 1407–1415.

47 The TRIUMPH Investigators. Effect of tilarginine acetate in patients with acute myocardial infarction and cardiogenic shock. The TRIUMPH Randomized Controlled Trial. *JAMA*, 2007; 297: 1657–1666.

48 Abdel-Wahab M, Saad M, Kynast J, et al. Comparison of hospital mortality with intra-aortic balloon counterpulsation insertion before versus after primary percutaneous coronary intervention for cardiogenic shock complicating acute myocardial infarction. *Am J Cardiol*, 2010; 105(7): 967–971.

49 Cheng JM, van Leeuwen MA, de Boer SP, et al. Impact of intra-aortic balloon pump support initiated before versus after primary percutaneous coronary intervention in patients with cardiogenic shock from acute myocardial infarction. *Int J Cardiol*, 2013; 168: 3758–3763.

10

Present Role of Thrombectomy in STEMI Interventions

Francesco Giannini MD, Azeem Latib MD, Antonio Colombo MD

Rationale for Thrombectomy in Acute Myocardial Infarction

Acute ST-segment elevation myocardial infarction (STEMI) is most often caused by plaque rupture with overlying thrombus formation in a coronary artery, for which the preferred treatment today is primary percutaneous coronary intervention (PPCI) [1,2]. PPCI is very effective in restoring epicardial flow in the infarct artery but a significant limitation is distal embolization of thrombus and obstruction of the microvasculature [3]. About one-third of patients treated with PPCI have impaired microvascular perfusion, despite restoration of normal epicardial flow, and they have a significantly increased mortality [4,5]. This phenomenon has been attributed to a combination of distal embolization of thrombus and plaque debris, vasoconstriction and reperfusion injury [6].

Thrombus burden during PPCI has been linked to mortality [7]. In an analysis of 812 consecutive STEMI patients, patients with large compared with small thrombus burden had higher mortality (12.9% vs. 7.8% at 1 year, $P = 0.025$), higher rates of stent thrombosis (8.2% vs. 1.3%, $P = 0.001$) and lower rates of myocardial blush grade (MBG) 3 (35% vs. 53%, $P < 0.001$) [7]. The use of glycoprotein (GP) IIb/IIIa inhibitors, either peripherally or intracoronarily, and of coronary vasodilators, such as verapamil and adenosine, has been shown to be effective in reducing such events [8]. However, the need to reduce such phenomena further and the fact that distal embolization seems to occur predominantly at the time of first balloon inflation and stent deployment has led to the development of devices for thrombus removal or trapping, to assist in improving clinical outcomes after PPCI. In addition, thrombectomy allows better visualization of the culprit lesion, and thrombus removal may decrease the risk of acute stent thrombosis by facilitating stent deployment and reducing thrombus burden. Removal of thrombus may also prevent late stent malapposition and subsequent late stent thrombosis.

Thrombectomy Devices

Thrombectomy devices currently in use vary in design and mechanism of action but can be broadly divided in two groups, depending on the presence or absence of a motorized system. Some common manual thrombectomy devices are shown in Figure 10.1 and some non-manual thrombectomy devices in Figure 10.2. The Excimer laser coronary angioplasty system can also be considered as a form of thrombectomy, as thrombus is highly susceptible to laser energy and the device has already been used as an adjunct therapy in PPCI. The characteristics of the main manual and mechanical thrombectomy devices are summarized in Table 10.1.

Manual of STEMI Interventions, First Edition. Edited by Sameer Mehta.
© 2017 John Wiley & Sons Ltd. Published 2017 by John Wiley & Sons Ltd.

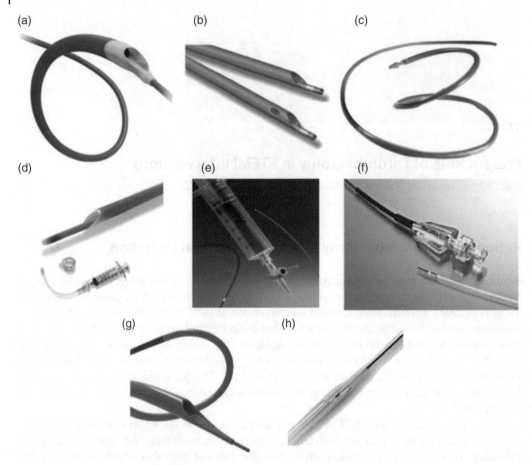

Figure 10.1 Manual thrombectomy devices: a) Export catheter. b) Diver CE catheter. c) Pronto catheter. d) QuickCat catheter. e) Fetch catheter. f) Thrombuster. g) Hunter catheter. h) Vmax catheter.

In clinical practice, thrombectomy is most commonly performed using a simple manual aspiration device. Manual devices are significantly less expensive and simpler to use than mechanical devices. Manual devices are composed of monorail catheters with a central lumen, which communicates with one or more holes located at the tip. The catheter is connected proximally to a syringe for manual aspiration. All of these devices operate on similar principles but differ in terms of catheter material and aspiration lumen size, with theoretical differences in deliverability and thrombus extraction. Non-manual thrombectomy devices vary in their working mechanism depending on their ability to actively fragment atherosclerotic thrombus material prior to aspiration. The AngioJet, X-sizer catheters and the Rinspirator system are capable of such active thrombus fragmentation. One significant limitation of manual aspiration is its inability to remove large-volume thrombi, so mechanical thrombectomy may be postulated to be particularly beneficial in cases of large thrombus burden. Tortuosity of the coronary artery, heavy calcification, and bifurcations are the main causes of failure of successful thrombectomy. Such failure has been observed in about 10% of cases [9]. However, the newest generation of aspiration catheters achieved improved deliverability by using a stylet-based system, such as the Export Advance system. Box 10.1 summarizes common recommendations for using manual thrombectomy devices.

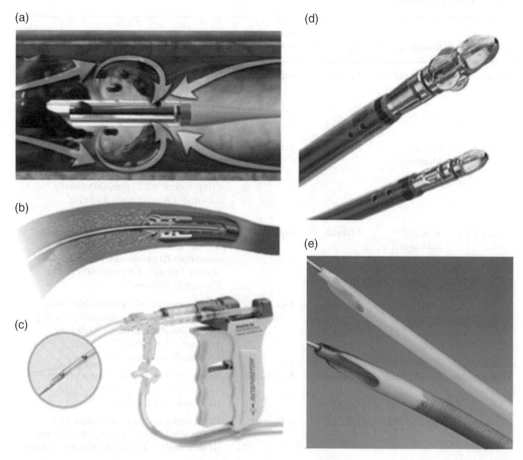

Figure 10.2 Mechanical thrombectomy devices: a) Angiojet system. b) X-sizer system. c) Rinspirator system. d) Rescue. e) TVAC system.

Evidence for Manual Thrombectomy

A number of randomized trials compared thrombectomy using manual devices with standard percutaneous coronary intervention (PCI; Table 10.2) [10–26]. In the first large study of manual thrombectomy, the single-center Thrombus Aspiration during Percutaneous Coronary Intervention in Acute Myocardial Infarction Study (TAPAS) [18], patients with 1071 STEMI were randomly assigned to receive manual aspiration thrombectomy ($n = 535$) prior to stenting using the Export device or to conventional PPCI and stenting ($n = 536$). All patients received standard therapy, including GP IIb/IIIa inhibitors unless contraindicated. The primary endpoint was myocardial blush grade (MBG) with ST-resolution and thrombolysis in myocardial infarction (TIMI) flow being secondary endpoints. Patients treated with thrombus aspiration had a higher MBG grade (grade 0/1 in 17% vs. 26.3%; grade 2 in 37.1% vs. 41.4%; grade 3 in 45.7% vs. 32.2%; $P < 0.001$), greater and more rapid reduction of ST-segment elevation (more than 70% in 56.6% vs. 44.2 %; 30–70% in 30.8% vs. 37.9 %; less than 30% in 12.6% vs. 17.9 %; $P < 0.001$), and fewer pathological Q waves ($P = 0.001$). Results showed that manual thrombectomy was associated with a lower incidence of cardiac death and nonfatal reinfarction at 1 year (cardiac death: 3.6% vs. 6.7%, $P = 0.020$; cardiac death or nonfatal reinfarction: 5.6% vs. 9.9%, $P = 0.009$) [19].

Table 10.1 Characteristics of the most common manual and mechanical thrombectomy devices compatible with 0.014-inch guide wires.

Device Name	Manufacturer	Type	Mechanism of Action	Description
Export	Medtronic	Manual	Aspiration	Rapid exchange. 6 Fr compatible. Dual-lumen catheter with an oblique aspiration tip design. OD proximally 1.35 mm, OD distally 1.70 mm. EA proximally 0.85 mm^2, EA distally 0.87 mm^2.
Diver CE	Invatec/ Medtronic	Manual	Aspiration	Rapid exchange. 6 Fr compatible. Dual-lumen catheter with hydrophilic coating and available with and without side holes. OD proximally 1.21 mm, OD distally 1.64 mm. EA proximally 0.77 mm^2, EA distally 1.12 mm^2.
Pronto V3	Vascular Solutions	Manual	Aspiration	Rapid exchange. 6 Fr compatible. Dual-lumen catheter with rounded atraumatic distal tip. OD proximally 1.64 mm, OD distally 1.65 mm. EA proximally 0.90 mm^2, EA distally 0.90 mm^2.
QuickCat	Spectranetics	Manual	Aspiration	Rapid exchange. 6 Fr compatible. Dual-lumen catheter with hydrophilic coating. OD proximally 1.26 mm, OD distally 1.50 mm. EA proximally 0.75 mm^2, EA distally 0.87 mm^2.
Thrombuster	Kaneka Medix	Manual	Aspiration	Rapid exchange and over the wire. 6 Fr compatible. Single-lumen catheter. ID 1.1 mm OD 1.7 mm.
Eliminate	Terumo Europe	Manual	Aspiration	Rapid exchange. 6 Fr compatible. OD proximally 1.40 mm, OD distally 1.70 mm. ID proximally 1.10 mm, ID distally 1.00 mm.
Hunter	IHT Cordynamic	Manual	Aspiration	Rapid exchange. 6 Fr compatible. Dual-lumen catheter. OD proximally 1.40 mm, OD distally 1.65 mm. EA proximally 1.04 mm^2, EA distally 0.95 mm^2.
Fetch 2	Medrad	Manual	Aspiration	Rapid exchange. 6 Fr compatible. OD 1.40 mm.
VMAX	Stron Medical	Manual	Aspiration	Rapid exchange. 6 Fr compatible. OD proximally 1.37 mm, OD distally 1.37 mm. ID proximally 1.1 mm, ID distally 0.53 mm
X-SIZER	Covidien	Mechanical	Disruption and extraction	Over the wire. 7 Fr compatible. Capable of active thrombus aspiration. Double-lumen catheter with a cutter at the tip that rotates at 2100 rpm driven by a handheld battery motor unit. 1 catheter lumen is connected a 250-ml vacuum bottle.
Rinspirator	FoxHollow technologies	Mechanical	Disruption and extraction	Rapid exchange. 6 Fr compatible. Allows detachment and aspiration of thrombotic debris. Capable of active thrombus aspiration. Double-lumen catheter for simultaneous aspiration and infusion of heparinized saline. Perforations located proximal to the aspiration hole of the catheter create turbulent flow that allows detachment and aspiration of thrombotic debris.

Table 10.1 (Continued)

Device Name	Manufacturer	Type	Mechanism of Action	Description
AngioJet	Medrad	Mechanical	Disruption and extraction	Rapid exchange and over the wire. 6 Fr compatible. Capable of active thrombus aspiration. Double-lumen catheter attached to a piston pump and drive unit. High-velocity heparinized jets enclosed in the catheter use the Bernoulli principle for capture and microfragmentation. The debris is aspirated using vacuum aspiration.
Rescue	Boston Scientific	Mechanical	Aspiration	Rapid exchange. 7 Fr compatible. Double-lumen catheter connected to an aspiration pump for vacuum formation and removal of thrombotic material.
TVAC	Nipro	Mechanical	Aspiration	Rapid exchange. 7 Fr compatible. Single-lumen catheter with a beak-shaped distal tip. The catheter is attached to an aspiration pump for vacuum formation and removal of thrombotic material.
Laser	Spectranetics	–	Physical dissolution	Ultraviolet light pulse hits tissue for 135 ns. 50-μm penetration. Billions of molecular bonds fractures per pulse. After 135 ns, laser energy is not emitted.
Low-frequency ultrasound	Vascular Solutions	–	Physical dissolution	Ultrasound transmission probe and electromechanical apparatus that uses ultrasonic energy (308-nm light) to eliminate blood clots.

EA, extraction area; ID, internal diameter; nm, nanometer; ns, nanosecond; OD, outside diameter.

Box 10.1   Recommendations for the Use of Manual Thrombectomy Devices

- Start aspiration before crossing the thrombotic lesion.
- Ensure adequate guide support to reach the target lesion with aspiration catheter.
- If suction stops suddenly during aspiration despite changing syringe, remove aspiration catheter and flush it outside the body, as tip may be obstructed by large thrombus.
- Ensure guide engagement in the coronary ostium when removing the thrombectomy catheter, to avoid thrombus embolization to cerebral vasculature and risk of stroke.
- Aspirate guide catheter after thrombectomy to remove air or residual thrombus, as thrombus embolization in non-infarct territory can be catastrophic.
- If you are not able to cross the lesion with the thrombectomy catheter, consider a small-diameter balloon dilation and then reattempt.

Although the TAPAS trial did not assess infarct size or left ventricular function, results clearly suggested that manual thrombectomy in STEMI patients improves myocardial perfusion and this seems to confer a survival benefit at 1-year follow-up. Subsequently, a number of meta-analyses that included smaller trials showed clinical benefit of manual thrombectomy, thus favoring its use [27–30]. This was reflected in practice guidelines, as manual thrombec-

Table 10.2 Randomized studies showing the effects of manual thrombus aspiration.

Study name or author [reference]	Year	Design	Thrombectomy device	Patients (n)	Endpoints	Results thrombectomy vs. standard PPCI
TOTAL [10]	2015	Multicenter, randomized trial	Export Catheter (Medtronic)	10,732	Composite outcome of: CV death, recurrent MI, cardiogenic shock or NYHA class IV failure within 180 days.	6.9% vs. 7.0%, (p = 0.86)
					Stroke within 30 days.	0.7% vs. 0.3%, (P = 0.02)
TROFI [11]	2013	Multicenter, randomized trial	Eliminate (Terumo) Export (Medtronic)	141	Minimum flow area post-procedure assessed by optical frequency domain imaging defined as (stent area + ISA area) − (intraluminal defect + tissue prolapse area).	7.08 vs. 6.51 mm, (P = 0.12)
TASTE [12]	2013	Multicenter RCT from the national comprehensive Swedish Coronary Angiography and Angioplasty Registry	Eliminate (Terumo), Export (Medtronic) and Pronto extraction (Vascular Solutions) recommended	7,244	All-cause mortality at 30 days.	2.8% vs. 3.0%, (P = 0.63)
					Hospitalization for recurrent myocardial infarction at 30 days.	0.5% vs. 0.9%, (P = 0.09)
					Stent thrombosis.	0.2% vs. 0.5%, (P = 0.06)
					Stroke/neurological complications.	No significant differences
MUSTELA [13]	2012	Multicenter RCT	Export Catheter (Medtronic) or the AngioJet Ultra catheter (Possis Medical)	208 with high thrombus burden	STRes	57% vs. 37%, (P = 0.004)
					3-month infarct size	20.4% vs. 19.3%, (P = 0.54)
INFUSE-AMI [14]	2012	Multicenter RCT	Export Catheter (Medtronic)	452 with anterior MI	Infarct size at 30 days (cardiac MRI).	17.0% vs. 17.3%, (P = 0.51)
					Absolute infarct mass.	median 20.3g vs. 21.0g, (P = 0.36)
PIHRATE [15]	2010	RCT	Diver CE (Invatec)	196	60 minutes STRes ≥ 70%.	53.7% vs. 35.1%, (P = 0.29)
					Combined angiographic endpoint of TIMI grade 3 flow + MBG 3.	72.7% vs. 54.2%, (P = 0.012)
					Cardiac death.	4% vs. 3.1%, (P = 0.74)
					Procedural complications.	16 vs. 24.2%, (P = 0.15)
					MBG grade 3.	76.1% vs. 57.8%, (P = 0.026)

Study	Year	Study type	Device	N	Endpoints	Results
EXPIRA [16]	2010	Mono-center RCT	Export (Medtronic)	175	Final MBG ≥ 2.	88% vs. 59%, (P < 0.001)
					STRes > 70%.	63% vs. 39%, (P < 0.001)
					9-month cardiac death.	0.0% vs. 4.6% (P = 0.023)
					2-year cardiac death.	0.0% vs. 6.8% (P = 0.012)
Liistro et al. [17]	2009	Mono-center RCT	Export (Medtronic)	111	STRes.	71% vs. 39% (P = 0.001)
					TIMI ≥ 2 flow.	93% vs. 71% (P = 0.006)
					Myocardial contrast echocardiography score index.	0.86 vs. 0.65 (P < 0.001)
					Improvement in LVEF at 6 months.	48% to 55% vs. 48% to 49% (P < 0.0001)
TAPAS [18]	2008	RCT	Export (Medtronic)	1071	Rate of a MBG 0–1 after procedure.	17.1% vs. 26.3% (P < 0.001)
					Complete STRes.	56.6% vs. 44.2% (P < 0.001)
					Death at 30 days.	2.1% vs. 4.0% (P = 0.07)
					Reinfarction at 30 days.	0.8% vs. 1.9% (P = 0.11)
1-year follow-up of TAPAS [19]	2008	RCT	Export (Medtronic)	1071	Cardiac death at 1 year.	3.6% vs. 6.7% (P = 0.020)
					Cardiac death and non-fatal reinfarction at 1 year.	5.6% vs. 9.9% (P = 0.009)
EXPORT study [20]	2008	Randomized multicenter study	Export (Medtronic)	249	MBG 3 and/or STRes > 50%	85.0% vs. 71.9% (P = 0.025)
					MBG grade 3	35.8% vs. 25.4% (P = 0.094)
					STRes > 50%.	73.5% vs. 64.8% (P = 0.218)
Chao et al [21]	2008	Mono-center RCT	Export (Medtronic)	74	Improvements in TIMI flow (delta TIMI).	2.2 vs. 1.5 (P = 0.014)
					Myocardial blush (delta MBG).	
Lipiecki et al. [22]	2009	Prospective controlled pilot study	Export (Medtronic)	44	Infarct size (SPECT).	2.3 vs. 1.0 (P < 0.001)
						30.6% vs. 28.5% (P < 0.05)
DEAR-MI [23]	2006	Mono-center RCT	Pronto aspiration extraction catheter (Vascular Solutions)	148 with TIMI 0/1 or visible thrombus	STRes ≥ 70%.	68% vs. 50% (P < 0.05)
					MBG of 3.	88% vs. 44% (P < 0.001)
					In-hospital death, reinfarction, LV failure, revascularization.	No statistical significance between groups

(Continued)

Table 10.2 (Continued)

Study name or author [reference]	Year	Design	Thrombectomy device	Patients (n)	Endpoints	Results thrombectomy vs. standard PPCI
De Luca et al. [24]	2006	Mono-center RCT	Diver CE (Invatec)	76	Blush grade 3.	36.8% vs. 13.1% ($P=0.03$)
					STRes.	81.6% vs. 55.3% ($P=0.02$)
					Development of LV dilatation.	19 patients vs. 15 patients ($P=0.006$)
					MACE.	No significant differences
REMEDIA [25]	2005	Mono-center RCT	Diver CE (Invatec)	100	Rate of MBG ≥ 2.	68% vs. 44% ($P=0.020$)
					STRes ≥ 70%.	58% vs. 36.7% ($P=0.034$)
					Rate of patients with MBG ≥ 2 and STRes ≥ 70%.	46% vs. 24.5% ($P<0.025$)
Noel et al. [26]	2004	Mono-center RCT	Export (Medtronic)	50	STRes.	50% vs. 12% ($P=0.037$)

CV, cardiovascular; ISA, incomplete stent apposition; LV, left ventricular; LVEF, left ventricular ejection fraction; MACE, major adverse cardiovascular events; MBG, myocardial blush grade; MI, myocardial; MRI, magnetic resonance imaging; NYHA, New York Heart Association; SPECT, single-photon emission computed tomography; STRes, ST-segment resolution; TIMI, thrombolysis in myocardial infarction.

tomy received a class IIa recommendation in both the European Society of Cardiology (ESC) and American College of Cardiology/American Heart Association guidelines published in 2012 and 2013, respectively [31,32].

The TAPAS trial led to the design of the Thrombus Aspiration in ST-Elevation Myocardial Infarction in Scandinavia (TASTE) trial ($n = 7244$), a registry-based randomized trial in Sweden, published in 2013 and 2014 (30-day and 1-year results, respectively) [12,33]. The primary outcome of mortality was no different (2.8% vs. 3.0%, $P = 0.63$), but there were trends toward reduction in rehospitalization for myocardial infarction (0.5% vs. 0.9%, $P = 0.09$) and stent thrombosis (0.2% vs. 0.5%, $P = 0.06$). There were no significant differences between the groups with respect to the rate of stroke or neurologic complications at the time of discharge ($P = 0.87$). Importantly, the trial had fewer deaths than anticipated (213 vs. 456), so the trial cannot exclude realistic but important reductions in mortality. The 1-year results showed no differences in death from any cause (5.3% vs. 5.6%, $P = 0.57$), rehospitalization for myocardial infarction (2.7% vs. 2.7%, $P = 0.81$) and stent thrombosis (0.7% vs. 0.9%, $P = 0.51$) (33). The TASTE trial design was based on national heart registries and on a secondary randomization that could introduce an initial bias. There were no reported procedural data, such as TIMI flow post-aspiration, MBG or ST-resolution. Finally, the frequency of thrombus score greater than 3 was very low (32%) in the total population.

The results of TASTE influenced practice guidelines as the ESC downgraded the class of recommendation for manual thrombectomy to IIb [34]. Interestingly, a subsequent meta-analysis on manual thrombectomy use that included TASTE continued to suggest an important clinically benefit, as it showed a reduced rate of late (6–12 months) mortality, reinfarction, stent thrombosis and major adverse cardiac events (MACE) in the thrombus aspiration group [35].

The Trial of Routine Aspiration Thrombectomy With PCI vs. PCI Alone in Patients With STEMI (TOTAL) trial was published in 2015, and is the largest randomized, controlled trial of manual thrombectomy to date [10]. The TOTAL trial enrolled 10,731 patients with STEMI and randomized them to upfront manual thrombus aspiration or PCI alone. Within 180 days, routine manual thrombectomy did not reduce the risk of cardiovascular death, recurrent myocardial infarction, cardiogenic shock or New York Heart Association class IV heart failure (composite primary endpoint: 6.9% in the thrombectomy group vs. 7.0% in the control group, $P = 0.86$). The rates of cardiovascular death (3.1% vs. 3.5%, $P = 0.34$) and the primary endpoint, plus stent thrombosis or target-vessel revascularization (9.9% vs. 9.8%, $P = 0.95$) were also similar. There was an increased rate of stroke within 30 days for the thrombectomy group (0.7% vs. 0.3%, $P = 0.02$).

Many reasons could explain the differences between the TASTE and TOTAL trials compared with TAPAS. Mainly, the event rates for the primary endpoints were lower than expected in both TASTE and TOTAL, potentially indicative of a selection bias toward a lower-risk population. There is also a possibility that the embolization of thrombus only plays a small part in the slow flow/no-reflow phenomenon. Aspiration catheters or techniques for using these catheters may also not be sufficient to remove the thrombus, or thrombus aspiration may only be beneficial in patients with a high risk of microembolization. Lastly, although TAPAS was successful, it was still a single-center study, which has to be confirmed in multicenter studies for the procedure to be broadly applicable.

Evidence for Mechanical Thrombectomy

A number of randomized trials have compared thrombectomy using mechanical devices with standard PCI (Table 10.3) [13,36–41,52,43–45].

Table 10.3 Randomized studies showing the effects of mechanical thrombus aspiration.

Study name or author [reference]	Date	Design	Thrombectomy Device	Patients (n)	Endpoints	Results: Thrombectomy vs. Standard PPCI
MUSTELA [13]	2012	Multicenter RCT	Export Catheter (Medtronic) or AngioJet Ultra catheter (Possis Medical)	208 with high thrombus burden	STRes.	57% vs. 37%, (P = 0.004)
					3-month infarct size.	20.4% vs. 19.3%, (P = 0.54)
Ciszewski et al. [36]	2011	Single-center RCT	RESCUE catheter (Boston Scientific/Scimed) and Diver CE (Invatec)	137 with thrombus score of ≥3	Myocardial salvage (SPECT imaging).	25.4% vs. 18.5%, (P = 0.02)
					In-hospital mortality.	3% vs. 4%, (P = 1.0)
JETSTENT [37]	2010	Multicenter, international, randomized, prospective study	AngioJet rheolytic thrombectomy system (Medrad Interventional/ Possis)	501 with evidence of thrombus grade 3–5	STRes.	85.8% vs. 78.8%, (P = 0.043)
					MACE at 6 months.	11.2% vs. 19.4%, (P = 0.011)
					1-year event-free survival rate.	85.2% vs. 75%, (P = 0.009)
VAMPIRE [38]	2008	Single-center RCT	Nipro's TransVascular Aspiration Catheter	355	Final TIMI <3.	12.4% vs. 19.4%, (P = 0.07)
					MBG 3.	46% vs. 20.5%, (P < 0.001)
Andersen et al. [39]	2007	Single-center RCT	RESCUE catheter (Boston Scientific/Scimed)	215	Left ventricular ejection fraction during follow-up.	No significant differences
					Systolic velocities.	Higher in thrombectomy group (P < 0.05)
					Diastolic function.	No significant differences
Kaltoft et al. [40]	2006	Single-center RCT	RESCUE catheter (Boston Scientific/Scimed)	215	Myocardial salvage (sestamibi SPECT), calculated as the difference between area at risk and final infarct size at 30 days.	13% vs. 18%, (P = 0.12)
					Final infarct size.	15% vs. 8%, (P = 0.004)
AIMI [41]	2006	Single-center RCT	Rheolytic thrombectomy a	480	Infarct size (sestamibi SPECT) at 14–28 days.	9.8% vs. 12.5%, (P = 0.03)
					Final TIMI 3 flow.	91.8% vs. 97.0%, (P < 0.02)
					Tissue myocardial perfusion blush.	No significant differences
					STRes.	No significant differences
					MACE at 30 days.	6.7% vs. 1.7%, (P = 0.01)

Study	Year	Study type	Device	Patients	Endpoints	Results
X AMINE ST [42]	2005	Prospective randomized multicenter study	X-Sizer (eV3)	201 with TIMI 0–1 flow	Magnitude of ST-segment resolution 1 hour after PCI. STRes > 50%. MBG grade 3.	7.5 vs. 4.9 mm, (P = 0.033); 68% vs. 53%; (P = 0.037); 30% vs. 31%; (P = NS)
Antoniucci et al. [43]	2004	Single-center RCT	Rheolytic thrombectomy	100	STRes. Corrected TIMI frame count. Infarct size.	90% vs. 72%, (P = 0.022); 18.2 vs. 22.5, (P = 0.032); 13% vs. 21.2, (P = 0.010)
Napodano et al. [44]	2003	Single-center RCT	X-Sizer catheter (EndiCOR Inc.)	92 with evidence of thrombus	Final TIMI 3. MBG 3. STRes > 50%.	93.5% vs. 95.7% (P = 0.39); 71.7% vs. 36.9%, (P = 0.006); 82.6% vs. 52.2% (P = 0.001)
Beran et al. [45]	2002	Single-center RCT	X-sizer	66	Final TIMI 3 flow. MBG and myocardial dye intensity.	90% vs. 84%, (P = NS) No significant differences

MACE, major adverse cardiovascular events; MBG, myocardial blush grade; PPCI, primary percutaneous coronary intervention; RCT, randomized controlled trial; SPECT, single-photon emission computed tomography; STRes, ST-segment resolution; TIMI, thrombolysis in myocardial infarction.

The AngioJet Rheolytic Thrombectomy System

The mechanism of the AngioJet rheolytic thrombectomy system (Medrad, Minneapolis, MN) involves the delivery of pressurized heparinized saline from the catheter where saline jets travel backwards creating a low pressure zone and thus a powerful vacuum effect. Thrombus as a result is drawn back into the catheter where it is fragmented by the saline jets prior to being evacuated from the body. A first study demonstrated a benefit in its use as compared to standard PPCI in terms of infarct size as assessed by Tc-99 m sestamibi scintigraphy and ST-resolution [43]. The larger, multicenter, randomized AiMI trial however failed to reproduce such results [41]. The discrepancy between the two studies could be explained to some extent by the complexity of the device and therefore the importance of operator experience in its use. Furthermore, angiographic evidence of thrombus was absent in a large percentage of both groups (25%) in the AiMI trial suggesting that the AngioJet device is perhaps best suited in cases with high thrombus burden. The JETSTENT trial aimed to answer the questions raised by the previous two conflicting studies [37]. It recruited 501 patients all of whom were treated with dual antiplatelet therapy and GP IIb/IIIa antagonists. The presence of thrombus as a prerequisite for entry into the study was an important difference between the JETSTENT and AiMI studies. Results showed that there was no significant difference in ST-resolution, angiographic endpoints or myocardial infarct size as assessed by 99-Tc-sestamibi scanning between the AngioJet and conventional treatment groups. However, a significant decrease in MACE was noted at 6 and 12 months in the AngioJet group primarily driven by a lower incidence of death and TVR. This was attributed to better myocardial perfusion and to better stent length and diameter assessment following rheolytic thrombectomy.

The X-sizer Device

The X-sizer device (eV3 Inc., MN) consists of a dual-lumen hydrophilic-coated catheter shaft connected to a handheld control module. Once the catheter is engaged the vacuum captures the thrombus and the helical cutter present inside the inner lumen and inside the distal tip shears this off. The efficacy of the X-sizer catheter in STEMI patients has been tested in several randomized trials and although it has been shown to improve ST-resolution post-PCI, achieve better angiographic flow, reduce no-reflow and distal embolization of atherosclerotic plaque debris, its use did not provide significant clinical benefit at 1 and 6 months (X-AMINE ST trial) [42,44,45]. Moreover, the routine use of the X-sizer catheter in PPCI is limited by its rigidity and thus inability to navigate tortuous and heavily calcified vessels as well as risk of vessel perforation.

The Rinspirator System

The Rinspirator system (eV3 Inc., MN) is a newer non-manual thrombectomy device consisting of three lumens. The first lumen allows passage over a standard coronary guidewire whereas the second lumen allows distal aspiration. The third lumen allows injection of a rinsing solution (heparinized saline) through perforations located proximal to the aspiration lumen and distributed circumferentially along a short length of the catheter. This generates turbulent flow that rinses the vessel wall, detaches any adherent thrombus and simultaneously evacuates the thrombotic material from the vessel. The efficacy of this device as an adjunct to PPCI has yet to be evaluated although data from an international registry suggest that delivery of this device is safe and its use does not seem to be associated with higher complication rates [46]. Whether it offers additional benefit over standard PPCI remains to be seen.

Vacuum Aspiration Devices

The Rinspirator, TVAC (Nipro, Japan) and Rescue (Boston Scientific, MA) devices do not offer active thrombus fragmentation but as they are connected to a vacuum motor unit they can be considered as mechanical thrombectomy devices. Only the former has shown some promise based on the results of a multicenter randomized trial (VAMPIRE) [38]. The VAMPIRE study showed a marginal benefit of thrombectomy on myocardial perfusion as assessed by final TIMI flow and MBG with the most benefit observed in patients presenting 6 hours after symptom onset. MACE rates were similar at 30-days to standard PPCI but a significant reduction in MACE was seen at 8 months in the thrombectomy group mainly as a result of lower rates of revascularization in the treatment group. This was attributed to the better TIMI flow following thrombectomy which may have facilitated better selection of stent diameter and length as well as to the removal of inflammatory thrombus material. The use of GP IIb/IIIa inhibitors and drug-eluting stents were not allowed in the VAMPIRE study and it may be that if these had been permitted the rate of future revascularization in the control group may have been more comparable to that of the treatment group. The Rescue system has not been shown to improve infarct size or myocardial salvage as measured by sestamibi SPECT or have a beneficial effect on ST-resolution, MBG and left ventricular ejection fraction in randomized trials. Equally important, it has been associated with a high rate of procedural failure in the randomized trial by Kaltoft et al. due to failure of the catheter to reach the culprit lesion [39,40,47,48].

Conclusions

With the published results of the TOTAL and TASTE trials, it seems certain that there is no clinical benefit of routine thrombus aspiration in patients with STEMI undergoing PPCI. Manual thrombectomy should be considered simply another tool in PPCI that might be useful in selected patients with large thrombus burden and as a bailout procedure. Based on the current evidence, mechanical thrombectomy remains a bailout option in cases of very high thrombus burden not responsive to manual thrombectomy or other measures.

References

1 Bentzon JF, Otsuka F, Virmani R, Falk E. Mechanisms of plaque formation and rupture. *Circ Res*, 2014; 114: 1852–1866.

2 Keeley EC, Boura JA, Grines CL. Primary angioplasty versus intravenous thrombolytic therapy for acute myocardial infarction: a quantitative review of 23 randomised trials. *Lancet*, 2003; 361: 13–20.

3 Henrique JP, Zijlstra F, Ottervanger JP, et al. Incidence and clinical significance of distal embolization during primary angioplasty for acute myocardial infarction. *Eur Heart J*, 2002; 23: 1112–1117.

4 Galasso G, Schiekofer S, D'Anna C, et al. No-reflow phenomenon: pathophysiology, diagnosis, prevention, and treatment. A review of the current literature and future perspectives. *Angiology*, 2014; 65: 180–189.

5 Prasad A, Stone GW, Holmes DR, et al. Reperfusion injury, microvascular dysfunction, and cardioprotection: the "dark side" of reperfusion. *Circulation* 2009; 120: 2105–2112.

6 Niccoli G, Burzotta F, Galiuto L, et al. Myocardial no-reflow in humans. *J Am Coll Cardiol*, 2009; 54: 281–292.

7 Sianos G, Papafaklis MI, Daemen J, et al. Angiographic stent thrombosis after routine use of drug-eluting stents in ST-segment elevation myocardial infarction: the importance of thrombus burden. *J Am Coll Cardiol*, 2007; 50: 573–583.

8 Haeck JD, Verouden NJ, Henriques JP, et al. Current status of distal embolization in percutaneous coronary intervention: mechanical and pharmacological strategies. *Future Cardiol*, 2009; 5: 385–402.

9 Vink MA, Kramer MC, Li X, et al. Clinical and angiographic predictors and prognostic value of failed thrombus aspiration in primary percutaneous coronary intervention. *JACC Cardiovasc Interv* 2011; 4: 634–642.

10 Jolly SS, Cairns JA, Yusuf S, et al. Randomized trial of primary PCI with or without routine manual thrombectomy; TOTAL trial. *N Engl J Med*, 2015; 372(15): 1389–1398.

11 Onuma Y, Thuesen L, van Geuns RJ, et al. Randomized study to assess the effect of thrombus aspiration on flow area in patients with ST-elevation myocardial infarction: An optical frequency domain imaging study; TROFI trial. *Eur Heart J*, 2013; 34: 1050–1060.

12 Fröbert O, Lagerqvist B, Olivecrona GK, et al. Thrombus aspiration during ST-segment elevation myocardial infarction; TASTE trial. *N Engl J Med* 2013; 369(17): 1587–1597.

13 De Carlo M, Aquaro GD, Palmieri C, et al. A prospective randomized trial of thrombectomy versus no thrombectomy in patients with ST-segment elevation myocardial infarction and thrombus-rich lesions: MUSTELA (MUltidevice Thrombectomy in Acute ST-Segment ELevation Acute Myocardial Infarction) trial. *JACC Cardiovasc Interv*, 2012; 5(12): 1223–1230.

14 Stone GW, Maehara A, Witzenbichler B, et al. Intracoronary abciximab and aspiration thrombectomy in patients with large anterior myocardial infarction: the INFUSE-AMI randomized trial. *JAMA*, 2012; 307(17): 1817–1826.

15 Dudek D, Mielecki W, Burzotta F, et al. Thrombus aspiration followed by direct stenting: a novel strategy of primary percutaneous coronary intervention in ST-segment elevation myocardial infarction. Results of the Polish–Italian–Hungarian Randomized ThrombEctomy Trial (PIHRATE Trial). *Am Heart J*, 2010; 160: 966–972.

16 Sardella G, Mancone M, Bucciarelli-Ducci C, et al. Thrombus aspiration during primary percutaneous coronary intervention improves myocardial reperfusion and reduces infarct size: the EXPIRA (thrombectomy with Export Catheter in infarct-related artery during primary percutaneous coronary intervention) prospective, randomized trial. *J Am Coll Cardiol*, 2009; 53: 309–315.

17 Liistro F, Grotti S, Angioli P, et al. Impact of thrombus aspiration on myocardial tissue reperfusion and left ventricular functional recovery and remodeling after primary angioplasty. *Circ Cardiovasc Interv* 2009; 2: 376–83.

18 Svilaas T, Vlaar PJ, van der Horst IC, et al. Thrombus aspiration during primary percutaneous coronary intervention; TAPAS trial. *N Engl J Med* 2008; 358: 557–67.

19 Vlaar PJ, Svilaas T, van der Horst IC, et al. Cardiac death and reinfarction after 1 year in the Thrombus Aspiration during Percutaneous Coronary Intervention in Acute Myocardial Infarction Study (TAPAS): a 1-year follow-up study. *Lancet*, 2008; 371: 1915–1920.

20 Chevalier B, Gilard M, Lang I, et al. Systematic primary aspiration in acute myocardial percutaneous intervention: a multicentre randomised controlled trial of the export aspiration catheter. *Euro Intervention*, 2008; 4: 222–228.

21 Chao CL, Hung CS, Lin YH, et al. Time-dependent benefit of initial thrombosuction on myocardial reperfusion in primary percutaneous coronary intervention. *Int J Clin Pract*, 2008; 62: 555–561.

22 Lipiecki J, Monzy S, Durel N, et al. Effect of thrombus aspiration on infarct size and left ventricular function in high-risk patients with acute myocardial infarction treated by percutaneous coronary intervention: results of a prospective controlled pilot study. *Am Heart J*, 2009; 157(583): e1–e7.

23 Silva-Orrego P, Colombo P, Bigi R, et al. Thrombus aspiration before primary angioplasty improves myocardial reperfusion in acute myocardial infarction: the DEAR-MI (Dethrombosis to Enhance Acute Reperfusion in Myocardial Infarction) Study. *J Am Coll Cardiol*, 2006; 48: 1552–1559.

24 De Luca L, Sardella G, Davidson CJ, et al. Impact of intracoronary aspiration thrombectomy during primary angioplasty on left ventricular remodelling in patients with anterior ST elevation myocardial infarction. *Heart*, 2006; 92: 951–957.

25 Burzotta F, Trani C, Romagnoli E, et al. Manual thrombus-aspiration improves myocardial reperfusion: the randomized evaluation of the effect of mechanical reduction of distal embolization by thrombus-aspiration in primary and rescue angioplasty (REMEDIA) trial. *J Am Coll Cardiol*, 2005; 46: 371–376.

26 Noël B, Morice MC, Lefèvre T, et al. Thromboaspiration in acute ST elevation myocardial infarction improves myocardial perfusion. *Circulation*, 2005; 112: 519.

27 De Luca G, Dudek D, Sardella G, et al. Adjunctive manual thrombectomy improves myocardial perfusion and mortality in patients undergoing primary percutaneous coronary intervention for ST-elevation myocardial infarction: a meta-analysis of randomized trials. *Eur Heart J*, 2008; 29(24): 3002–3010.

28 Costopoulos C, Gorog DA, Di Mario C, et al. Use of thrombectomy devices in primary percutaneous coronary intervention: a systematic review and meta-analysis. *Int J Cardiol*, 2013; 163(3): 229–241.

29 De Luca G, Navarese EP, Suryapranata H, et al. A meta-analytic overview of thrombectomy during primary angioplasty. *Int J Cardiol*, 2013; 166(3): 606–612.

30 Bavry AA, Kumbhani DJ, Bhatt DL, et al. Role of adjunctive thrombectomy and embolic protection devices in acute myocardial infarction: a comprehensive meta-analysis of randomized trials. *Eur Heart J*, 2008; 29(24): 2989–3001.

31 Steg PG, James SK, Atar D, et al. ESC Guidelines for the management of acute myocardial infarction in patients presenting with ST-segment elevation. *Eur Heart J*, 2012; 33(20): 2569–2619.

32 O'Gara P, Kushner F, Ascheim D, et al. 2013 ACCF/AHA guidelines for the management of ST-elevation myocardial infarction. *J Am Coll Cardiol*, 2013; 61(4): e78–e140.

33 Lagerqvist B, Fröbert O, Olivecrona GK, et al. Outcomes 1 year after thrombus aspiration for myocardial infarction. *N Engl J Med*, 2014; 371: 1111–1120.

34 Windecker S, Kolh P, Alfonso F, et al. 2014 ESC/EACTS Guidelines on myocardial revascularization. *Eur Heart J*, 2014; 35(37): 2541–2619.

35 Kumbhani D, Bavry A, Desai M, et al. Aspiration thrombectomy in patients undergoing primary angioplasty: totality of data to 2013. *Catheter Cardiovasc Interv*, 2014; 84: 973–977.

36 Ciszewski M, Pregowski J, Teresińska A, et al. Aspiration coronary thrombectomy for acute myocardial infarction increases myocardial salvage: Single center randomized study. *Catheter Cardiovasc Interv*, 2011; 78: 523–531.

37 Migliorini A, Stabile A, Rodriguez AE, et al. Comparison of AngioJet rheolytic thrombectomy before direct infarct artery stenting with direct stenting alone in patients with acute myocardial infarction. The JETSTENT trial. *J Am Coll Cardiol*, 2010; 12(56): 1298–1306.

38 Ikari Y, Sakurada M, Kozuma K, et al. Upfront thrombus aspiration in primary coronary intervention for patients with ST-segment elevation acute myocardial infarction: Report of the VAMPIRE (VAcuuM asPIration thrombus REmoval) trial. *JACC Cardiovasc Interv*, 2008; 1: 424–431.

39 Andersen NH, Karlsen FM, Gerdes JC, et al. No beneficial effects of coronary thrombectomy on left ventricular systolic and diastolic function in patients with acute S-T elevation myocardial infarction: a randomized clinical trial. *J Am Soc Echocardiogr*, 2007; 20: 724–730.

40 Kaltoft A, Bøttcher M, Nielsen SS, et al. Routine thrombectomy in percutaneous coronary intervention for acute ST-segment elevation myocardial infarction: a randomized, controlled trial. *Circulation* 2006; 114: 40–47.

41 Ali A, Cox D, Dib N, et al. Rheolytic thrombectomy with percutaneous coronary intervention for infarct size reduction in acute myocardial infarction: 30-day results from a multicenter randomized study. *J Am Coll Cardiol* 2006; 48: 244–52.

42 Lefèvre T, Garcia E, Reimers B, et al. X-sizer for thrombectomy in acute myocardial infarction improves ST-segment resolution: results of the X-sizer in AMI for negligible embolization and optimal ST resolution (X AMINE ST) trial. *J Am Coll Cardiol*, 2005; 46: 246–252.

43 Antoniucci D, Valenti R, Migliorini A, et al. Comparison of rheolytic thrombectomy before direct infarct artery stenting versus direct stenting alone in patients undergoing percutaneous coronary intervention for acute myocardial infarction. *Am J Cardiol*, 2004; 15(93): 1033–1035.

44 Napodano M, Pasquetto G, Saccà S, et al. Intracoronary thrombectomy improves myocardial reperfusion in patients undergoing direct angioplasty for acute myocardial infarction. *J Am Coll Cardiol*, 2003;42:1395–1402.

45 Beran G, Lang I, Schreiber W, et al. Intracoronary thrombectomy with the X-sizer catheter system improves epicardial flow and accelerates ST-segment resolution in patients with acute coronary syndrome: a prospective, randomized, controlled study. *Circulation*, 2002; 105: 2355–2360.

46 De Carlo M, Wood DA, Webb JG, et al. Adjunctive use of the Rinspiration system for fluidic thrombectomy during primary angioplasty: the Rinspiration international registry. *Catheter Cardiovasc Interv*, 2008; 72: 196–203.

47 Dudek D, Mielecki W, Legutko J, et al. Percutaneous thrombectomy with the RESCUE system in acute myocardial infarction. *Kardiol Pol*, 2004; 61: 523–533.

48 Kunii H, Kijima M, Araki T, et al. Lack of efficacy of intracoronary thrombus aspiration before coronary stenting in patients with acute myocardial infarction: A multicenter randomized trial. *J Am Coll Cardiol*, 2004; 43: 245A.

11

Choice of Stent in STEMI Interventions

Roopa Salwan MD

           "Choices are journeys not destinations."

Introduction

The urgent restoration of blood flow to the culprit coronary artery is vital after a sudden thrombotic obstruction causes a myocardial infarction with ST-segment elevations on the electrocardiogram. The duration and location of the coronary obstruction and the existence of collateral vessels to the affected myocardial region are the main factors affecting the size of myocardial necrosis and eventually the prognosis of these patients. Since the 1990s, numerous randomized trials have been performed to define the optimal reperfusion therapy in patients with acute ST-elevation myocardial infarction. Primary percutaneous coronary intervention (PPCI) is the preferred treatment, owing to improved vessel patency, decreased infarct size, lower rates of reinfarction and improved survival compared with pharmacological reperfusion, if provided in a timely manner by experienced teams.

Historical Perspective

Primary angioplasty was first performed by Hartzler et al. in 1980 [1]. The first 41 patients reported were treated with PCI either following intracoronary lytic (29 patients with occlusion) or directly (12 patients with subtotal occlusions) with a clinical success rate of 98%. The same group reported results in 1000 consecutive patients, with 94% recanalization rate and 7.8% in-hospital mortality, stroke in 0.5% and major bleeding in 2.8% [2]. Subsequent clinical trials examined the utility of immediate PCI following lytic therapy, found that this strategy was associated with a higher incidence of death, reinfarction and emergency bypass surgery. These results highlighted the complexity of the interaction between mechanical trauma to the vessel wall, a highly thrombogenic milieu, enhanced platelet activation following fibrinolytic therapy, and stimulated intense research into adjunctive pharmacotherapy.

    While relatively small series of PPCI were reporting excellent results in specialized centers, large trials of fibrinolytic therapy were establishing that strategy as the cornerstone of reperfusion therapy in acute myocardial infarction. The first trials randomizing patients to PCI compared with intravenous thrombolytic therapy were not published until 1993 [3–5]. A meta-analysis of 23 studies comparing PPCI to thrombolysis in 7739 patients with ST-elevation

Manual of STEMI Interventions, First Edition. Edited by Sameer Mehta.
© 2017 John Wiley & Sons Ltd. Published 2017 by John Wiley & Sons Ltd.

myocardial infarction (STEMI) demonstrated a clear advantage. PPCI was better than thrombolytic therapy at reducing overall 30-day death (7% vs. 9% $P = 0.0002$), non-fatal reinfarction (3% vs. 7% $P < 0.0001$), stroke (1% vs. 2% $P = 0.0004$), and the combined endpoint of death, non-fatal reinfarction, and stroke (8% vs. 14% $P < 0.0001$) [6].

Overall, the results of PPCI in the first 15 years of fibrinolytic therapy use indicated significant progress in the ability to recanalize acutely occluded arteries, excellent initial outcomes, ability to treat patients who could not be treated with or who would not benefit from fibrinolytic therapy.

Stents in STEMI Interventions: How it all Started

The survival benefit of percutaneous transluminal coronary angioplasty (PTCA) over thrombolytic therapy derives from the higher rates of antegrade epicardial thrombolysis in myocardial infarction (TIMI) grade 3 blood flow, as well as from lower rates of reinfarction and stroke. However, dissection and residual luminal narrowing after PTCA was associated with an incidence of reinfarction of 3–5%, 10% reocclusion rate and a 40% rate of restenosis. With respect to early recurrent ischemia, the Primary Angioplasty in Myocardial Infarction-1 (PAMI-1) investigators have shown that a suboptimal angiographic result after successful primary PTCA is a strong predictor of early major adverse events [2]. However, an acute optimal angiographic result (i.e., the largest minimum luminal diameter achievable) is assumed to be inversely related to late restenosis or reocclusion. It was believed that stent implantation, by mechanical stabilization of the unstable plaque, would give a more predictable initial result of angioplasty and would reduce acute complications. At the same time, there were concerns that implantation of a metallic device within a thrombotic environment, such as that of plaque disruption resulting in myocardial infarction, would be likely to precipitate stent thrombosis, with resultant vessel reocclusion.

The first report of bailout stenting in acute myocardial infarction (AMI) was published in 1991, and the first studies showing the feasibility and efficacy of stenting in patients with AMI with suboptimal results after conventional coronary angioplasty appeared in 1996 [7–11]. At that time, stent thrombosis, with a rate that could be as high as 20% in bailout procedures, had been dramatically reduced to less than 2% by improvement in stent deployment techniques and advances in antiplatelet therapy, allowing a prompt reassessment of the role of stenting in AMI [12,13]. In the Stent PAMI trial, although stenting did reduce the rates of recurrent ischemia and restenosis, the percentage of patients with TIMI grade 3 flow rate was unexpectedly lower after stenting than after PTCA (89.4 %, vs. 92.7% in the angioplasty group; $P = 0.10$), resulting in a strong trend toward increased 6-month mortality rates (4.2 % in the stent group vs. 2.7 % in the angioplasty group ($P = 0.27$) and late mortality rates (1-year mortality 5.8% in stent arm vs. 3.1% in balloon angioplasty arm; $P = 0.07$) [14]. This finding of slower antegrade flow after stenting than after balloon angioplasty was at least partly attributable to the extrusion of thrombus through the stent struts, followed by distal embolization. Because of concern about the possibility of reduced epicardial flow and increased mortality rates, routine stenting in patients with acute myocardial infarction was recommended only for those with suboptimal PTCA results.

At the same time, several randomized trials comparing primary infarct artery stenting with PPCI started. The Florence Randomised Elective Stenting in Acute Coronary Occlusion (FRESCO) trial compared optimal coronary angioplasty with primary infarct artery stenting [15]. After successful primary PTCA, 150 patients were randomly assigned to elective stenting or no further intervention. At 6 months, the recurrent ischemia rate was 9% in the stent group and 28% in the PTCA group ($P = 0.003$). The incidence of restenosis or reocclusion was 17% in the stent group and 43% in the PTCA group ($P = 0.001$). The benefit of stenting was evident both in the early phase (1 month recurrent ischemia rate 3% in stent arm and

15% in angioplasty arm) and the late phase (1–6-month recurrent ischemia rate 7% in stent arm and 16% in angioplasty arm) [15].

In the STENTing in Acute Myocardial Infarction 2 (STENTIM-2) trial, patients with AMI were randomized to a strategy of either systematic or provisional stenting [16]. Results showed that systematic stenting was associated with a significantly lower (25.3% vs. 39.6%) re-stenosis rate. Repeat revascularization rates were 16.8% vs. 26.4% at 6 months and 17.8% vs. 28.2% at 1 year (*P* = 0.1), cross over to stenting was required in 36.4% of patients in the balloon angioplasty group (*P* = 0.0001) [16].

Adjuvant Pharmacotherapy to Optimize Outcomes

Since the thromboemboli that occur after mechanical intervention are rich in platelets, block-ade of glycoprotein IIb/IIIa receptors was believed to have synergistic effect when paired with stent implantation. This was observed in the Abciximab before Direct Angioplasty and Stenting in Myocardial Infarction Regarding Acute and Long-Term Follow-up (ADMIRAL) trial [17], in which abciximab therapy during stenting resulted in improved distal microcirculatory flow capacity with a corresponding improvement in the early recovery of myocardial function. The relative contribution of pharmacotherapy and devices was evaluated in the Controlled Abciximab and Device Investigation to Lower Late Angioplasty Complications (CADILLAC) trial; 2082 patients with acute myocardial infarction were randomized to undergo PTCA alone (518 patients), PTCA plus abciximab therapy (528 patients), stenting alone with the MultiLink stent (512 patients), or stenting plus abciximab therapy (524 patients) [18]. Normal flow was restored in the target vessel in 94.5–96.9% of patients and did not vary according to the reper-fusion strategy. At 6 months, the primary endpoint (a composite of death, reinfarction, disa-bling stroke, and ischemia driven revascularization of the target vessel) had occurred in 20% of patients after PTCA, 16.5% after PTCA plus abciximab, 11.5% after stenting, and 10.2% after stenting plus abciximab (*P* < 0.001). The difference in the incidence of the primary endpoint was entirely due to differences in the rates of target vessel revascularization (ranging from 15.7% after PTCA to 5.2% after stenting plus abciximab, *P* < 0.001). The rate of angiographically established restenosis was 40.8 percent after PTCA and 22.2 percent after stenting (P < 0.001), and the respective rates of reocclusion of the infarcted- related artery were 11.3 percent and 5.7 percent (P = 0.01), both independent of abciximab use.(18) With the lower-profile stents, with better adjunct pharmacotherapy, and possibly better operator technique, the CADILLAC trial removed concerns on increased mortality with stents reported in earlier trials. Routine admin-istration of a thienopyridine (ticlopidine or clopidogrel) and heparin in the emergency room, which has been associated with increased rates of TIMI grade 3 flow before PTCA is likely to have contributed to improve patient outcomes.

After the encouraging results of these studies, BMS quickly became the standard of care for AMI patients. Randomised AMI trials showed a benefit of primary stenting in terms of decreased incidence of early and late target vessel revascularization (TVR) and re-stenosis, but stents did not reduce mortality or improve ventricular function. In-stent re-stenosis (ISR) due to neointimal hyperplasia remained the Achilles heel of the procedure.

Re-stenosis

The incidence and the time course of re-stenosis after bare-metal coronary stenting is similar to that reported for conventional PTCA. The incidence of re-stenosis (defined as a diameter stenosis greater than 50%) was 22% at 3 months, 31.9% at 6 months, and 33.2% at 12 months [19].

Coronary lumen dimensions demonstrated a peak at 3 months. Late loss is generally complete by 9–12 months, after which there is stabilization and often regression of late loss [20].

ISR is not a benign process, and presentation as AMI has been reported in 3.5–20% of patients [21,22]. The mechanism of late myocardial infarction associated with ISR is multi-factorial. A silent occlusive re-stenosis can be difficult to differentiate from a thrombotic event. In addition, a highly stenotic ISR lesion may also promote local non-occlusive thrombosis and lead to a clinical presentation of non-STEMI or troponin-positive unstable coronary syndrome. In the bare-metal stent (BMS) era, ISR has been reported to occur an average of 5.5 months after stent implantation, with a shorter interval for patients presenting with myocardial infarction than those presenting with recurrent angina. Furthermore, diffuse ISR was more frequent in patients with myocardial infarction and correlated with early ISR presentation [23].

Great Expectations: First-Generation Drug-Eluting Stents in STEMI

In the 2000s, drug-eluting stents (DES) emerged as tremendous tools to combat issues related to neointimal hyperplasia and restenosis. The re-stenosis rates with BMS reported to be between 16% and 44% were reduced to single digit with DES, and off-label the benefit was extended to patients with STEMI undergoing PPCI. Reduced rates of target-lesion revascularization with DES, as compared with BMS, in patients with STEMI have been reported in small-to-moderate-size randomized trials; none, however, was powered for safety endpoints, and the routine performance of follow-up angiography may have exaggerated the benefits of DES in many of these studies.

The largest randomized trial was the Harmonizing Outcomes with Revascularization and Stents in Acute Myocardial Infarction (HORIZON AMI) study [24]. This was a prospective, randomized, multicenter trial comparing bivalirudin monotherapy with heparin plus a glyco-protein IIb/IIIa inhibitor and paclitaxel-eluting stents with bare-metal stents in patients with STEMI undergoing a PPCI. Between March 2005 and May 2007, 3606 patients with STEMI undergoing PPCI were randomly allocated to receive either a paclitaxel-eluting stent (PES; 2257 patients, 75%) or a BMS (749 patients, 25%). Patients who received PES had significantly lower 12-month rates of ischemia-driven target lesion revascularization compared with those who received BMS (4.5% vs. 7.5%; $P = 0.002$) and TVR (5.8% vs. 8.7%; $P = 0.006$). The 12-month rates of the primary safety endpoint of major adverse cardiovascular events were similar between patients who received PES and those who received BMS (8.1% and 8.0%, respectively). Patients treated with PES and those treated with BMS had similar 12-month rates of death (3.5% and 3.5%, respectively; $P = 0.98$) and stent thrombosis (3.2% and 3.4%, respectively; $P = 0.77$). The 13-month rate of binary restenosis was significantly lower with paclitaxel-eluting stents than with bare-metal stents (10.0% vs. 22.9; $P < 0.001$). There were no significant differences in the rates of reocclusion of the infarct related artery (TIMI flow grade of 0 or 1), ulceration, ectasia, or aneurysm formation between the stent groups. At 3-year follow-up, compared with the 749 patients who received a BMS, the 2257 patients who received a PES had lower rates of ischemia-driven target lesion revascularization (9.4% vs. 15.1%, $P < 0.0001$), with no significant differences in the rates of death, reinfarction, stroke, or stent thrombosis. Stent thrombosis was high ($\geq 4.5\%$) in both groups [24].

Previous randomized studies in which patients were followed-up beyond 1 year have reported conflicting data for the late safety profile of DES in STEMI [25–31]. However, all these studies were underpowered to examine low frequency adverse event rates, thus increasing the likelihood for false negative (or false positive) findings. These trials included low-risk patients: Exclusion of screened patients was 65% in TYPHOON (trial to assess the use of the CYPHer sirolimus-eluting coronary stent in acute myocardial infarction treated with BallOON angio-plasty) [25], 40% in the Paclitaxel Eluting Stent Versus Conventional Stent in ST-segment Elevation Myocardial Infarction (PASSION) trial [26] and 25% in the SESAMI trial [28]. No significant differences in cardiac death or stent thrombosis were noted between PES and BMS at 5 years in 619 patients in the PASSION trial [26] or between the sirolimus-eluting stent (SES) and BMS at 4 years in 501 patients in the TYPHOON trial [27]. By contrast, cardiac mortality was increased at 3 years in patients with DES rather than BMS in the 626 patients in the DEDICATION trial [31], despite non-significant differences in stent thrombosis and total mortality, and a robust reduction in late target lesion revascularization with DES.

Reality Check: The Shadow of Late Stent Thrombosis

Since the "European Society of Cardiology firestorm" in September 2006, thrombosis of DES has become an important topic for interventional cardiologists and clinicians, despite several analyses showing that the increase of stent thrombosis with DES is modest, with no rise in major events such as death or myocardial infarction (Figure 11.1).

The Drug Eluting Stents in Primary Angioplasty (DESERT) Cooperation was a pooled patient level meta-analysis of randomized trials to evaluate the long-term safety (mortality) and effectiveness (reinfarction, stent thrombosis and TVR) of DES compared with BMS in patients undergoing PPCI for STEMI. Individual patient data were obtained from 11 trials, including a total of 6298 patients, of which 3980 (63.2%) were randomized to DES (99% sirolimus-eluting or paclitaxel-eluting stents) and 2318 (36.8%) to BMS [32]. At long-term follow-up (3.3 ± 1.2 years), a total of 432 patients had died. No significant difference in mortality was observed with DES compared with BMS implantation (8.5% vs. 10.2%, respectively; hazard ratio, HR, 0.85, 95% confidence interval, CI, 0.70–1.04; $P = .11$). There were no differences in cardiac mortality between DES and BMS implantation (5.7% vs. 6.8%, respectively; HR 0.84, 95% CI 0.65–1.09; $P = .19$).

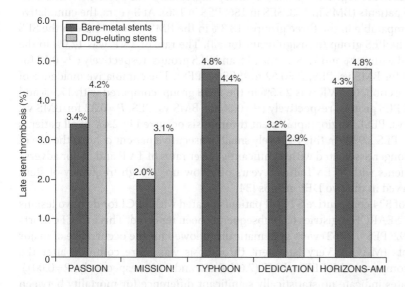

Figure 11.1 Definite or probable late stent-thrombosis after primary percutaneous coronary intervention with either bare-metal or drug-eluting stents in major clinical trials. Stent thrombosis rates were at 5 years for the PASSION trial, at 3 years for MISSION!, 4 years in TYPHOON, 3 years in DEDICATION, and 3 years in HORIZONS-AMI [5].

Reinfarction was observed in a total of 350 patients. No significant difference in reinfarction was observed between DES and BMS implantation (9.4% vs. 5.9%, respectively; HR 1.1, 95% CI 0.88–1.41; P = .36), the hazard ratio changed across time, suggesting that at long-term follow-up (after 2 years from the beginning of the study) the reinfarction rate increased significantly for the DES group compared with the BMS group (HR 2.06, 95% CI 1.22–3.49; P = .03).

Stent thrombosis, according to the Academic Research Consortium definition, was observed in a total of 267 patients (219 definite and 48 probable), the long-term rate of stent thrombosis was not significantly different between DES and BMS implantation (5.8% vs. 4.3%, respectively; HR 1.13, 95% CI 0.86–1.47; P = .38), the hazard ratio changed across time, suggesting that at long-term follow-up (after 2 years from the beginning of the study), the rate of stent thrombosis increased significantly for the DES group compared with the BMS group (HR 2.81, 95% CI 1.28–6.19; P = .04). A total of 837 patients underwent a repeated intervention of the target vessel. DES use significantly reduced the occurrence of TVR compared with BMS use (12.7% vs. 20.1%, respectively; HR 0.57, 95% CI 0.50–0.66; P < .001). Similar findings were observed in terms of target lesion revascularization (10.1% DES vs. 17.9% BMS; HR 0.54, 95% CI 0.45–0.64; P < .001) Reductions in TVR were noted with DES in both the early and very late periods. However, a significantly higher occurrence of very late reinfarction and stent thrombosis was seen with DES compared with BMS.

Registry data have results that differ from randomized studies and have raised very important safety concerns. A so-called "real-world registry" can also reveal the influence of human biases and perception in influencing stent choice. This trend may be evident in the Cleveland Clinic experience, in which the use of DES for PPCI rose rapidly to about 75% of cases after its commercial availability in March 2003, and then fell to only 15% in 2007 – a dramatic turnaround [33]. The reasons for this rapid shift from extreme enthusiasm to extreme caution are unclear, but the reversal serves to remind us of the myriad of factors that influence clinical practice.

The 3-year clinical efficacy of SES and PES compared with BMS in AMI was assessed in the RESEARCH and T-SEARCH registries [34,35]. Primary angioplasty was performed in a consecutive group of 505 patients (BMS in 183, SES in 186, PES in 136). At 3 years, the cumulative mortality rate was comparable in the three groups: 13.3% in the BMS group, 11.5% in the SES group, and 12.4% in the PES group (nonsignificant for all). The rate of TVR was 12.0% in the BMS group, compared with 8.0% and 7.7% in the SES and PES groups, respectively (P = 0.12 for BMS vs. SES, P = 0.30 for BMS vs. PES, P = 0.62 for SES vs. PES). The cumulative incidence of death, myocardial infarction, or TVR was 25.5% in the BMS group, compared with 17.9% and 20.6% in the SES and PES groups, respectively (P = 0.06 for BMS vs. SES, P = 0.32 for BMS vs. PES, P = 0.45 for SES vs. PES). Angiographic stent thrombosis occurred in 2.4% of all patients (BMS 1.6%, SES 2.7%, PES 2.9%). In this relatively small consecutive patient cohort, the use of SES and PES was no longer associated with significantly lower rates of TVR and major adverse cardiac events in patients with STEMI after 3 years of follow-up. A high frequency of stent thrombosis was observed in the two DES groups [34].

A 6-year follow up of 334 consecutive STEMI patients treated with PPCI for de novo lesions in RESEARCH and T-SEARCH registries has subsequently been reported. Three PPCI cohorts (BMS n = 80; SES n = 92; PES n = 162) were systematically followed for the occurrence of major adverse cardiac events (MACE). Very late stent thrombosis was more common after the implantation of SES compared with PES or BMS (7.6%, 0.6%, and 0.0%, respectively; P = 0.001). Kaplan–Meier estimates indicate no statistically significant difference for mortality between the three stent types at 6 years (BMS 25%; SES 15%; PES 21%; log-rank P = 0.2). After adjustment for differences in baseline characteristics, mortality, mortality/myocardial infarction, and MACE rates were significantly lower for SES compared with BMS, but not for PES (adjusted

HR 0.41, 95% CI 0.17–0.98; adjusted HR 0.44, 95% CI 0.21–0.96; adjusted HR 0.35, 95% CI 0.17–0.72, respectively). The use of SES was still associated with a higher rate of very late stent thrombosis compared with PES and BMS at 6 years; however, no events were noted beyond 4 years of follow-up in the three cohorts. The rate of MACE was significantly lower in the SES patients compared with BMS patients, driven primarily by a lower mortality rate at 6 years. No difference was observed in terms of TVR between the three stent types [35].

In an all-inclusive clinical setting, Brodie et al. followed 1640 consecutive patients who underwent PCI for STEMI from 1995 to 2009 for 1–15 years, to evaluate the predictors of stent thrombosis. This population had a high risk profile with Killip class III–IV in 11.5% of patients and STEMI due to stent thrombosis in 10.2% of patients; 1147 were treated with BMS and 410 with DES (366 DES I, 44 DES II). Clinical follow-up was complete to at least 4 years in 85% of patients, with a mean follow-up of 3.7 years. Stent thrombosis continued to increase to at least 11 years with BMS and to at least 4.5 years with DES. The cumulative frequency of stent thrombosis was 2.7% at 30 days, 5.2% at 1 year and 8.3% at 5 years. Stent thrombosis rates with BMS compared with DES were similar at 1 year (5.1% and 4.0%, respectively) but increased more with DES after the first year (1.9%/year vs. 0.6%/year, respectively; Figure 11.2). Landmark analysis (> 1 year) found that DES had a higher frequency of very late stent thrombosis ($P < 0.001$) and reinfarction ($P < 0.003$). DES was the only significant independent predictor of very late stent thrombosis (HR 3.79, 95% CI 1.64–8.79, $P < 0.002$) [36,37].

Stent Thrombosis

The frequency of stent thrombosis after stent implantation for STEMI is relatively high and implantation of stents for STEMI is one of the strongest independent predictors of subsequent stent thrombosis. In addition, the cumulative frequency of stent thrombosis continues to increase out to 3–5 years and beyond [38,39]. Stent thrombosis, although infrequent, remains catastrophic and occupies a central place in the risk benefit equation of DES in PPCI.

The pathophysiology of stent thrombosis is related to the stent, including its geometry (strut thickness, polymer and drug), procedure (including residual dissection and incomplete stent expansion) and patient (including clinical presentation and comorbid conditions), the duration and extent of antiplatelet therapy, and the patient's response to this therapy. Early events may be related to residual target lesion thrombus or dissection, stasis, stent under expansion or a combination of these.

Early stent thrombosis is related to pronounced activation of platelets and the coagulation cascade in the milieu of acute coronary thrombosis. In this context, the permanent polymers of first generation DES (SES and PES) were noted to induce granuloma, hypersensitivity reactions, fibrin deposition, and resulting thrombogenic reactions. Thick stent struts are also associated with increased thrombogenicity related to build up of thrombus in the vicinity of the protruding strut.

Late stent thrombosis is thought to be a chronic process because of delayed arterial healing and vessel remodeling resulting from continual local inflammation from persistence of durable polymers and the long-term effects of eluted drugs. Histopathological and invasive imaging studies following stent thrombosis identify that DES deployment in yellow, vulnerable or ruptured plaque is associated with incomplete endothelialization, less neointima formation, and greater risk for late stent thrombosis. The presence of endothelial coverage may not confer functional integrity and chronic vascular/endothelial dysfunction may contribute to very late stent thrombosis.

In an autopsy study, Nakazawa et al. compared 25 specimens of patients treated for AMI with an underlying necrotic core and a ruptured fibrous cap with 26 specimens of stable angina patients with thick-cap fibroatheroma serving as controls [40]. Histomorphometric analyses

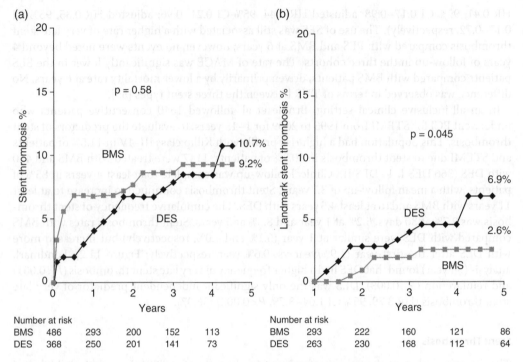

Figure 11.2 Kaplan–Meier estimates of cumulative stent thrombosis rates After primary percutaneous coronary intervention bare-metal (BMS) or drug-eluting stents (DES) for STEMI in the DES Era. A cumulative frequency of ST B landmark analysis showing the cumulative frequency of very late stent thrombosis (> 1 year) comparing BMS and DES.

were performed in those 17 and 18 patients, respectively, who died over 30 days after stent implantation. Late stent thrombosis was significantly more frequent in AMI compared with stable patients (41% versus 11%; $P < 0.04$). The histopathological correlates for this finding were a significantly lower neointimal thickness in AMI patients, with a higher prevalence of stent struts not covered by endothelial cells (49% vs. 9% in stable patients; $P < 0.01$), more fibrin deposits, and more inflammatory cells [40]

The notion of a differential healing response between DES and BMS among STEMI patients is further substantiated in the optical coherence tomography substudy of HORIZON-AMI [41], which observed a higher rate of uncovered and malapposed strut among DES-treated lesions at 13 months. Late acquired stent malapposition (LASM) was more common among DES (31%) than BMS (8%) 13 months after PCI in the intravascular ultrasound substudy of the HORIZON-AMI study [42]. LASM may be related to jailed thrombus. Subsequent resolution or vessel remodeling in response to the drug or polymer is presumably caused by extensive inflammation elicited by DES and highly prevalent among patients presenting with very late stent thrombosis (75%). Because LASM is a dynamic process that appears over time, it may be clinically apparent only during very long-term follow-up. The true cause and effect relationship between imaging findings and clinical outcomes is not clear [42].

In-Stent Re-stenosis in Drug-Eluting Stents

In one study of 39 cases of in-stent re-stenosis (ISR) associated with DES, Lee et al. [43] showed that the mean time from PCI to ISR detection was approximately 12 months. Antiproliferative drugs can delay the biologic response to injury. The time frame to re-stenosis after DES may indeed be longer than that after BMS. The presentation of DES ISR is similar to that of BMS ISR, with approximately 16–66% of patients presenting with unstable angina and 1–20% with myocardial infarction.

In-Stent Neoatherosclerosis

Neoatherosclerotic changes in BMS and DES have been described in an autopsy study of 406 implants. The incidence of neoatherosclerosis was significantly greater in DES lesions (31%) than in BMS lesions (16%; $P < 0.001$). The underlying plaque morphology was different, with unstable lesions (i.e., ruptured plaques and thin-cap fibroatheroma) more commonly found in DES compared with BMS. However, fibrocalcific and pathologic intimal thickening were significantly more frequent in BMS than DES. Nearly one-half the DES lesions with neoatherosclerosis (31 of 64 lesions, 48%) contained peristrut foamy macrophage clusters, and the other half showed fibroatheromas. The median stent duration with neoatherosclerosis was shorter in DES than BMS (DES 420 days, interquartile range, IQR, 361–683 days; BMS, 2160 days, IQR 1800–2880 days], $P < 0.001$). The earliest implant duration showing early atherosclerotic change characterized by foamy macrophage clusters was observed at 70 days for PES and 120 days for SES, whereas its occurrence in BMS was found much later, at 900 days. Similarly, the earliest implant durations for lesions with necrotic cores were relatively short in DES: 270 days and 360 days for SES and PES, respectively, whereas the earliest duration for necrotic core formation in BMS was longer, 900 days. Independent determinants of neoatherosclerosis identified by multiple logistic regression included younger age ($P < 0.001$), longer implant durations ($P < 0.001$), SES use ($P < 0.001$), PES usage ($P < 0.001$), and underlying unstable plaques ($P < 0.004$) [44].

Dawn of a New Era: Second-Generation Drug-Eluting Stents

Very late stent thrombosis rates are indeed higher with DES compared with BMS, but the benefit of reduced re-stenosis with DES might not be worth the increased risk of very late stent thrombosis. New strategies to prevent this complication have been developed, including better deployment techniques, new-generation DES with biocompatible and biomimetic polymers or bioabsorbable polymers, bioabsorbable platforms, and better antiplatelet therapies.

Second-generation DES, such as Xience (everolimus-eluting stent, EES), Endeavor (zotarolimus-eluting stent, ZES), Resolute (ZES-R), have polymers that induce less inflammation because they are biomimetic. They contain phosphatidylcholine (ZES and ZES-R), a component of the cell wall, or are biocompatible, containing acrylic and fluorinated polymers (Xience V and EES), and the biolimus-eluting stent (BES) has a biodegradable polymer. In addition, DES-II have a much thinner coating of permanent polymer and strut thickness than DES-I, making them much more deliverable and allowing for complete endothelial coverage. There are stents with an abluminal coating, with a drug and bioabsorbable polymer likely to promote early and complete endothelization. These changes in polymer may be most beneficial in patients at the highest risk for stent thrombosis – those with STEMI treated by PPCI, and two randomized trials have compared these with BMS [45,46].

Data from Randomized Trials

The EXAMINATION trial was the first trial to compare a second-generation DES with BMS during PPCI. This study was a multicenter, multinational, prospective, randomized, single-blind, controlled trial, held between December 2008 and May 2010; 1498 patients with STEMI treated by PPCI were randomized to receive EES ($n = 751$) or BMS ($n = 747$). Most of the patients included were STEMI less than 12 hours (84.6%). Rescue PCI involved 6.5% of patients, PCI early after successful thrombolysis in 2.3% and, 6.5% were latecomers. At 1 year, the primary endpoint was similar in both groups (11.9% in the EES group vs. 14.2% in the BMS group; difference −2.34, 95% CI −5.75 to 1.07; $P = 0.19$).) [45]. Rates of all-cause mortality (3.5% for EES vs. 3.5% for BMS, $P = 1.00$), cardiac death (3.2% for EES vs. 2.8% for BMS, $P = 0.76$), or myocardial infarction (1.3% vs. 2.0%, $P = 0.32$) did not differ between groups at 2-year follow-up. The patient-oriented endpoint occurred in 17.3% patients in the BMS group and 14.4% patients in the EES group ($P = 0.11$). No significant differences were observed between groups in the rates of all-cause (4.3% for EES vs. 5% for BMS) and cardiac death 3.7% for EES vs. 3.7% for BMS) and any recurrent myocardial infarction (1.9% for EES vs 2.4% for BMS) [46].

At 1 year, rates of target lesion and vessel revascularization were significantly lower in the EES group (2.1% vs. 5.0%, $P = 0.003$, and 3.7% vs 6.8%, $P = 0.0077$, respectively). At two years, rate of target lesion and TVR continued to be significantly lower in the EES group than in the BMS group (2.9% vs. 5.6%; $P = 0.009$, and 4.8% vs. 7.9%; $P = 0.014$ respectively). At 1 year, stent thrombosis rates were significantly lower in the EES group (definite stent thrombosis 0.5% for EES vs. 1.9% for BMS, and definite or probable stent thrombosis 0.9% for EES vs. 2.5% for BMS; both $P = 0.019$). At 2-year follow-up, the rate of definite stent thrombosis remained significantly reduced in the EES group compared with the BMS group (0.8% vs. 2.1%; $P = 0.03$). Overall, the rate of definite or probable stent thrombosis was also reduced in the EES group at 2 years (1.3% vs. 2.8%; $P = 0.04$). There were three episodes of very late definite or probable stent thrombosis in the EES arm and two in the BMS arm. Landmark analyses between 1- and 2-year follow-up did not demonstrate any significant differences in the patient-oriented endpoint ($P = 0.461$), clinically driven target lesion revascularization ($P = 0.511$), or probable/definite stent thrombosis ($P = 0.672$) [45,46].

The Comparison of Biolimus Eluted From an Erodible Stent Coating With Bare Metal Stents in Acute ST-Elevation Myocardial Infarction (COMFORTABLE-AMI) trial was a prospective, randomized, single-blinded, controlled trial of patients presenting with STEMI between September 2009 and January 2011. A total of 1161 patients were randomly assigned to receive BES with biodegradable polymer (578 patients) or BMS (583 patients). At 1 year, the primary endpoint of MACE (cardiac death, target vessel-related reinfarction, and ischemia driven target-lesion revascularization) occurred in 4.3% of patients receiving BES and 8.7% of patients receiving BMS (HR 0.49, 95% CI 0.30–0.80; $P = .004$). The difference was driven by a lower risk of target vessel-related reinfarction (0.5% vs. 2.7%, HR 0.20, 95% CI 0.06–0.69; $P = .01$) and ischemia-driven target-lesion revascularization (1.6% vs. 5.7%, HR 0.28, 95% CI 0.13–0.59; $P < .001$) in patients receiving BES compared with those receiving BMS. Rates of cardiac death were not significantly different (2.9% vs. 3.5%, $P = .53$). Definite stent thrombosis occurred in five patients (0.9%) treated with BES and 12 patients (2.1%, HR 0.42, 95% CI 0.15–1.19; $P = .10$) treated with BMS. Differences between stent types with respect to the primary outcome emerged early and continued throughout the study period. The risk of target vessel-related reinfarction associated with stent thrombosis or re-stenosis was lower among patients treated with BES compared with BMS (HR 0.22, 95% CI 0.06–0.75; $P = .02$). This trial showed better clinical outcomes in terms of MACE of a stent releasing biolimus from a biodegradable polymer compared with a BMS for the treatment of patients with STEMI [47].

Pooled Data from EXAMINATION and COMFORTABLE-AMI

Individual patient data for 2665 STEMI patients enrolled in the EXAMINATION and COMFORTABLE-AMI trials comparing newer-generation DES with BMS were pooled: 1326 patients received a newer-generation DES (EES or biolimus A9-eluting stent), whereas the remaining 1329 patients received a BMS. Pre-specified endpoints of this analysis were the device-oriented composite endpoint of cardiac death, TVR and ischemia-driven target-lesion revascularization, and the patient-oriented endpoint of all-cause death, any myocardial infarction, and any revascularization. DES reduced the device-oriented composite endpoint by 42% compared with BMS (HR 0.58, 95% CI 0.43–0.79; $P < 0.001$). Similarly, the patient-oriented endpoint was significantly reduced with DES (HR 0.76, 95% CI 0.61–0.96; $P = 0.02$). Differences in favor of newer-generation DES were driven by both a lower risk of repeat revascularization of the target lesion (HR 0.32, 95% CI 0.20–0.52; $P < 0.001$) and a lower risk of TVR (HR 0.36, 95% CI 0.14–0.91; $P = 0.032$). No differences were found between groups in terms of all-cause mortality (HR 0.90, 95% CI 0.60–1.35; $P = 0.613$) or cardiac mortality (HR 0.98, 95% CI 0.63–1.51 $P = 0.921$). The risk of either definite or definite/probable stent thrombosis was lower among patients treated with DES than BMS (HR 0.35, 95% CI 0.16–0.75; $P < 0.01$; HR 0.53, 95% CI 0.29–0.95; $P < 0.03$, respectively. The benefit was particularly evident within the first 30 days after implantation. It is interesting to note that a reduction in acute/subacute stent thrombosis was able to reduce target vessel reinfarction but not cardiac mortality. Although the former is strictly dependent on the type of stent implanted, the latter is multifactorial in a STEMI population [48].

The Swedish Coronary Angiography and Angioplasty Register

All consecutive patients in Sweden with STEMI undergoing PPCI from January 2007 to January 2013 were included in the Swedish Coronary Angiography and Angioplasty Register (SCAAR). The new-generation DES group (n-DES) included the Endeavor Resolute, the Xience V and Xience Prime, Promus and Promus Element stents. The old-generation DES group (o-DES) included the Cypher and Cypher Select, Taxus Express and Taxus Liberté, and Endeavor. The BMS group included the Multilink Vision, Multilink MiniVision, Multilink 8, and Multilink Flexmaster, Driver, Micro Driver, and Integrity, Liberté, Coroflex Blue, and Chrono stents. The choice of stent type was at the operator's discretion. In all, 34,147 patients with STEMI were treated by PCI with n-DES ($n = 4811$), o-DES ($n = 4271$), or BMS ($n = 25,065$). A landmark analysis with a pre-specified landmark set at 1 year to provide separate descriptions of the early/late (up to 1 year) and very late risks of ST (later than 1 year) events. Cox regression landmark analysis adjusted by propensity score showed a significantly lower risk of early and late stent thrombosis in the n-DES and o-DES groups. Cox regression analysis showed no statistically significant impact of bivalirudin use (HR 1.17, 95% CI, 0.93–1.46), glycoprotein IIb/IIIa inhibitors (HR 0.95, 95% CI 0.74–1.22), and ticagrelor (HR 1.09, 95% CI 0.49–2.39) on the early stent thrombosis risk up to 30 days. There was no significant difference in the risk of very late stent thrombosis between the n-DES group and the BMS group, whereas a higher risk of very late stent thrombosis was observed in the o-DES group compared with the BMS group. The risk of death was significantly and constantly lower in the n-DES (adjusted HR 0.55, 95% CI 0.48–0.62) and o-DES (adjusted HR 0.58, 95% CI 0.52–0.65) groups compared with the BMS group. A significantly lower risk of stent thrombosis in both the n-DES and o-DES groups was observed only during the first year after PCI, with a rate at 1 year of 0.9% in the n-DES group compared with 1.1% in the o-DES group and 1.5% in the BMS group. The rate in the o-DES group increased by 0.6% during the second year and by 0.4% during the third year of follow-up. The very late stent thrombosis risk up to 3 years was more than doubled in the o-DES group compared with the BMS group (Figure 11.3).

During the first year, the use of second-generation DES was associated with substantial reduction in risk for stent thrombosis: 64% at 30 days and 51% between 31 days and 1 year.

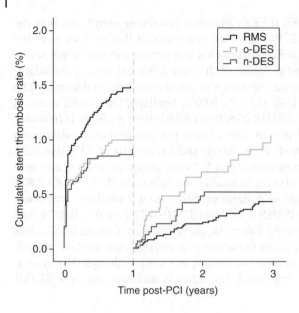

Figure 11.3 Landmark analysis of definite stent thrombosis up to 3 years in the Swedish Coronary Angiography and Angioplasty Register.

In addition, there were significantly lower rates of TVR and myocardial infarction at 1 year with the use of second-generation DES compared with BMS. There were no differences in the overall mortality at 30 days or 1 year with the use of either stent platform for PPCI [49].

Network meta-analysis is a statistical method that is particularly relevant when there are multiple treatment evidence structures with limited direct evidence addressing the research question at hand. A network meta-analysis allows to create a cyclic evidence network where indirect evidence can augment evidence from direct comparisons. Philip et al. used network meta-analysis to pool direct (comparison of second-generation DES to BMS) and indirect (first-generation DES with BMS and second-generation DES) evidence from the randomized trials (Figure 11.4). Twenty-one trials comparing all stents types, including 12,866 patients randomly assigned to treatment groups, were analyzed [50].

There was a significant 64% reduction in the incidence of early stent thrombosis and a 51% reduction in the incidence of late stent thrombosis with the use of second-generation DES when compared with BMS (30 days odds ratio, OR, 0.36, 95% CI 0.15–0.82, and between 31 days and 1 year OR 0.49, 95% CI 0.30–0.79). Second-generation DES was associated with significantly lower incidence of stent thrombosis at 1 year (OR 0.3, 95% CI 0.11–0.83) and myocardial infarction (OR 0.3, 95% CI 0.17–0.54) and TVR at 1 year (OR 0.54, 95% CI 0.80–0.98) when compared with BMS. There was no difference in mortality at 30 days (OR 0.84, 95% CI 0.45–1.59) or 1 year (OR 0.80, 95% CI 0.56–1.14) with the use of second-generation DES versus BMS. After exclusion of patients from Asia (where reported rates of stent thrombosis are low) and the COMFORTABLE-AMI trial (not a Federal Drug Administration approved stent), there was still a significantly lower incidence of stent thrombosis with second-generation DES when compared with BMS (OR 0.20, 95% CI 0.34–0.78). After excluding the EXAMINATION trial, a nonsignificant 43% reduction in the incidence of stent thrombosis (OR 0.57, 95% CI 0.30–1.0) at 1 year was noted (Figure 11.5).

In another network meta-analysis, Banglore et al. studied 14,740 patients with STEMI from 28 randomized clinical trials with 34,068 patient-years of follow-up (Table 11.1) [51]. When compared with BMS, DES (SES, PES, EES, ZES) were associated with a statistically significant reduction in rate of TVR. There was no increase in the risk of death, myocardial infarction, or stent thrombosis

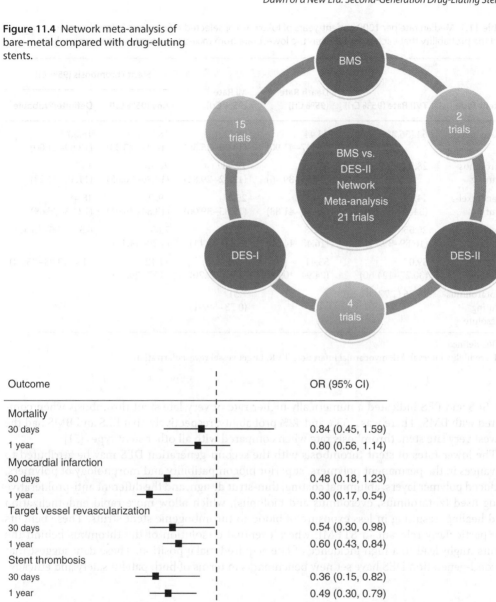

Figure 11.4 Network meta-analysis of bare-metal compared with drug-eluting stents.

Outcome		OR (95% CI)
Mortality		
30 days		0.84 (0.45, 1.59)
1 year		0.80 (0.56, 1.14)
Myocardial infarction		
30 days		0.48 (0.18, 1.23)
1 year		0.30 (0.17, 0.54)
Target vessel revascularization		
30 days		0.54 (0.30, 0.98)
1 year		0.60 (0.43, 0.84)
Stent thrombosis		
30 days		0.36 (0.15, 0.82)
1 year		0.49 (0.30, 0.79)

0 — Favors DES II   1 — Odds ratio   2 — Favors BMS

Figure 11.5 Pooled odds ratio (OR) of outcomes of all the randomized trials in the network meta-analysis (BMS, bare-metal stent; CI, confidence interval; DES, drug-eluting stent) [49].

with any DES compared with BMS. EES was associated with statistically significant lower rate of any stent thrombosis when compared with SES (62% reduction) and PES (61% reduction). There was a 74% probability that EES had the lowest rate of any stent thrombosis when compared with all other stent types (no data on ZES Resolute). There was no increase in very late stent thrombosis with EES versus BMS (RR 0.89, 95% CI 0.09–8.67). However, the point estimate

Table 11.1 Median rate per 1000 patient-years of follow-up of selected efficacy and safety outcomes and the probability that each stent type has the lowest rate from mixed treatment comparison analysis.

Stent Type	TVR Rate (95% CrI)	Death Rate (95% CrI)	MI Rate (95% CrI)	Stent Thrombosis (95% CI)	
				Any (95% CrI)	Definite/Probable[a]
Bare metal	64 (56.31–72.42)	35.44 (29.47–41.90)	19.77 (14.39–25.59)	18.54 (14.44–23.33)	16.60 (12.69–21.00)
Sirolimus-eluting	28.93 (23.26–35.5)	31.33 (24.55–39.46)	19.93 (12.72–29.84)	20.20 (14.86–26.65)	15.75 (11.43–21.23)
Paclitaxel-eluting	44.38 (34.45–56.16)	32.67 (25.37–41.88)	25.37 (15.85–39.06)	19.70 (13.84–26.64)	18.46 (12.25–26.69)
Everolimus-eluting	26.55 (16.89–39.71)	27.38 (16.43–44.50)	12.22 (5.32–27.11)	7.65 (4.20–14.15)	6.54 (2.95–13.42)
Zotarolimus-eluting	59.07 (30.27–124.60)	53.41 (24.94–105.80)	7.76 (1.94–27.20)	11.12 (3.77–29.54)	11.41 (3.88–25.34)
Zotarolimus-eluting Resolute	14.76 (1.77–81.13)	–	7.51 (0.73–59.91)	–	–

[a] ARC defined.

CrI, credibility interval; MI, myocardial infarction; TVR, target vessel revascularization.

for SES and PES indicated a numerically higher rate of very late stent thrombosis when compared with BMS. There was a 53% and 42% probability, respectively, that EES and BMS had the lowest very late stent thrombosis rate when compared with all other stent types [51].

The lower rates of stent thrombosis with the second-generation DES may be attributed to advances in the permanent polymers, superior biocompatibility and morphology of polymers, reduced polymer layers, abluminal coating, thin-strut design, and the different anti-proliferative drug used (zotarolimus, everolimus and biolimus), which allow more rapid endothelization and healing, resulting in less exposure of blood to thrombogenic stent struts. These benefits are particularly relevant in STEMI, where eventual dissolution of the thrombus behind the struts might lead to a high incidence of late acquired malapposition. These data suggest that second-generation DES have set new benchmarks in terms of both patient safety and efficacy.

The Emperor's New Clothes

Self-Expanding Drug-Eluting Stent

Stent malapposition has been demonstrated as a contributor to clinical events on follow.up. A self-expanding SES (STENTYS Self-Apposing®) was designed to overcome this limitation of balloon-expandable stents, with the hope that correct stent sizing and elimination of malapposition after PPCI would improve the long-term outcome for patients. The unique self-apposing technology enables full vessel apposition in thrombus-laden lesions when vessel sizing is unclear. Complete apposition allows effective elution of the drug into the vessel wall, minimizing late lumen loss without compromising healing. The polymer, polysulfone, is a hemocompatible, noninflammatory and nonthrombogenic polymer, allows for a more rapid re-endothelialization of the vessel. The drug, sirolimus, is mixed into the excipient $(1.4\,\mu g/mm^2)$, and is released as the excipient dissolves. This stent maintains full apposition with the vessel wall in situations such as STEMI, where there is significant change in the vessel after an acute procedure; that is, it accommodates early changes in the vessel caused by thrombus dissolution and resolution of vessel spasm. The reference vessel has shown a 19% increase in lumen area distal to the occlusion at 3 days in STEMI patients.

In the APPOSITION IV trial, patients were randomized to self-expanding SES ($n = 90$) or the balloon-expandable ZES ($n = 62$) and were evaluated at 4 months and 9 months by optical coherence tomography [51]. The mean lumen diameter was larger at 4 months and 9 months in the SES self-expanding stent group and late lumen loss was 0.08 mm at 4 months and 0.04 mm at 9 months compared with 0.18 mm and 0.17 mm in the ZES group. However, clinically driven TLR was greater (4.7% vs. 1.7%), rates of stent thrombosis (definite/probable) were higher (3.4% vs. 1.8%) and overall MACE tended to be higher (8% vs. 4.9%). These numbers were not statistically significant in view of small sample size, nevertheless they are important observations [52].

Balloon-Expandable Mesh-Covered Stent

During PPCI, distal embolization of thrombus and friable atheromatous debris leading to impaired myocardial perfusion are ubiquitous and contribute to a decrease in stent thrombosis resolution, and an increase in infarct size and mortality. Although conventional stent implantation appeared to be superior to balloon angioplasty in STEMI patients, there has been no evidence of improved myocardial flow, decreased embolization, or improvement in left-ventricular function.

The MGuard Prime™ stent is a balloon-expandable cobalt–chromium stent with a strut thickness of 80 μm, crossing profile of 1.0–1.2 mm, covered with polyethylene terephthalate mesh (20 μm fiber width with net aperture size 150–180 μm) on its outer surface, which is designed to trap and exclude thrombus against the wall of the artery, thereby preventing distal embolization.

The MASTER Trial randomized patients to MGuard ($n = 217$) or BMS/DES ($n = 216$). The primary end point of ST-resolution at 60–90 minutes post procedure was significantly improved in those randomized to the MGuard stent (57.8% vs. 44.7%, $P = 0.008$). In core laboratory analysis, the MGuard stent also resulted in superior rates of TIMI 3 flow (91.7% vs. 82.9% $P = 0.006$), with comparable rates of MBG 2 or 3 (83.9% vs. 84.7%). At 30 days, for patients receiving MGuard stent, reinfarction and thrombosis rates were 1.4% compared with 0.9%, and ischemia-driven TVR were found in 2.8% compared with 0.5%. Among the patients in whom cardiac MRI was performed, there was no significant difference in infarct size or microvascular obstruction between the two groups.

Thirty-day results from the MASTER II trial, which enrolled 310 of a planned 1114 patients, have been presented. The trial was suspended in October 2014 as a result of a corporate shift in strategy to a next-generation MGuard DES platform. MASTER II did not show a difference in ST-segment resolution between MGuard and control stents (FDA-approved BMS or DES; 56.9% vs. 59.3%; $P = 0.68$). Pooled data between MASTER I and MASTER II for ST-resolution continued to favor MGuard (57.5% vs. 50.7% for the control group; $P = 0.07$). Thirty-day mortality results for the MGuard in the MASTER II trial remained low (0.6% vs. 1.9%, $P = 0.62$), consistent with all previous MGuard trials and registries, and the rate of overall MACE was favorable for MGuard (2.6% vs. 4.5%; $P = 0.36$). Pooled mortality data for MASTER I and II showed a statistically significant reduction in mortality with MGuard (0.3% vs. 1.9%; $P = 0.04$). Infarct size, another important indicator of mortality, showed a positive trend for MGuard in MASTER II (mean 22.60% vs. 27.48%; $P = 0.16$), as well as in the pooled analysis (mean 18.80% vs. 22.24%; $P = 0.26$) [53].

In the REWARD MI study, 262 patients were included from a single center, of which 35.9% had an MGuard stent implanted. The mean follow-up was 321 ± 12.94 days. There was no difference in mortality (7.6% in both groups) or non-fatal myocardial infarction (6.3% in both groups), but target-lesion revascularization was significantly higher in the MGuard group (11.4% vs. 1.3%; $P < 0.01$) [54].

Bioresorbable Vascular Scaffold in acute Myocardial Infarction

The concept of a stent that supports the vessel wall in the acute stage to prevent abrupt closure, and at the same time eluting an anti-proliferative agent to prevent re-stenosis, and later dissolving when its job is done so that there is no long-term risk of late stent thrombosis, was realized in form of Absorb™ bioresorbable vascular scaffold (BVS).

The Bioresorbable Vascular Scaffold: A Clinical Evaluation of Everolimus Eluting Coronary Stents in the Treatment of Patients With ST-segment Elevation Myocardial Infarction (BVS-EXAMINATION) trial [55] included 290 consecutive STEMI patients treated by BVS, compared with either 290 STEMI patients treated with EES or 290 STEMI patients treated with BMS from the EXAMINATION trial. The cumulative incidence of device-oriented endpoints, including cardiac death, target vessel myocardial infarction, and target-lesion revascularization, did not differ between the BVS and EES or BMS groups either at 30 days (3.1% vs. 2.4%, $P = 0.593$ vs. 2.8%, $P = 0.776$, respectively) or at 1 year (4.1% vs. 4.1%, $P = 0.994$; vs. 5.9%, $P = 0.306$, respectively). Definite and probable BVS thrombosis rate was numerically higher either at 30 days (2.1% vs. 0.3%, $P = 0.059$ vs. 1%, $P = 0.324$, respectively) or at 1 year (2.4% vs. 1.4%, $P = 0.948$ vs. 1.7%, $P = 0.825$, respectively), as compared with EES or BMS [55].

The present generation BVS is a bulky device with 150 μm struts that protrude further into the vessel wall, so theoretically flow disturbances and resulting endothelial shear stress may further promote a prothrombotic milieu in the setting of STEMI. BVS, because of its bulky structure, may not be the ideal stent in the AMI setting, especially in large thrombus lesions, but the concept of the bioresorbable scaffold holds promise. Refinement in stent design and large-scale clinical outcome studies are required, however, before these devices can be recommended.

Conclusion

Stenting of the infarct-related artery during PPCI allows an optimal restoration of flow and improves patient outcomes. BMS have been considered the benchmark for safety for patients with STEMI. Initial registry studies and clinical trials showed no benefit of DES in preventing restenosis in patients with STEMI, and a numeric excess of stent thrombosis when compared with BMS. The 2013 American College of Cardiology/American Heart Association guidelines for the management of patients with STEMI list a class IIa recommendation for the use of DES as an alternate to BMS for PPCI in STEMI [56]. Randomized trial and registry data in the past few years have conclusively shown that second-generation DES are more effective and potentially safer than BMS during PPCI in STEMI. In view of these data, in the 2014 European Society of Cardiology/European Association for Cardio-Thoracic Surgery guidelines on myocardial revascularization, new-generation DES are recommended over BMS in PPCI (class Ia recommendation) [57]. It is time to extend these benefits to all patients with STEMI treated by PPCI. In addition to the optimal use of stents, secondary prevention as adjunctive therapy to revascularization is crucial to improving patient-related outcomes.

References

1 Hartzler GO, Rutherford, McConahay DR, et al. Percutaneous transluminal angioplasty with and without thrombolytic therapy for treatment of acute myocardial infarction. *Am Heart Journal*, 1983; 106: 965–73.

2 O'Keef JH, Jr Bailey WL, Rutherford BD, et al. Primary angioplasty for acute myocardial infarction in 1000 consecutive patients. Results in an unselected population and high risk subgroups. *Am J Cardiol*, 1993; 72: 107G–115G.

3 Grines CL, Browne KR, Marco J, et al. A comparison of primary angioplasty with thrombolytic therapy for acute myocardial infarction. *N Engl J Med*, 1993; 328: 673–679.

4 Zijlstra F, DeBoer MJ, Hoorntje JCA. A comparison of immediate coronary angioplasty with intravenous streptokinase in acute myocardial infarction. *N Engl J Med*, 1993; 328: 680–684.

5 Gibbons RJ, Holmes DR, Reeder GS, et al. Immediate angioplasty compared with the administration of a thrombolytic agent followed by conservative treatment for myocardial infarction. *N Engl J Med*, 1993; 328: 685–691.

6 Keeley EC, Boura JA, Grines CL. Comparison of primary angioplasty and intravenous thrombolytic therapy for acute myocardial infarction: a quantitative review of 23 randomised trials. *Lancet*, 2003; 361: 13–20.

7 Cannon AD, Roubin GS, Macander PJ, et al. Intracoronary stenting as an adjunct to angioplasty in acute myocardial infarction. *J Invasive Cardiol*, 1991; 3: 255–258.

8 Garcia-Cantu E, Spaulding C, Corcos T, et al. Stent implantation in acute myocardial infarction. *Am J Cardiol*, 1996; 77: 451–454.

9 Rodriguez AE, Fernandez M, Santaera O, et al. Coronary stenting in patients undergoing percutaneous coronary angioplasty during acute myocardial infarction. *Am J Cardiol*, 1996; 77: 685–689.

10 Antoniucci D, Valenti R, Buonamici P, et al. Direct angioplasty and stenting of the infarct-related artery in acute myocardial infarction. *Am J Cardiol*, 1996; 78: 568–571.

11 Saito S, Hosokawa G, Kunikane K, et al. Primary stent implantation without coumadin in acute myocardial infarction. *J Am Coll Cardiol*, 1996; 28: 74–81.

12 Colombo A, Hall P, Nakamura S, et al. Intracoronary stenting without anticoagulation accomplished with intravascular ultrasound guidance. *Circulation* 1995; 91: 1676–88.

13 Leon MB, Baim DS, Popma JJ, et al. A clinical trial comparing three anti thrombotic drug regimens after coronary artery stenting. *N Engl J Med*, 1998; 339: 1665–1671.

14 Grines CL, Cox DA, Stone GW, et al. Coronary angioplasty with or without stent implantation for acute myocardial infarction. Stent Primary Angioplasty in Myocardial Infarction Study Group. *N Engl J Med*, 1999; 341: 1949–1956.

15 Antonuucci D, Santoro GM, Bolognese L, et al. A clinical trial comparing primary stenting of the infarct-related artery with optimal primary angioplasty for acute myocardial infarction results from the Florence Randomized Elective Stenting in Acute Coronary Occlusions (FRESCO) Trial. *J Am Coll Cardiol*, 1998; 31: 1234–1239.

16 Maillard L, Hamon M, Khalife K, et al. A comparison of systematic stenting and conventional balloon angioplasty during primary percutaneous transluminal coronary angioplasty for acute myocardial infarction. STENTIM-2 Investigators. *J Am Coll Cardiol*, 2000; 35(7): 1729–1736.

17 Montalescot G1, Barragan P, Wittenberg O, et al. Abciximab before direct angioplasty and stenting in myocardial infarction regarding acute and long-term follow-up. Platelet glycoprotein IIb/IIIa inhibition with coronary stenting for acute myocardial infarction. *N Engl J Med*, 2001; 344(25): 1895–1903.

18 Stone GW, Grines CL, Cox DA, et al.Comparison of angioplasty with stenting, with or without abciximab in acute myocardial infarction. *N Engl J Med*, 2002; 346: 957–966.

19 Kastrati A, Schomig A, Dietz R, et al. Time course of restenosis during the first year after emergency coronary stenting. *Circulation*, 1993; 87: 1498–1505.

20 Kimura T, Yokoi H, Nakagawa Y, et al. Three-year follow-up after implantations of metallic coronary artery stents. *N Engl J Med*, 1996; 334: 561–566.

21 Bossi I, Klersy C, Black AJ, et al. In-stent restenosis: long-term outcome and predictors of subsequent target lesion revascularization after repeat balloon angioplasty. *J Am Coll Cardiol*, 2000; 35: 1569–1576.

22 Chen MS, John JM, Chew DP, et al. Bare metal stent restenosis is not a benign clinical entity. *Am Heart J*, 2006; 151: 1260–1264.

23 Nayak AK, Kawamura A, Nesto RW, et al. Myocardial infarction as a presentation of clinical in-stent restenosis. *Circ J*, 2006; 70: 1026–1029.

24 Stone GW, Witzenbichler B, Guagliumi G, et al. Heparin plus a glycoprotein IIb/IIIa inhibitor vs. bivalirudin monotherapyand paclitaxel-eluting stents vs. bare-metal stents in acute myocardial infarction (HORIZONS-AMI): final 3-year results from a multicentre, randomised controlled trial. *Lancet*, 2011; 377(9784): 2193–2204.

25 Valgimigli M, Campo G, Percoco G, et al. Comparison of angioplasty with infusion of tirofi ban or abciximab and with implantation of sirolimus-eluting or uncoated stents for acute myocardial infarction: the MULTISTRATEGY randomized trial. *JAMA*, 2008; 299: 1788–1799.

26 Vin MA, Dirksen MT, Suttorp MJ, et al. 5-year follow-up after primary percutaneous coronary intervention with a paclitaxel-eluting stent versus a bare-metal stent in acute ST-segment elevation myocardial infarction. *J Am Coll Cardiol Interv*, 2011; 4: 24–29.

27 Spaulding C, Teiger E, Commeau P, et al. Four-year follow-up of TYPHOON (trial to assess the use of the cypher sirolimus-eluting coronary stent in acute myocardial infarction treated with balloon angioplasty). *J Am Coll Cardiol Interv*, 2011; 4: 14–23.

28 Violini R, Musto C, De Felice F, et al. Maintenance of long-term clinical benefit with sirolimus-eluting stents in patients with ST-segment elevation myocardial infarction 3-year results of the SESAMI (sirolimus-eluting stent versus bare-metal stent in acute myocardial infarction) trial. *J Am Coll Cardiol*, 2010; 55: 810–814.

29 Di Lorenzo E, Sauro R, Varricchio A, et al. Long-term outcome of drug-eluting stents compared with bare metal stents in ST-segment elevation myocardial infarction: results of the paclitaxel- or sirolimus-eluting stent versus bare metal stent in Primary Angioplasty (PASEO) Randomized Trial. *Circulation*, 2009; 120: 964–972.

30 Atary JZ, van der Hoeven BL, Liem SS, et al. Three-year outcome of sirolimus-eluting versus bare-metal stents for the treatment of ST-segment elevation myocardial infarction (from the MISSION Intervention Study). *Am J Cardiol*, 2010; 106: 4–12.

31 Kaltoft A, Kelbaek H, Thuesen L, et al. Long-term outcome after drug-eluting versus bare-metal stent implantation in patients with ST-segment elevation myocardial infarction: 3-year follow-up of the randomized DEDICATION (Drug Elution and Distal Protection in Acute Myocardial Infarction) Trial. *J Am Coll Cardiol*, 2010; 56: 641–645.

32 De Luca G, Dirksen MT, Spaulding C, et al. Drug eluting versus bare metal stent in primary angioplasty for the drug eluting stent in primary angioplasty (DESERT) Cooperation. *Arch Intern Med*, 2012; 172(8): 611–621.

33 Shishehbor MH, Amini R, Oliveria LPJ, et al. Comparison of drug-eluting stents versus bare-metal stents for treating ST-segment elevation myocardial infarction. *J Am Coll Cardiol Interv*, 2008; 1: 227–232.

34 Daemen J, Tanimoto S, Garcia-Garcia HM, et al. Comparison of three-year clinical outcome of sirolimus- and paclitaxel-eluting stents versus bare-metal stents in patients with ST-segment

elevation myocardial infarction (from the RESEARCH and T-SEARCH Registries). *Am J Cardiol*, 2007; 99: 1027–1032.

35 Simsek C, Magro M, Boersma E, et al. Comparison of six-year clinical outcome of sirolimus- and paclitaxel-eluting stents to bare-metal stents in patients with ST-segment elevation myocardial infarction: an analysis of the RESEARCH (rapamycin-eluting stent evaluated at Rotterdam cardiology hospital) and T-SEARCH (taxus stent evaluated at Rotterdam cardiology hospital) registries. *J Invasive Cardiol*, 2011; 23(8): 336–341.

36 Brodie B, Pokharel Y, Fleishman N, et al. Very late stent thrombosis after primary percutaneous coronary intervention with bare-metal and drug-eluting stents for ST-segment elevation myocardial infarction: A 15-year single-center experience. *J Am Coll Cardiol Interv*, 2011; 4: 30–38.

37 Brodie B, Pokharel Y, Garg A, et al. Predictors of early, late, and very late stent thrombosis after primary percutaneous coronary intervention with bare-metal and drug-eluting stents for ST-segment elevation myocardial infarction. *J Am Coll Cardiol Interv*, 2012; 5: 1043–1051.

38 Lagerqvist B, Carlsson J, Fröbert O. Stent thrombosis in sweden a report from the Swedish Coronary Angiography and Angioplasty Registry. *Circ Cardiovasc* Interv, 2009; 2: 401–408.

39 Kukreja N, Onuma Y, Garcia-Garcia HM, et al. The risk of stent thrombosis in patients with acute coronary syndromes treated with bare-metal and drug-eluting stents. *J Am Coll Cardiol Interv*, 2009; 209: 534–541.

40 Nakazawa G, Finn AV, Joner M, et al. Delayed arterial healing and increased late stent thrombosis at culprit sites after drug-eluting stent placement for acute myocardial infarction patients: an autopsy study. *Circulation*, 2008; 118: 1138–1145.

41 Guagliumi G, Costa MA, Sirbu V, et al. Strut coverage and late malapposition with paclitaxel eluting stents compared with bare metal stents in acute myocardial infarction: optical coherence tomography substudy of HORIZON-AMI Trial. *Circulation*, 2011; 123: 274–281.

42 Choi SY, Witzenbichler B, Maehara A, et al. Intravascular ultrasound findings of early stent thrombosis after primary percutaneous intervention in acute myocardial infarction: a Harmonizing Outcomes with Revascularization and Stents in Acute Myocardial Infarction (HORIZONS-AMI) substudy. *Circ Cardiovasc Interv*, 2011; 4(3): 239–2347.

43 Lee MS, Pessegueiro A, Zimmer R, et al. Clinical presentation of patients with in-stent restenosis in the drug-eluting stent era. *J Invasive Cardiol*, 2008; 20: 401–403.

44 Nakazawa G, Otsuka F, Nakano M, et al. The pathology of neoatherosclerosis in human coronary implants bare-metal and drug-eluting stents. *J Am Coll Cardiol*, 2011; 57: 1314–1322.

45 Sabate M, Cequier A, Iniguez A, et al. Everolimus-eluting stent versus bare-metal stent in ST-segment elevation myocardial infarction (EXAMINATION): 1 year results of a randomised controlled trial. *Lancet* 2012; 380: 1482–1490.

46 Sabaté M, Brugaletta S, Cequier A, et al. The EXAMINATION Trial (Everolimus-Eluting Stents Versus Bare-Metal Stents in ST-Segment Elevation Myocardial Infarction) 2-year results from a multicenter randomized controlled trial. *J Am Coll Cardiol Interv*, 2014; 7: 64–71.

47 Raber L, Kelbaek H, Ostojic M, et al. Effect of biolimus-eluting stents with biodegradable polymer vs. bare-metal stents on cardiovascular events among patients with acute myocardial infarction: the COMFORTABLE AMI randomized trial. *JAMA*, 2012; 308(8): 777–787.

48 Sabate M, Raber L, Heg D, et al. Comparison of newer-generation drug-eluting with bare-metal stents in patients with acute st-segment elevation myocardial infarction: a pooled analysis of the EXAMINATION (clinical Evaluation of the Xience-V stent in Acute Myocardial INfArc-TION) and COMFORTABLE-AMI (Comparison of Biolimus Eluted From an Erodible Stent Coating With Bare Metal Stents in Acute ST-Elevation Myocardial Infarction) trials. *JACC Cardiovasc Interv*, 2014; 7(1): 55–63.

49 Sarno G, Lagerqvist B, Nilsson J, et al. Stent thrombosis in new-generation drug-eluting stents in patients with stemi undergoing primary PCIA, report from SCAAR. *J Am Coll Cardiol*, 2014; 64: 16–24.

50 Philip F, Agarwal S, Bunte MC, et al. Stent thrombosis with second-generation drug-eluting stents compared with bare-metal stents network meta-analysis of primary percutaneous coronary intervention trials in ST-segment-elevation myocardial infarction. *Circ Cardiovasc Interv*, 2014; 7: 49–61.

51 Bangalore S, Amoroso N, Fusaro M, et al. Outcomes with various drug-eluting or bare metal stents in patients with ST-segment-elevation myocardial infarction a mixed treatment comparison analysis of trial level data from 34,068 patient-years of follow-up from randomized trials. *Circ Cardiovasc Interv* 2013; 6(4): 378–390.

52 van Geuns RJ, Tamburino C, Fajadet J, et al. Self-expanding versus balloon-expandable stents in acute myocardial infarction: results from the APPOSITION II Study: Self-expanding stents in ST-segment elevation myocardial infarction. *JACC Cardiovasc* Interv, 2012; 5(12): 1209–1219.

53 Stone GW, Abizaid A, Silber S, et al. Prospective, randomized, multicenter evaluation of a polyethylene terephthalate micronet mesh-covered stent (MGuard) in ST-segment elevation myocardial infarction: The MASTER trial. *J Am Coll Cardiol*, 2012; 60(19): 1975–1984.

54 Fernández-Cisnal A, Cid-Álvarez B, Álvarez-Álvarez B, et al. Real world comparison of the MGuard Stent versus the bare metal stent for ST elevation myocardial infarction (the REWARD-MI study). *Catheter Cardiovasc* Interv, 2015; 85(1): e1–e9.

55 Brugaletta S, Gori T, Low AF, et al. Absorb bioresorbable vascular scaffold versus everolimus-eluting metallic stent in ST-segment elevation myocardial infarction: 1-year results of a propensity score matching comparisonThe BVS-EXAMINATION study (Bioresorbable Vascular Scaffold-A Clinical Evaluation of Everolimus Eluting Coronary Stents in the Treatment of Patients With ST-segment Elevation Myocardial Infarction). *J Am Coll Cardiol* Interv, 2015; 8:189–197.

56 Anderson JL, Jacobs AK, Halperin JL, et al. 2013 ACCF/AHA Guideline for the management of ST-elevation myocardial infarction: A Report of the American College of Cardiology Foundation/American Heart Association Task Force on Practice Guidelines. *J Am Coll Cardiol*, 2013; 61(4): e80–e140.

57 Windecker S, Kolh P, Alfonso F, et al., Task Force on Myocardial Revascularization of the European Society of Cardiology (ESC) and the European Association for Cardio-Thoracic Surgery (EACTS). 2014 ESC/EACTS Guidelines on myocardial revascularization. *Eur Heart J*, 2014; 35: 2541–2619.

12

Illustrated STEMI Procedures I – Basic STEMI Skills

Sameer Mehta MD, Tracy Zhang BS, Michael Schweitzer MD, Alexandra Ferré MD,
Daniella Nacad MD, Landy Luna Diaz MD, Alicia Henao Velasquez MD

Introduction

Based upon the feedback from four previous textbooks that we have written on ST-elevation myocardial infarction (STEMI) interventions, readers have found illustrated cases to be the most educational. Combining these illustrated procedures is the hardest task of writing this textbook. We are also presenting these in a previously proven format – at the top of each case are the pre- and post-intervention STEMI electrocardiograms (EKG), followed by images of the cineangiograms. Finally, a detailed case description is submitted, which highlights the teaching points of the case. In this book, we present 50 illustrated STEMI procedures. These have been meticulously selected from over 1600 procedures recorded in the SINCERE (Single Individual Community Experience Registry) database. We emphasize that all these procedures were performed by a single operator, who completed the entire procedure without assistance by fellows or other interventional cardiologists. These 50 cases have been divided into three sections – basic skills (this chapter), management of thrombus (Chapter 13), and complex STEMI procedures (Chapter 14). Of course, there are numerous overlaps. However, this is a deliberate strategy to emphasize and reemphasize the special teaching tips that may be required to perform STEMI interventions.

In this chapter, the fundamental tenets of STEMI intervention are addressed. Primarily, the paramount focus is on identifying the culprit lesion and on successfully mandating our four recommended parameters of STEMI success: The relief of chest pain, ST-segment resolution, thrombolysis in myocardial infarction (TIMI) flow 3, and myocardial blush grade 3.

Each of the illustrated procedures has a common denominator: A mandated strategy of short door-to-balloon time. Although we recognize the numerous limitations of door-to-balloon time, we firmly believe that short and shorter treatment times are critical for performing STEMI interventions.

Finally, we apologize that some images do not have optimal resolution. The illustrated procedures have been accumulated from five different institutions and have varying imaging quality.

Manual of STEMI Interventions, First Edition. Edited by Sameer Mehta.
© 2017 John Wiley & Sons Ltd. Published 2017 by John Wiley & Sons Ltd.

Case 1

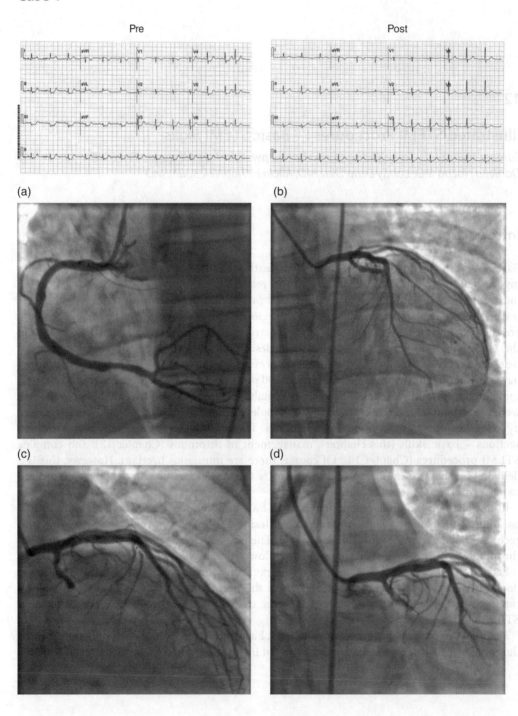

Pre

Post

(a)

(b)

(c)

(d)

(e)

(f)

(g)

(h)

(i)

(j)

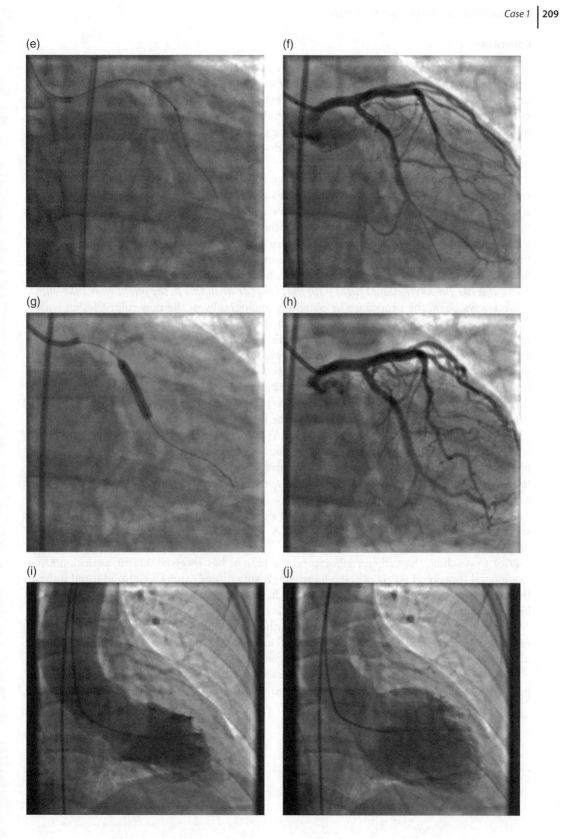

Comments

A straightforward STEMI intervention. However, even this simple case illustrates STEMI principles effectively. It begins with identification of the culprit lesion – this case was an emergency medical services transport with pre-hospital alert. It was challenging for a 2 a.m. presentation, but the early and accurate alert and the technical ease of the procedure enabled a good outcome with a very short door-to-balloon time of 62 minutes – not bad for a 2 a.m. case!

Various other tips can be learned from this first, simple procedure – the first for the book, not our first case.

We believe that it is critical to know the entire coronary history of the patient, prior to proceeding with the STEMI intervention. It provides a better understanding of the entire case – any additional disease, and the angiographic characteristics and collateral circulation, is useful information to have in advance of addressing the culprit lesion. These details can affect the STEMI interventional decision in several important ways, including consideration for additional staged percutaneous coronary intervention (PCI), surgery, choice of stents, the need to limit the contrast dose, even the speed with which the procedure should be accomplished. *To us, it is like the navigational flight path that is made available to the pilot before take-off.*

We always begin the procedure by obtaining angiography of the non-culprit lesion with a diagnostic catheter and then proceeding with the guiding catheter to perform the STEMI intervention. With rare exceptions, we use 6 Fr introducer sheaths, 6 Fr diagnostic and 6 Fr guide catheters. In the entire SINCERE database, in an experience spanning over 6 years of performing short door-to-balloon STEMI interventions, we have used the equipment we preselected in 92% of all cases. Most operators are similarly comfortable with equipment of their choice and we strongly encourage them to pull that equipment out before the case, as it can save those precious few minutes that may be lost in searching for the equipment.

Thus, for a culprit right coronary artery (RCA) lesion, we pull out the following equipment, which is opened and placed on the table – a diagnostic 6 Fr JL4, a JR4 guide catheter, a hydrophilic wire and the inflation kit. A 2.5/12 balloon catheter and an aspiration catheter are pulled out *but not opened* and the AngioJet and intra-aortic balloon pump are outside the room or in a corner.

For assessing the non-culprit lesion in the left anterior descending coronary artery (LAD), we suggest two orthogonal views and for the RCA, a single left anterior oblique view with the diagnostic catheter.

Prior to reaching the catheter laboratory, the patient has received 325 mg aspirin, 300 mg clopidogrel (prasugrel 60 mg is being increasingly substituted) and a weight-adjusted unfractionated heparin bolus. Once arterial access has been obtained, we administer a bolus of bivalirudin and begin an intravenous drip that is continued for 2 hours post-procedure.

Numerous subsequent cases will highlight other teaching points – but these are the bare essentials from the SINCERE database and incorporate the essentials of culprit lesion identification and compulsive thrombus management.

For this patient, a hydrophilic wire easily crossed the lesion; aspiration thrombectomy was performed and a 3.5 mm bare-metal stent (BMS) was used.

Case 2

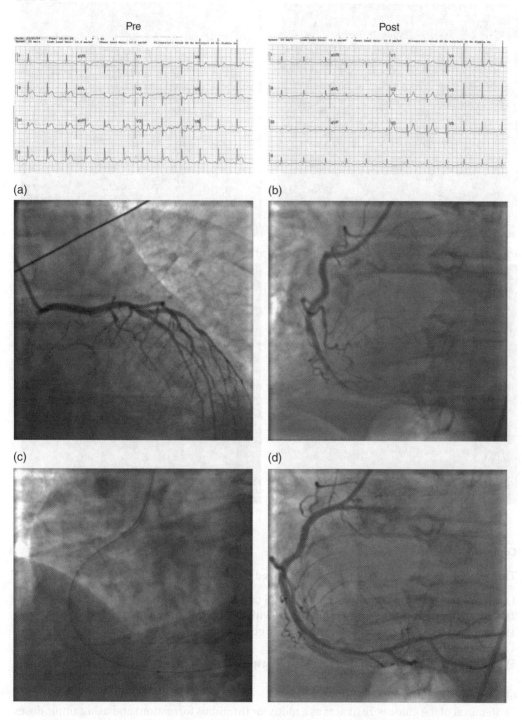

Pre

Post

(a)

(b)

(c)

(d)

(e)   (f)

(g)   (h)

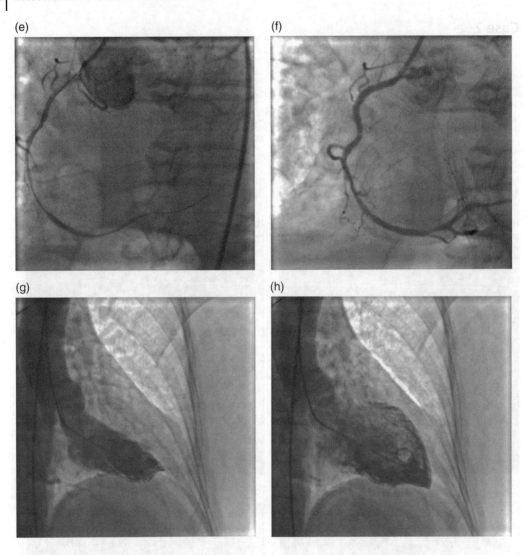

Comments

This procedure is performed in our standardized fashion, with the following steps:

1) Identification of the culprit lesion with EKG correlation – the RCA, in this case.
2) Cineangiography of the non-culprit vessel with a diagnostic 6 Fr catheter.
3) Cannulation of the culprit vessel with a 6 Fr guide catheter.
4) Crossing the lesion with a hydrophilic wire.
5) Selective strategy for thrombus removal – aspiration thrombectomy done with an Export catheter.
6) Stenting – a 3.0 mm BMS was used here.
7) Removal of the guide wire (it acts as a nidus for thrombus formation) and using ample doses of intracoronary nitroprusside to augment the distal, microvasculature flow.
8) Left ventriculography.
9) Removal of the arterial sheath with use of closure devices if technically feasible.

Case 3

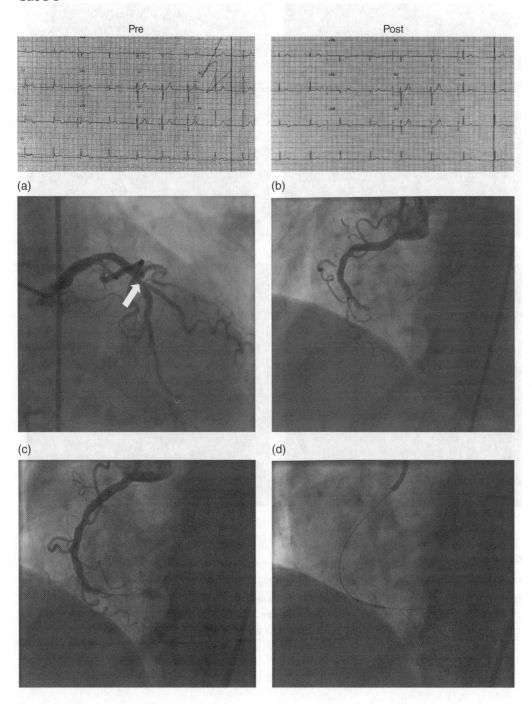

Pre

Pre

Post

(a)

(b)

(c)

(d)

(e) (f) (g) (h)

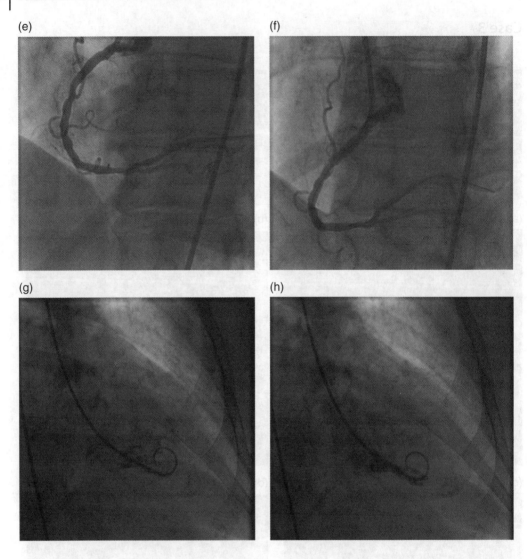

Comments

Several important lessons can be learned from this case. The RCA is the culprit and there is no reason, whatsoever, to treat the moderate disease in the LAD. It is not certain that the wire is in the true lumen, so a quick, very low pressure inflation is performed with a 2-mm balloon catheter. This is followed by aspiration (panel E) and then stenting with a BMS.

Case 4

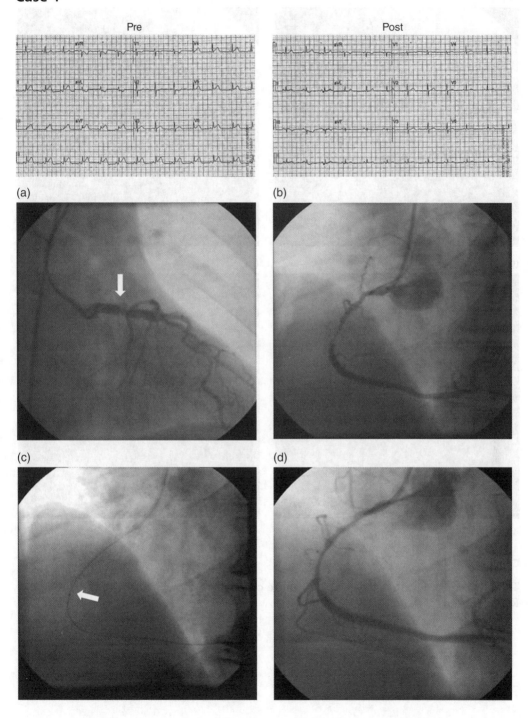

(a)

(b)

(c)

(d)

Pre

Post

(e)

(f)

(g)

(h)

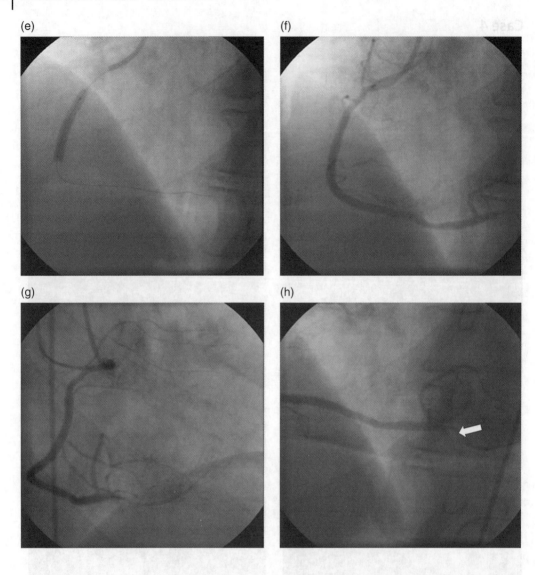

Comments

The detailed comments follow after the entire case – here successful PCI of the thrombotic RCA has been achieved.

(i)

(j)

(k)

(l)

(m)

(n)

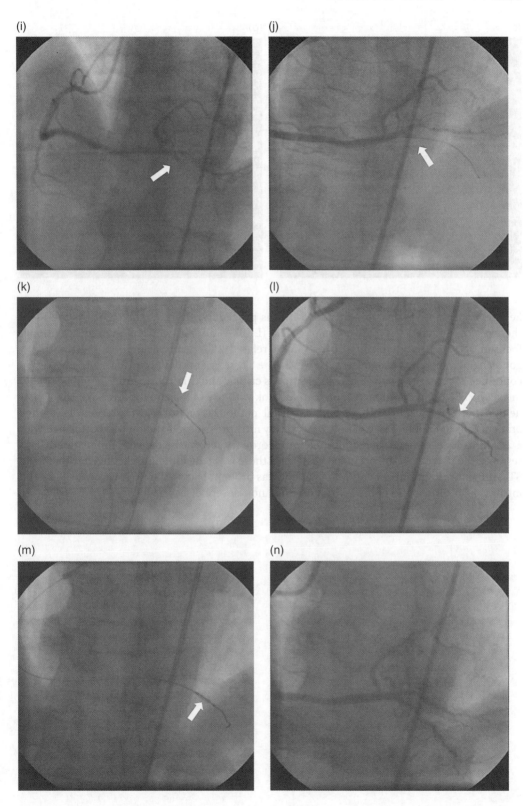

(o)   (p)

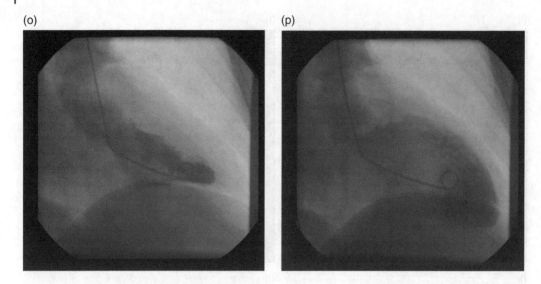

Several important lessons are embedded in this procedure. By EKG, the culprit is the RCA; there is also moderate left main coronary artery (LMCA) disease, which is ignored; attention is focused on rapid recanalization of the infarct-related RCA. After aspiration and stenting, a good angiographic result is present. However, the ST-segments did not resolve and the patient continued to have chest pain. This observation is critical and this information should be sought in every STEMI intervention. A more careful look with use of the anteroposterior cranial view demonstrates occlusion with thrombus (distal embolization) of the posterior descending branch. This did not improve with intracoronary nitroprusside. Dilatation was performed with a 2-mm balloon catheter, and additional intracoronary nitroprusside was administered. This restored the patency of the occluded vessel and there was concomitant relief of chest pain and ST-segment resolution. On day 3, the patient was brought back – the RCA was widely patent; intravascular ultrasound of the LMCA revealed non-severe disease.

Case 5

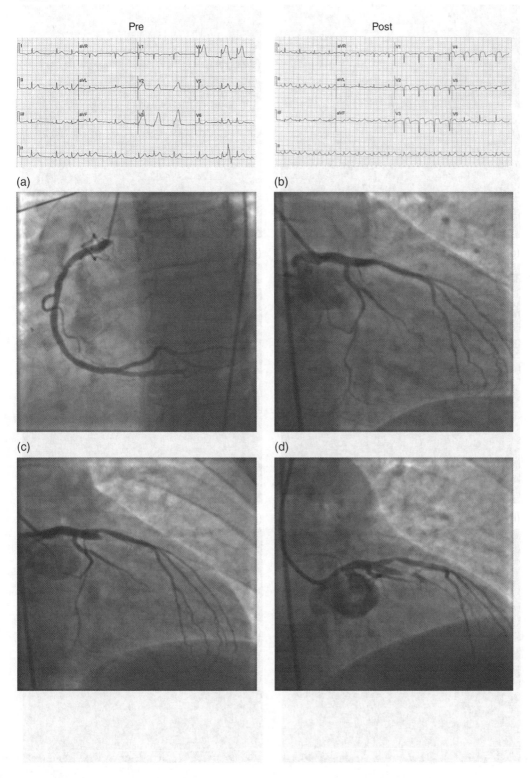

Pre

Post

(a)

(b)

(c)

(d)

(e)

(f)

(g)

(h)

(i)

(j)

Comments

The next several cases reiterate the importance of using good basic PCI skill for STEMI interventions, such as obtaining optimal views for performing STEMI interventions. Most STEMI lesions are soft and crossing with a guide wire, and in particular with a hydrophilic guide wire, is fairly easy. However, the operator gets just one shot at it in most cases – if the guide wire tracks subintimally, it is much harder to recross a thrombotic lesion which may additionally have dissection planes from the subintimal guide wire passage. This is all the more crucial when the STEMI lesion is totally occluded.

The other situation that can be treacherous for crossing with a guide wire is a thrombotically occluded segment, distal to a severe tortuosity (several cases have been selected and will be presented later in the illustrated cases to highlight this important teaching point). In such conditions, it is imperative to obtain the optimal view prior to crossing with a guide wire. This view should clearly demonstrate the nipple of the occlusion and this view should be freeze-framed on the screen as guide wire passage is attempted.

As described elsewhere in this book, we use a rapid, to-and-fro rotating movement to advance the hydrophilic guide wire, which tends to seek the lumen. The tip of the hydrophilic guide wire often doubles up after crossing the lesion. It is then completely safe and provides ample support. In practice, while exchanging catheters, we monitor the tip of the guide wire under fluoroscopy.

We would also like to mention here some impressive statistics from the SINCERE database – in 600 short door-to-balloon STEMI interventions, there have been no perforations, no emergency cardiothoracic surgery and almost all cases have been performed using a monorail technique. With rare exceptions where a low profile over the balloon may be needed to exchange wires or catheters, we strongly believe that STEMI interventions are more efficiently done using monorail, single-operator technique. In addition, except for uncommon situations where there was severe peripheral vascular disease and ileofemoral tortuosity, or where we needed to upsize to the very effective 7 Fr Export® thrombectomy catheter, almost all cases have been done with a 6 Fr system.

In this case, a casual review, such as panel B, shows no disease, and one could recklessly conclude that there is either no culprit or that the vessel has recanalized. Obviously, this is incorrect, as the next views demonstrate the occluded segment. Attention is then focused on obtaining the most optimal view to cross with the guide wire, as explained above.

Addendum: Just at this text was going to press, we experienced our first coronary perforation. This was a small, guide wire-induced, type A dye leak which occurred in a late-presenting STEMI lesion involving a severely tortuous, very proximal left circumflex artery (LCX) occlusion. An option was to place a covered stent in the LMCA across the LCX – but the leak was small and the patient was stable. Bivalirudin was stopped, and the patient was monitored on the table for 30 minutes. The dye leak disappeared and no pericardial effusion was seen on echocardiography. The echo imaging was repeated 6 hours later and it was unchanged. The patient was medically treated for myocardial infarction, and she left the hospital in a stable condition.

13

Illustrated STEMI Procedures II – Basic STEMI Skills

Sameer Mehta MD, Tracy Zhang BS, Michael Schweitzer MD, Alexandra Ferré MD, Daniella Nacad MD, Landy Luna Diaz MD, Alicia Henao Velasquez MD

Introduction

This chapter covers the Mehta strategy for treatment of thrombus in STEMI lesions. It encapsulates our strategy of direct stenting for low-grade thrombus, manual aspiration for moderate lesions, and mechanical thrombectomy for hybrid thrombus. In addition to this strategy, we employ the AngioJet® for late-presenting thrombus, where anatomy is suitable for using this device.

Manual of STEMI Interventions, First Edition. Edited by Sameer Mehta.
© 2017 John Wiley & Sons Ltd. Published 2017 by John Wiley & Sons Ltd.

Case 6

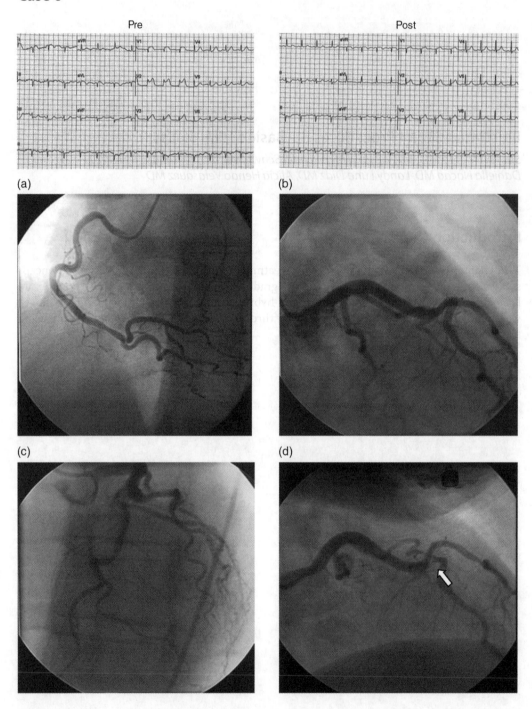

Pre

Post

(a)

(b)

(c)

(d)

(e)

(f)

(g)

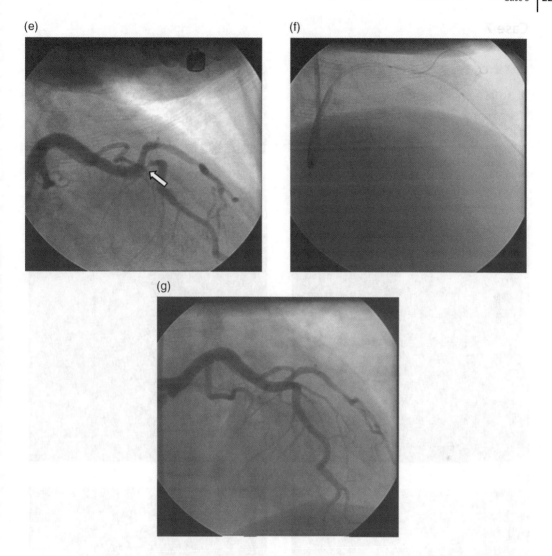

Comments

Just as in Case 11 (Chapter 14), this case demonstrates the basic principles of percutaneous coronary intervention and use of non-traditional views when a culprit lesion has not been identified – note the dramatic anterior wall EKG changes. The four traditional views did not demonstrate any lesion till the steeply, angulated view in Panel D demonstrated the severe lesion. A double-wire technique was used; the LAD was pre dilated and stented with a 3.5 mm DES with an excellent result and without compromise to the diagonal branch. The guide wire was removed from the diagonal prior to stent deployment. D2B Time 66 minutes – 'on hours'.

Case 7

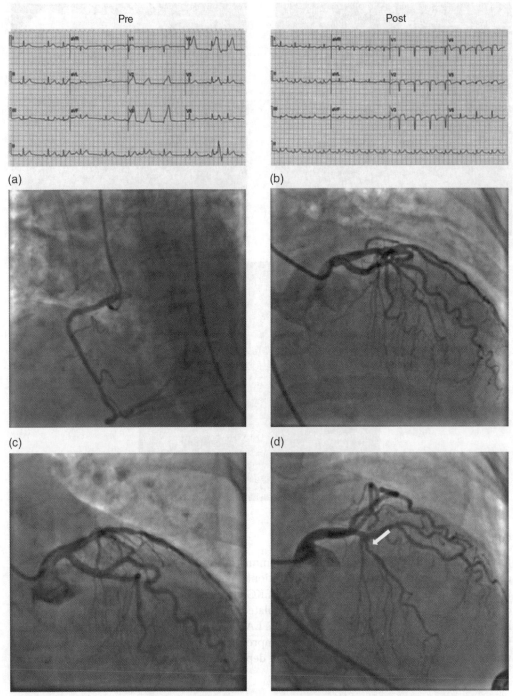

Pre

Post

(a)

(b)

(c)

(d)

(e)

(f)

(g)

(h)

(i)

(j)

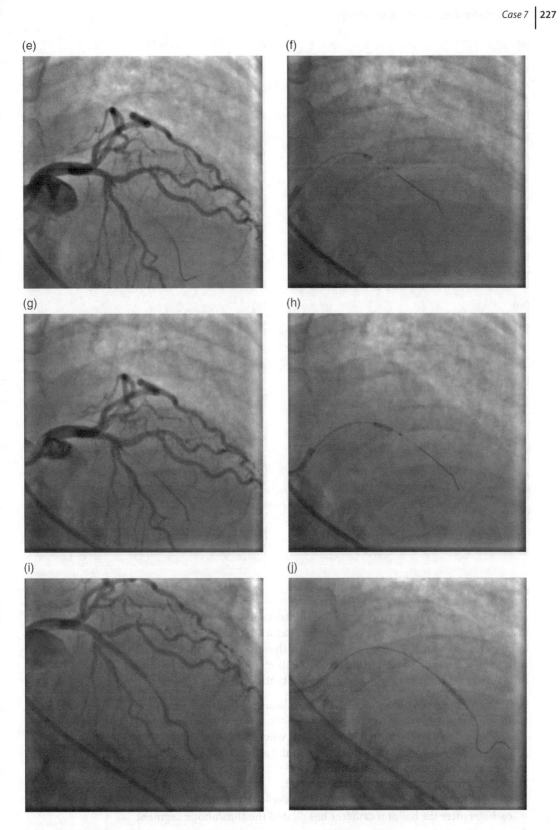

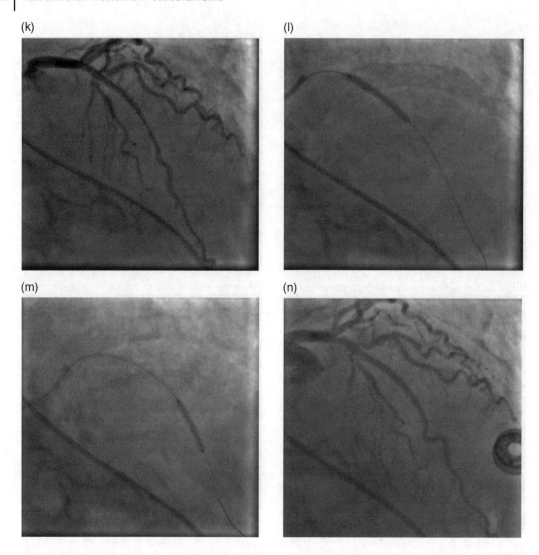

(k)   (l)

(m)   (n)

Comments

As a global strategy for performing STEMI interventions, we limit the use of balloon catheters, instead employing thrombectomy catheters as a first-line device. This fundamental belief is influenced by the hypothesis that balloon catheters will cause distal embolization. However, with as much fervor as restricting balloon catheters, we strongly advocate the use of balloon catheters in three distinct situations. These situations are:

1) To verify that the guide wire is in the true lumen.
   In several situations, it is extremely unclear that the wire has traversed the thrombus and is positioned in the true lumen. In situations where we have a doubt, we will put a small 2-mm balloon catheter and gently dilate to about 4 atmospheres. A quick dye spurt will confirm the presence of the wire in the lumen.
2) Inability to advance the aspiration catheter.
   In this situation, we will pre-dilate but persist with thrombectomy, advancing the aspiration catheter after the balloon catheter has dilated the thrombotic segment.

3) In calcified, tortuous, or distal lesions.

   Once again, balloon angioplasty is followed by thrombectomy whenever possible. In this case, a 2-mm balloon catheter was employed, as we were unsure that the guide wire was in the true lumen. After verifying luminal passage, the remaining procedure is routine.

Another highlight of this case is meticulous angiography analysis, often in multiple projections, to search scrupulously for an occluded segment. A casual inspection, as shown in panels B and C, could miss the lesion that is identified in panel D (see arrow) by this detailed search.

Case 8

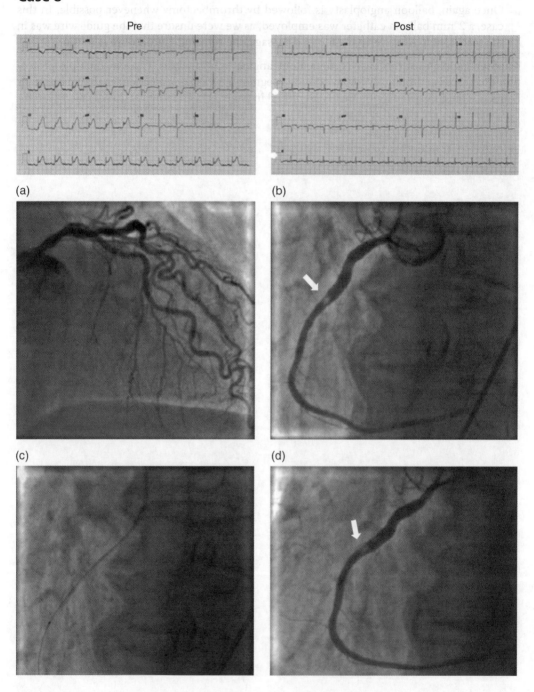

Pre

Post

(a)

(b)

(c)

(d)

(e)

(f)

(g)

(h)

(i)

(j)

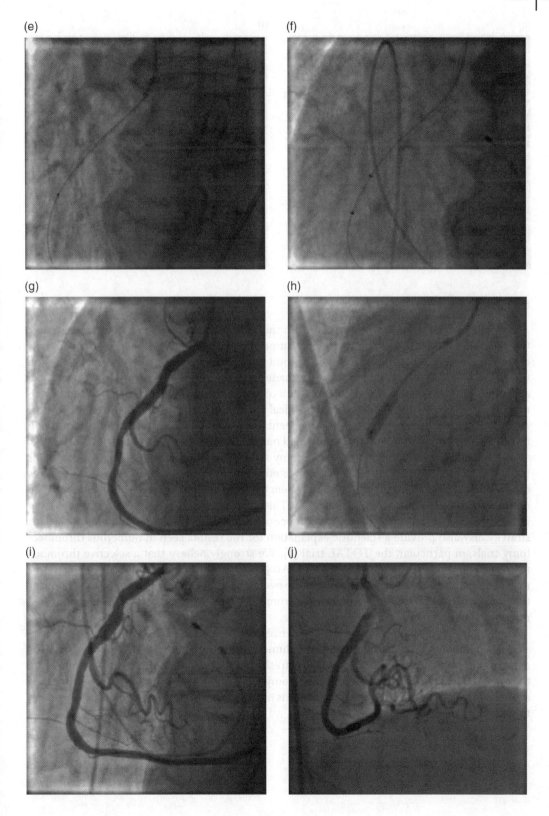

(k)   (l)

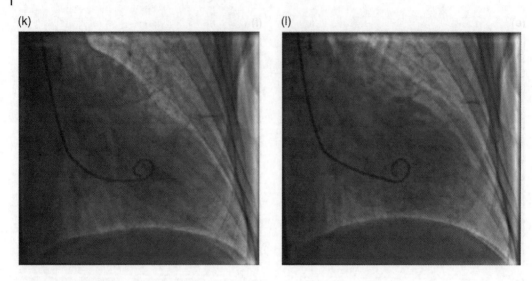

Comments

A few important lessons can be learned from this case. Although, unless angioscopy is used, the precise composition of the thrombus cannot be ascertained, we believe that this case represents a dense, organized and red thrombus. It is resistant to the use of aspiration thrombectomy where several passes were made with no improvement in the angiographic appearance of the thrombus and no extraction of visible thrombus. This is a large right coronary artery (RCA) with no tortuosity and ideal for the use of the AngioJet®. Panel G, post AngioJet, demonstrates dramatic improvement over Panel D, which was post aspiration thrombectomy. It is such cases that confirmed our belief and trust in the AngioJet.

We reaffirm our fundamental thrombectomy strategy as one that uses selective thrombus management employing multiple devices targeted at the thrombus grade. Low-grade thrombus can be directly stented; moderate thrombus benefits from aspiration; and large thrombus with optimal anatomy benefits from the AngioJet. This pragmatic methodology has now been used in the SINCERE database for over 1000 consecutive short door-to-balloon interventions. This strategy may also provide a scientific explanation for the results seen in numerous thrombectomy trials, in particular, the TOTAL trial [1]. We strongly believe that a selective thrombus management strategy, if applied to the TOTAL [1], TASTE [2], and TAPAS [3] populations, may demonstrate marked improvement in the overall results with low rates of distal embolization and superior ST-segment resolution, thrombolysis in myocardial infarction 3 flow, and myocardial blush grade.

The Mehta Selective Thrombus Management Strategy, as used in SINCERE for over a decade, has pathophysiological rationale and volumetric thrombectomy as mechanisms to treat dynamic thrombus. Based on this strategy, fresh, friable thrombus presenting as moderate thrombus benefits from aspiration thrombectomy. Conversely, dense, organized, red thrombus aggregates with large thrombus burden, which is maximally impacted by mechanical thrombectomy such as the AngioJet.

Case 9

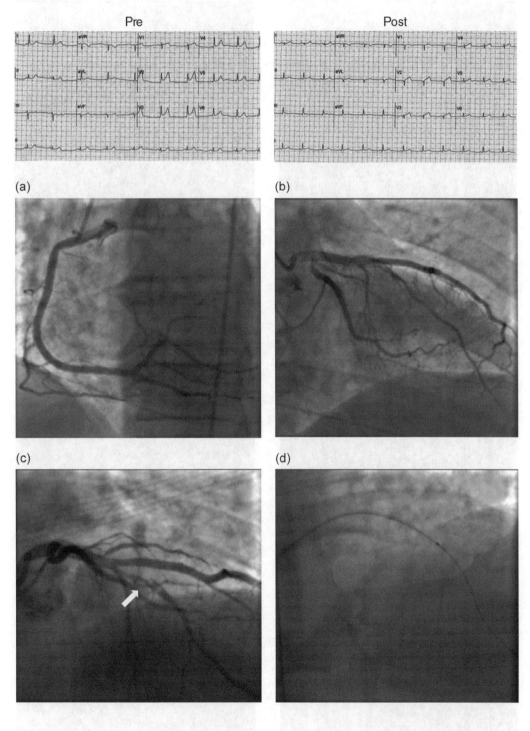

Pre

Post

(a)

(b)

(c)

(d)

(e)

(f)

(g)

(h)

(i)

(j)

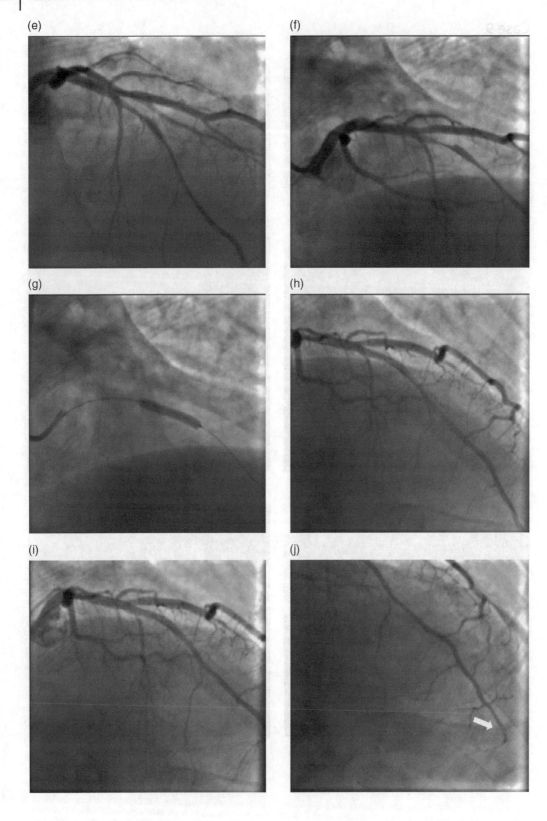

This is a relatively simple case from which key important lessons about thrombus visualization can be learned. In panel B, there appears to be a thrombotic lesion in the left main. Additionally, there is severe disease in the ostium of the left circumflex. However, this is simply streaming of the dye and not thrombus. Panel C is a better angiographic projection, and it demonstrates no thrombus in the left main but a clear, well-defined thrombus in the mid portion of the left anterior descending (LAD) coronary artery. Aspiration thrombectomy and stenting provides an excellent result, but with migration of minimal thrombus into the very apical portion of the LAD as shown in panel J, this was deliberately left alone, and the patient had an excellent clinical outcome.

Case 10

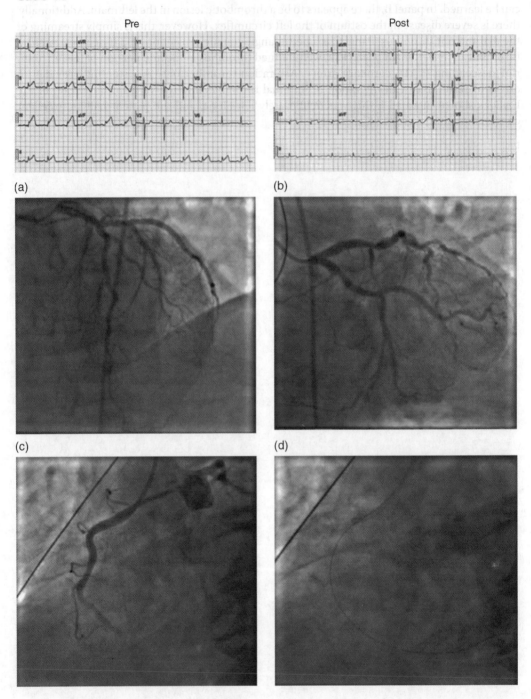

Pre

Post

(a)

(b)

(c)

(d)

(e)

(f)

(g)

(h)

(i)

(j)

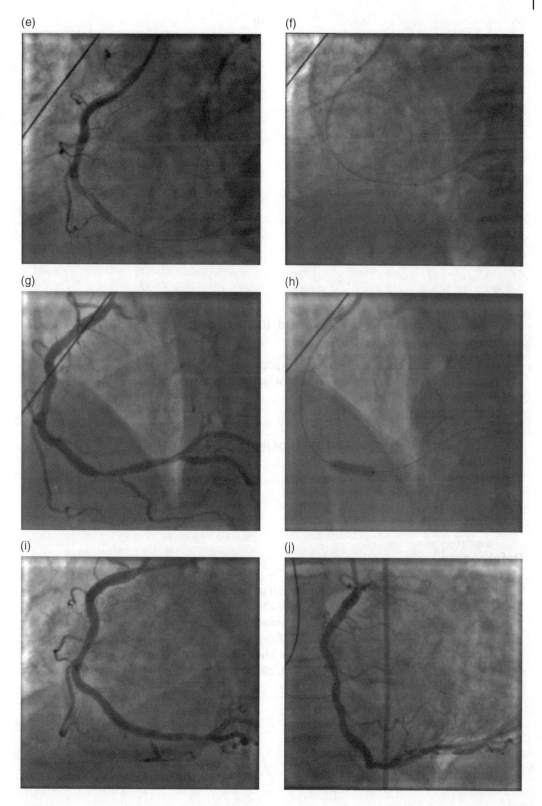

(k)   (l)

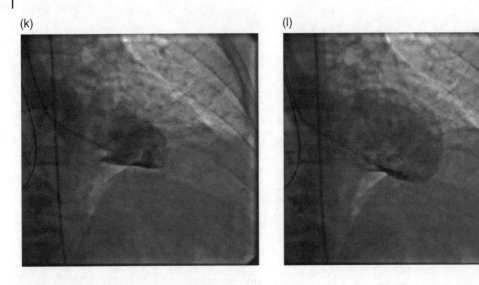

Comments

This is one of the most simple, straightforward, 10-minute STEMI intervention – performed in our traditional 10-step strategy:

1) Femoral or wrist access, depending on expertise.
2) Begin with angiography of the non-culprit lesion.
3) 6 Fr access sheath.
4) Hydrophilic guide wires.
5) Assess thrombus grade.
6) Aspiration thrombectomy as a default first device.
7) Drug-eluting or bare-metal stent.
8) Intracoronary vasodilators.
9) Left ventricular analysis.
10) Removal of vascular sheath.

References

1 Jolly S, Cairns J, Yusuf S, et al. Randomized trial of primary PCI with or without routine manual thrombectomy. *N Engl J Med*, 2015; 372:1389–1398.
2 Svilaas T, Vlaar PJ, van der Horst IC, et al. Thrombus aspiration during primary percutaneous coronary intervention. *N Engl J Med*, 2008; 358(6): 557–567.
3 Fröbert O, Lagerqvist B, Olivecrona GK, et al. Thrombus aspiration during ST-segment elevation myocardial infarction. *N Engl J Med*, 2013; 369(17): 1587–1597.

14

Illustrated STEMI Procedures III – Basic STEMI Skills

Sameer Mehta MD, Tracy Zhang BS, Michael Schweitzer MD, Alexandra Ferré MD, Daniella Nacad MD, Landy Luna Diaz MD, Alicia Henao Velasquez MD

Introduction

This chapter covers complex STEMI interventions. This group comprises several patients with cardiogenic shock and subsets such as left main intervention, saphenous vein graft lesions, multivessel disease, and complex anatomy.

Manual of STEMI Interventions, First Edition. Edited by Sameer Mehta.

Case 11

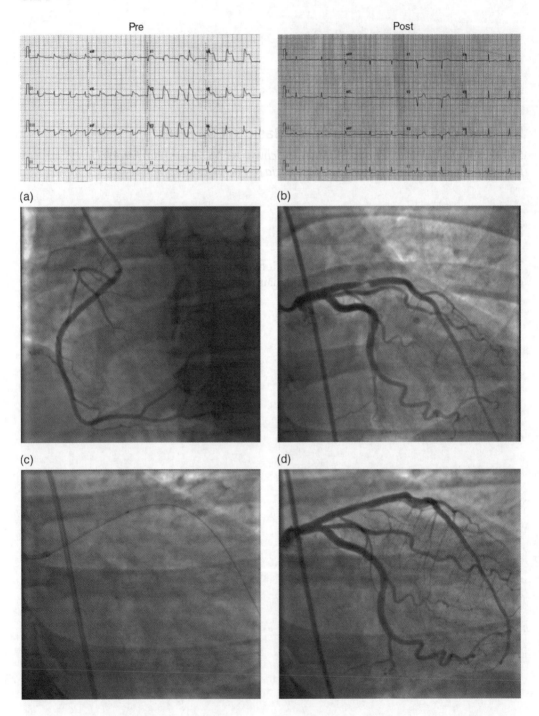

Pre

Post

(a)

(b)

(c)

(d)

(e)

(f)

(g)

(h)

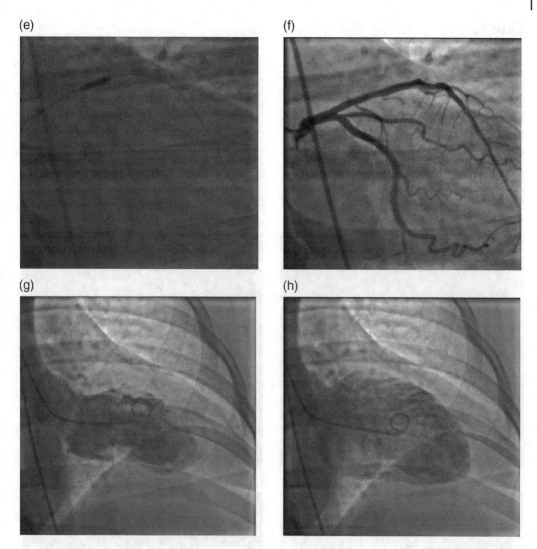

Comments

This is classic demonstration of thrombus (observe the angiographic appearance of the smooth, convex "meniscus" of the thrombus) and effective thrombus management with thromboaspiration in STEMI lesions. A drug-eluting stent (DES) is employed in this situation – we always use a DES for treating most left anterior descending (LAD) and diabetic lesions, as well as for long lesions and small vessels.

Case 12

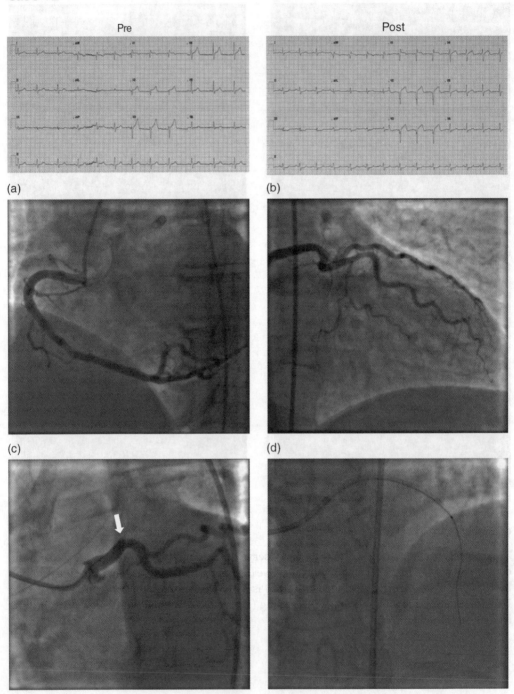

Pre

Post

(a)

(b)

(c)

(d)

(e)

(f)

(g)

(h)

(i)

(j)

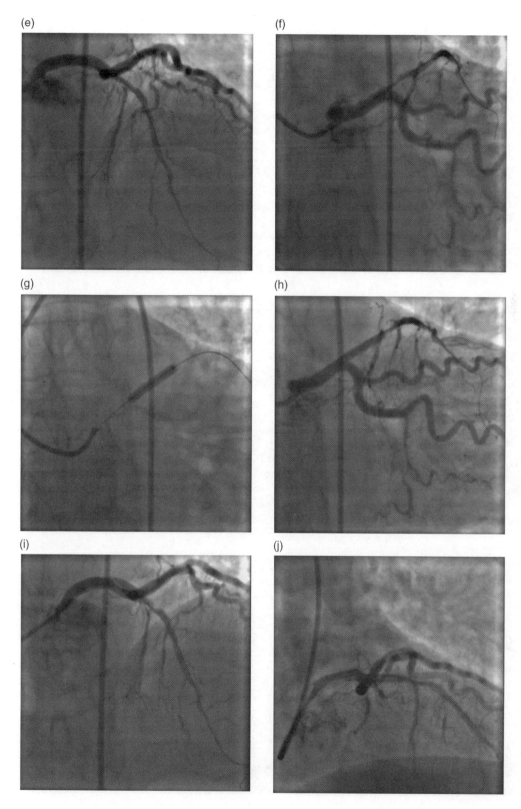

(k)

(l)

(m)

(n)

(o)

(p)

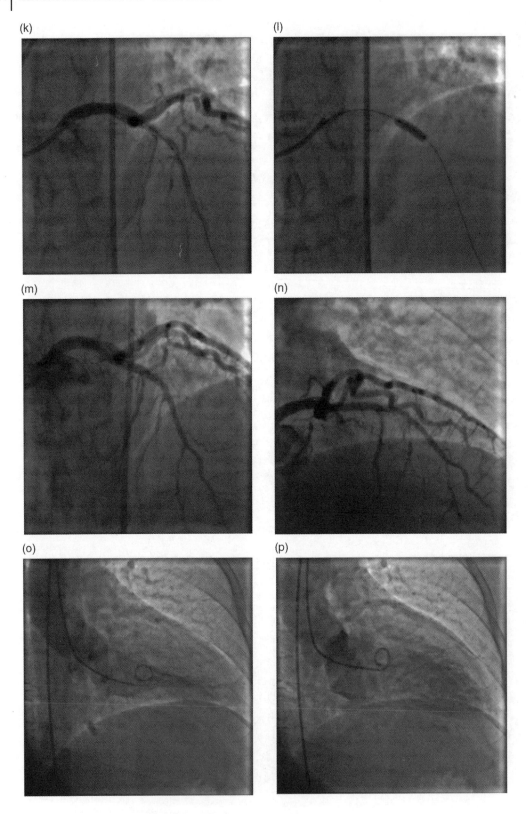

Comments

Good basic angiographic skills are paramount to performing STEMI interventions. A casual inspection of panel B will completely miss the coronary lesion. However, a left anterior oblique caudal projection demonstrates the ostial LAD lesion shown in panel C, highlighted by the arrow. Percutaneous coronary intervention (PCI) is performed in the usual fashion, with thrombectomy and DES. ST-segment resolution and left ventricular function is normal.

Case 13

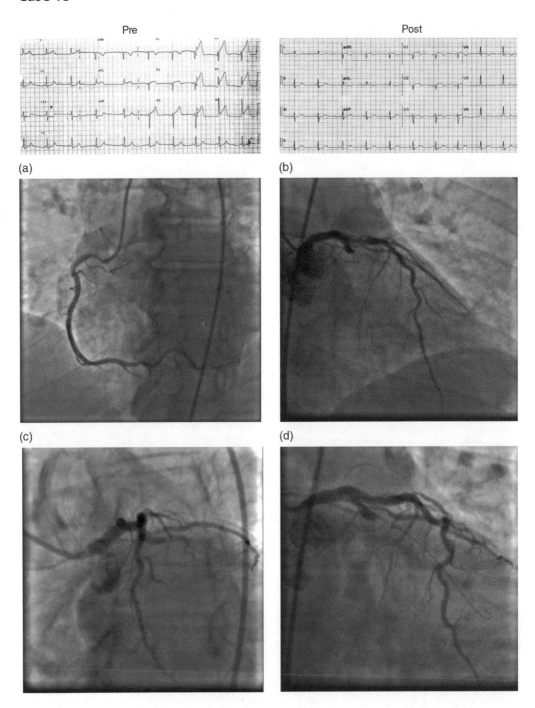

Pre

(a)

Post

(b)

(c)

(d)

(e)

(f)

(g)

(h)

(i)

(j)

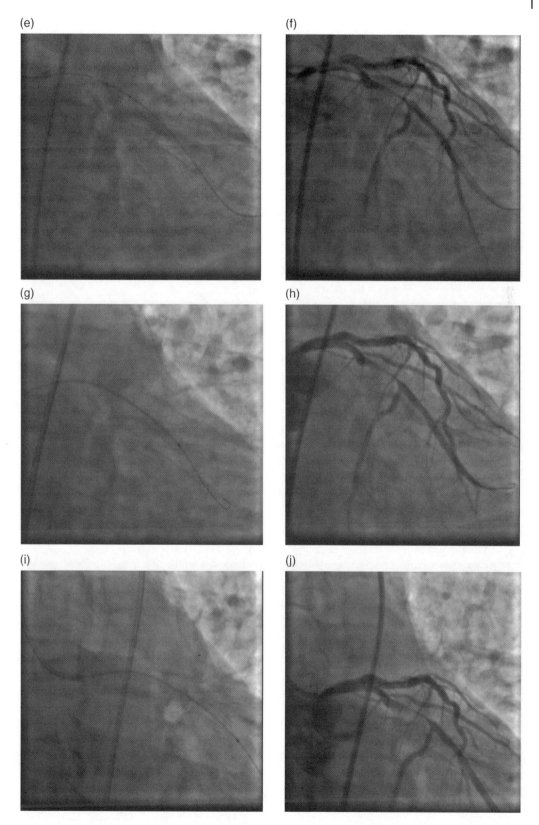

(k)

(l)

(m)

(n)

(o)

(p)

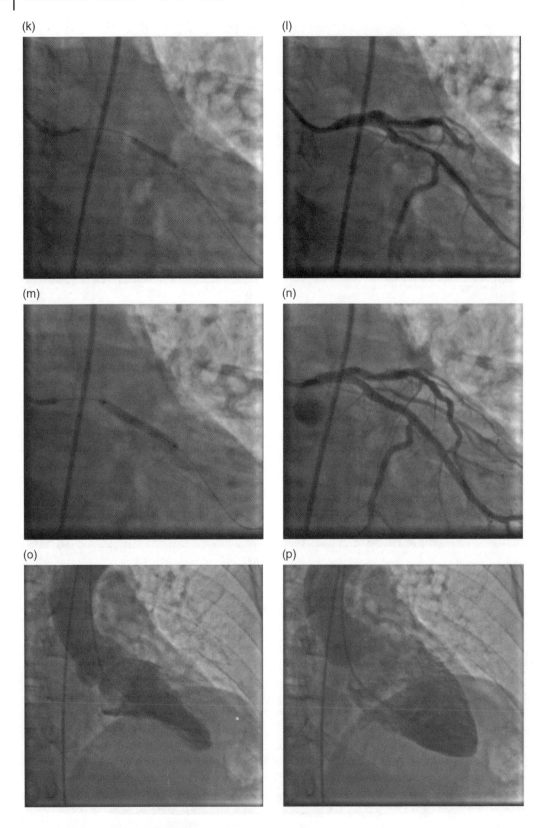

Comments

This is another simple STEMI intervention which provides dramatic results. The large occluded left circumflex artery is crossed with the hydrophilic wire. A 2-mm balloon catheter dilates for 4 atmospheres to permit passage of the aspiration catheter. Stenting is performed with a 3-mm DES. Procedure time was 9 minutes and door-to-balloon time was 42 minutes. Complete ST-segment resolution, relief of chest pain, thrombolysis in myocardial infarction (TIMI) grade 3, myocardial blush grade (MBG) 3 and preserved left ventricular function are achieved.

Case 14

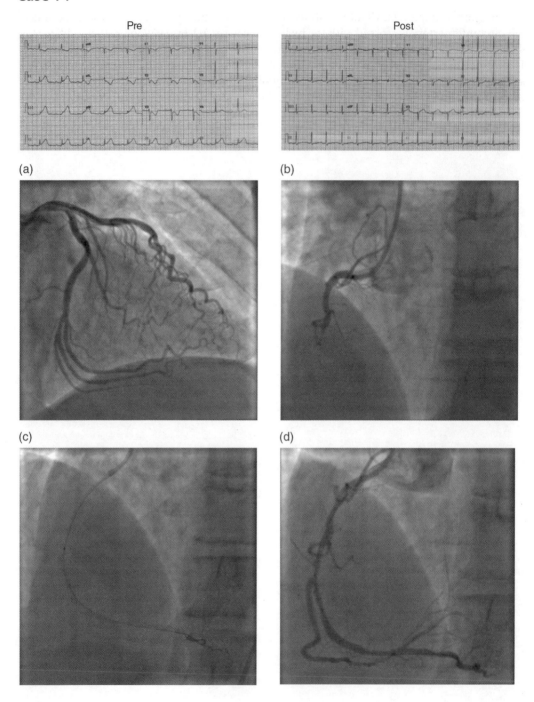

(a)

(b)

(c)

(d)

Pre

Post

(e)

(f)

(g)

(h)

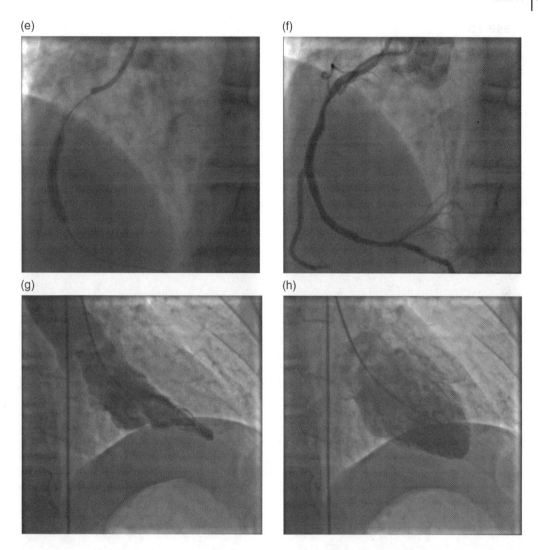

Comments

This is one of the simplest cases – irrespective, it aborted a STEMI in 6 minutes and preserved left ventricular function. An electrocardiogram normalizes post-procedure. We have found maximal benefit for STEMI interventions in large occluded arteries in patients presenting very early. To reiterate, we define STEMI success as:

1) Relief of chest pain.
2) ST-segment resolution.
3) TIMI grade 3 flow.
4) MPG 3.

Case 15

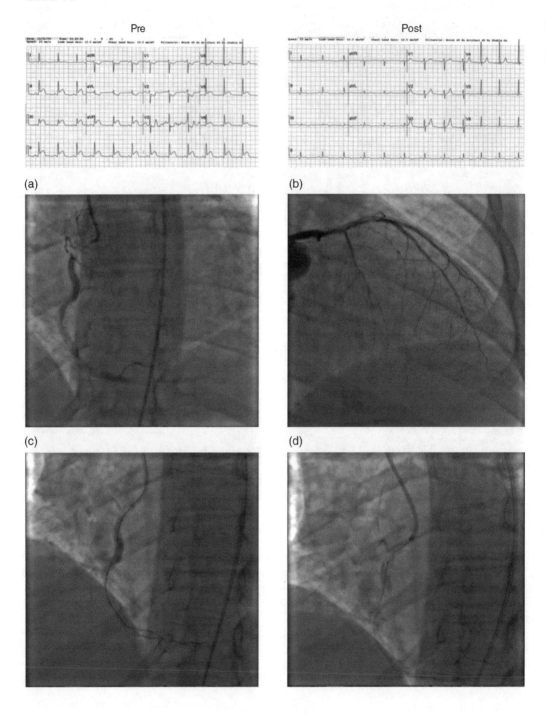

Pre

Post

(a)

(b)

(c)

(d)

(e)

(f)

(g)

(h)

(i)

(j)

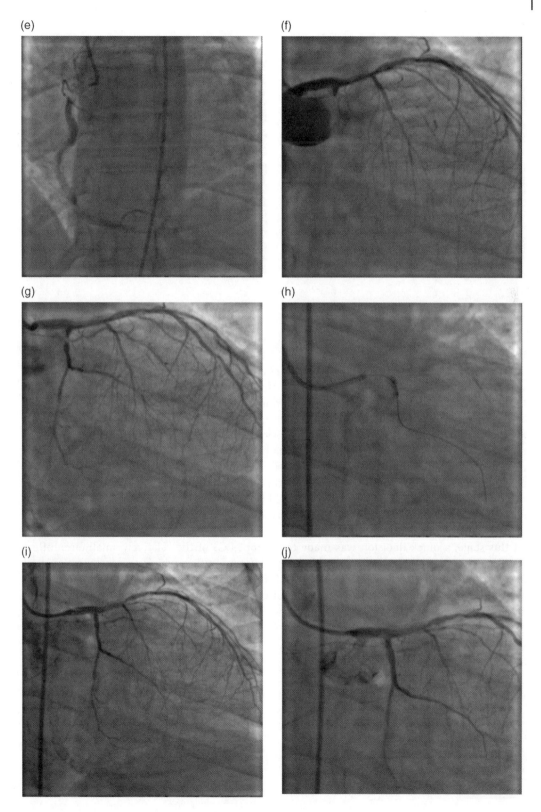

(k)　　　　　　　　　　　　　　　　　(l)

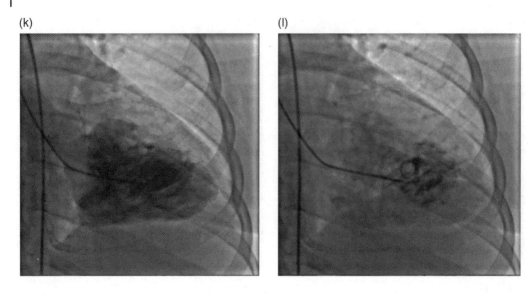

Comments

A STEMI EKG can often be confounding and the identification of the culprit lesion challenging. In particular, circumstances surrounding STEMI cases will require considerable maturity: at 4 a.m., with an exhausted team, such intellectual ability is compromised. Although an overwhelming number of STEMI cases will demonstrate a pristine culprit lesion corresponding to the EKG changes, in some cases, this presentation is blurred.

In the presenting case, the patient demonstrated infralateral EKG changes. Coronary cineangiography demonstrated two possible culprit lesions, those of the large, dominant right coronary artery (RCA) and the relatively small circumflex. In view of the larger RCA and demonstration of probable thrombus, we redirected our intervention to RCA. The lesion was easily crossed with the guide wire, but balloon dilation even with the 1.5 mm catheter was not possible. Additional angiography suggested probable calcification and not thrombus. Of course, evaluation through intravascular ultrasound could have differentiated thrombus and calcification, but with a crashing STEMI patient such intellectual curiosity is not our practice. At this stage, a quick decision was made to attempt PCI of the relatively small circumflex. A 6 Fr GL4 guide catheter easily cannulated the left circumflex, which was easily cannulated by the wire. The lesion was dilated with a 2.5 mm balloon catheter and easily stented with a 2.5 mm DES. Angiographic success, relief of chest pain, and ST-segment resolution were achieved.

15

Remote Ischemic Conditioning for Acute Myocardial Infarction

Hans Erik Bøtker MD PhD FACC FESC, Gerd Heusch MD FACC FESC FRCP

Introduction

Reperfusion Injury

The process leading to myocardial reperfusion in acute myocardial infarction (AMI) continues to improve with timely and effective coronary intervention enabled by early on-site diagnosis and optimized transportation directly to the catheterization facilities [1]. Added to this, optimized procedural techniques and improved antiplatelet and antithrombotic therapy maintain the patency of the infarct-related artery. However, in the chain of efforts required to accomplish optimal treatment benefit and outcome (Figure 15.1), the importance of reperfusion injury has been increasingly clear [2,3].

Reperfusion injury is the tissue damage caused by the return of blood supply to the tissue after a period of ischemia or oxygen deprivation. The absence of blood-borne oxygen and nutrients during the ischemic period creates a condition in which the restoration of circulation results in inflammation and oxidative damage by induction of oxidative stress rather than restoration of normal function (Figure 15.2) [4]. Reperfusion of ischemic tissues is associated with microvascular injury, particularly due to increased permeability of capillaries and arterioles, which leads to increased diffusion and fluid filtration across the tissues. Reintroduction of oxygen in cells suffering from metabolic disarrays established during prolonged ischemia and reperfusion results in molecular oxygen being converted into highly reactive superoxide and hydroxyl radicals that damage cellular proteins, DNA, and the plasma membrane, and act indirectly in redox signaling to turn on apoptosis. Affected endothelial cells produce an excess of reactive oxygen species but less nitric oxide during reperfusion. The imbalance results in an inflammatory response, which contributes the damage of reperfusion injury.

Clinical Implications of Reperfusion Injury

Reperfusion injury may contribute up to 50% of the final infarct size in experimental studies [2]. In the clinical setting, reperfusion injury is thought to play a significant role in the development of heart failure after AMI because 1-year mortality has decreased less than 30-day mortality [5,6]. The decline in the incidence of heart failure after AMI has not reached the expectations from clinical trial data and the prevalence is increasing [5]. Survival and quality of life in patients with heart failure following AMI remain poor, and worsened between 2007 and 2010, demonstrating that challenges still remain for the treatment of this high-risk condition [7]. Thus, the reduction of reperfusion injury is considered the next major target for improving outcome after AMI.

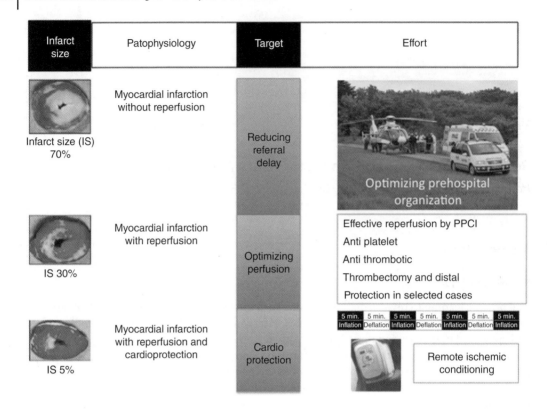

Figure 15.1 Chain of efforts during treatment of acute ST-elevation myocardial infarction to secure infarct reduction and optimal outcome. PPCI, primary percutaneous coronary intervention.

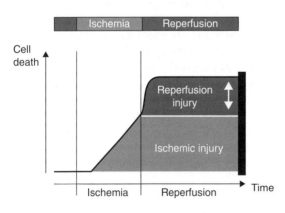

Figure 15.2 Reperfusion injury adds to the injury developed during initial ischemia. Protective procedures, such as drugs (e.g. cyclosporine, glucagon-like peptin 1 analogs and beta blockers), mild hypothermia and remote conditioning can modify the extent of reperfusion injury, when applied before onset of reperfusion.

The Concepts of Ischemic Conditioning

Remote ischemic conditioning (RIC) is a phenomenon by which brief, reversible episodes of ischemia and reperfusion applied in one vascular bed, tissue or organ confer a global, protective phenotype and make remote tissues and organs resistant to ischemia/reperfusion injury. Most tissues can be trained to enhance resistance against ischemic injuries. This intriguing biological observation was first described in the myocardium by Murry et al. in 1986 as local ischemic preconditioning, whereby brief periods of ischemia by repetitive cycles of occlusion and opening of a coronary artery before a sustained ischemic insult with eventual reperfusion, afford potent protection against ischemia-reperfusion injury [8].

Although the method was translated into clinical scenarios such as predictable ischemia during cardiac surgery [9], the technique has inherent limitations, as it requires interruption of blood flow to the target organ, and thus can be only achieved in the operating room or during coronary angioplasty. Furthermore, additional time for the preconditioning procedure is required before surgery or other intervention. Preconditioning itself might cause deterioration of organ function or cause complications, such as emboli of atheroma, because of the intermittent aortic clamping or intermittent coronary balloon inflation. Hence, local ischemic preconditioning has not found widespread clinical use [10].

Two important modifications of ischemic preconditioning provided the way for clinical applicability. Firstly, the discovery in experimental models that the stimulus could be delayed until the time of reperfusion – local ischemic postconditioning – and still preserve most of its protective effect, made it theoretically possible to use this method in situations involving acute or unpredictable ischemia. Local ischemic postconditioning can be performed by repeated brief inflations of an angioplasty balloon in the culprit lesion in the coronary artery immediately following primary percutaneous coronary intervention (PCI). However, the results of clinical trials using local ischemic postconditioning have been ambiguous [11,12] and the relevance of its clinical applicability remains to be clarified.

Secondly, and most likely with a broader clinical potential, is the concept of RIC. In 1993, Przyklenk et al. reported that brief coronary artery occlusions preconditioned the myocardium, not only within but also outside its perfusion territory [13]. Subsequently, it was shown that this remote cardioprotection could also be achieved from other organs or tissue beds; for example, by intermittent occlusion of a mesenteric or renal artery. The potential clinical utility became apparent when Kharbanda et al. demonstrated that repeated brief limb ischemia induced similar protection against myocardial ischemia-reperfusion injury [14]. Transient leg or arm ischemia in patients (achieved by intermittent inflation of a blood pressure cuff or an automatic device) has now become the far most widely used method to induce RIC. Owing to its noninvasive nature and easy applicability, RIC has found widespread interest. Since 2000, a large number of experimental and clinical studies have demonstrated a broad array of systemic effects of RIC [15–20].

Temporal Variants: Remote Pre-, Per-, and Postconditioning

In the initial discovery of RIC, the remote conditioning stimulus was administered prophylactically, similar to conventional ischemic preconditioning; that is, in the approximately 30–40-minute period before the onset of sustained myocardial ischemia. Pretreatment is not, however, a requirement for RIC-induced cardioprotection. Reduction of infarct size has also been described with concurrent application of the remote ischemic stimulus during sustained coronary occlusion (remote ischemic perconditioning) or at the time of reperfusion (remote ischemic postconditioning) [21].

Reduction of Myocardial Infarct Size by Remote Ischemic Conditioning

Cardioprotection with RIC was first demonstrated in swine [22,23] and subsequently confirmed in other models including rabbit and rat [24,25]. The results were subsequently translated into the clinical setting using limb ischemia applied with a blood pressure cuff on the upper arm during transport to hospital of patients with suspected STEMI [26]. RIC is thought to confer cardioprotection in early and delayed phases similar to local ischemic preconditioning. The first is immediate and lasts for 2–4 hours [27], while the second window of protection occurs at least 24 hours following the initial sublethal ischemic insult and has been shown to last up to 72 hours in certain species [28].

Mechanisms of Remote Ischemic Conditioning

Activation of the Remote Effector Organ

By definition, RIC is initiated by a brief ischemic stimulus. Although one clinical study has suggested that one occlusion cycle induces protection during elective PCI [29], the majority of experimental and clinical data indicate that the number and duration of inflations determine the cardioprotective efficacy, rather than the tissue volume exposed to intermittent short-lasting ischemia. We have tested several remote conditioning protocols experimentally in terms of one compared with two hind legs, fewer or more cycles, and duration of cycles, in a mice model. Occlusion of two limbs does not add further protection beyond that achieved by one limb. Maximum protection was achieved by four cycles, while an additional number of cycles did not induce further protection. In mice, a maximum protective effect was reached with 2 minutes of occlusion, while no additional protection was gained by longer periods [30]. In clinical practice, none has shown convincing superiority to the originally proposed algorithm of four times 5 minutes of limb ischemia in humans.

Growing evidence implies that transient ischemia or interruption of blood flow is not a requisite trigger for remote protection. Notably, several stimuli mimic the infarct-sparing effect of RIC, including physical exercise [31], peripheral nociception [32], direct peripheral nerve stimulation [33], as well as noninvasive transcutaneous nerve stimulation [34] and electro-acupuncture [35]. Accordingly, local anesthesia with lidocaine [36] or a sensory nerve blocker [33] and transection of the peripheral nerve [37–39] abrogated the protection by remote ischemic preconditioning.

Signal Transfer from the Remote Effector Organ to the Heart

The organ-protective effects of RIC are partially mediated through release of endogenous substances into the bloodstream, as plasma from RIC-treated animals and humans is cardioprotective [31,40,41]. The same plasma can be dialyzed and the dialysate applied to a naïve, isolated heart to achieve cardioprotection equal in strength to cardioprotection in hearts from RIC-treated animals [38]. Similarly, in a cardiac transplant model, RIC of a recipient animal reduces ischemia reperfusion injury in the subsequently transplanted (denervated) donor heart, again suggesting the presence of a powerful humoral component to the RIC stimulus [17].

The exact nature of the factor(s) remains elusive. Studies have identified putative contributors to the cardioprotective response. The shear stress-related release of nitric oxide, secondary to reactive hyperemia induced by transient limb ischemia, is expected to increase plasma nitrite in the blood, and increased endogenous plasma nitrite levels are known to be cardioprotective [42]. Adenosine and bradykinine may be involved but their specific mode of action is unknown. Opioids seem to be involved as the cardioprotective response can be attenuated by naloxone [31]. Stromal derived factor-1α is a small chemokine that fulfills the criteria for a putative circulating effector [43] and is cardioprotective via its interaction with its chemokine receptor 4.

Most recently, exosomes have been shown to have a role in the preconditioning effect of transient limb ischemia/reperfusion [44–46]. Their content of lipoprotein complexes and specific carriage proteins, such as argonaute [47] and microRNAs, render these extracellular vesicles ideal compounds of interorgan communication because their composition prevents digestion of mircroRNA by circulating RNase. Indeed, microRNA-144 levels are increased in mouse myocardium after RIC, markedly reduced after ischemia/reperfusion injury and the effect of RIC is completely abrogated by a specific antagomir to microRNA-144 [48]. Although nitric oxide, opioids, stromal derived factor-1α and microRNA-144 are humoral transfer signals, they are insufficient to explain the full RIC phenomenon, and other humoral factors remain to be identified.

Signal Transduction of Remote Ischemic Conditioning in the Heart

Specific cardioprotective pathways are identified and include the endothelial nitric oxide synthase (eNOS)-protein kinase G, the reperfusion injury salvage kinase (RISK) and the survivor-activating factor enhancement (SAFE) pathways (Figure 15.3). Activation of these pathways is associated with increased myocardial glycolytic flux and post-translational modification of proteins by O-linked β-N-acetylglucosamine (O-GlcNAc), which seems to be involved in cardioprotection by RIC [49]. The pathways interact and converge on the mitochondria to modify membrane integrity by inhibiting the opening of the membrane permeability transition pore. The pore is closed during myocardial ischemia but opens during reperfusion, causing mitochondrial swelling, loss of function and, potentially, cellular necrosis. Inhibition of the mitochondrial permeability transition pore appears to act as the dominating final effector in the cascade of events triggered by RIC [10,50–52].

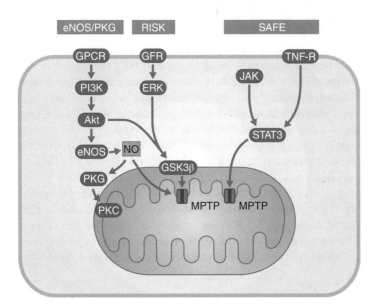

Figure 15.3 Simplified schematic presentation of the cytosol pathways that converge to prevent mitochondrial permeability transition pore (MPTP) opening in cardioprotection. eNOS/PGK: the nitric oxide dependent G-protein coupled receptor-eNOS-protein kinase G pathway; RISK: the reperfusion-injury salvage kinase pathway based on protein kinase B; PI3K-Akt and glycogen synthase kinase 3β; and SAFE: the survivor activating factor enhancement signaling pathway involving the JAK-STAT system and TNF-alpha receptors. eNOS, endothelial nitric oxide synthase; ERK, extracellular regulated kinase; GFR, growth factor receptor (insulin-like growth factor-1 and fibroblast growth factor-2); GPCR, G-protein-coupled receptor; GSK3-β: glycogen synthase kinase 3β.

Extracardiac Effects of Remote Ischemic Conditioning

In addition to the intracardiac signaling cascades, RIC seems to act in concert with inhibition of platelet [15] and neutrophil activation [19], other anti-inflammatory effects [16], endothelial function [14], and vascular functions [18]. These effects have not yet been integrated into a more complex and comprehensive scheme. However, they seem to play a significant role for the effect of RIC.

Measuring Myocardial Injury in the Clinic

Most clinical studies of infarct size after coronary revascularization have used indirect estimates of tissue damage, such as release of biomarkers and resolution of ST-segment elevation. These surrogate endpoints have predictive power in large cohorts, but their usefulness in the individual patient and small-sized study cohorts is moderate. Direct visualization of the area-at-risk and final infarct size to calculate the salvage index (proportion of salvaged area-at-risk) can be achieved by myocardial perfusion imaging using 99-technetium-sestamibi single photon emission computed tomography (SPECT). Final infarct size by SPECT correlates with histopathological estimates of infarct size. Final infarct size and salvage index are predictors of death. Once bound to viable myocardium, 99-technetium-sestamibi does not redistribute, such that the area-at-risk can be assessed by tracer injection before angioplasty. The isotope half-life of 6 hours allows subsequent SPECT imaging up to 8 hours after revascularization. SPECT visualization includes tissue perfusion by coronary collaterals. Assessment of final infarct size by SPECT requires repeated imaging in the stable post-infarction state. SPECT allows no distinction between previous and new infarction.

Because of the logistical challenges, cost and radiation exposure, efforts to assess area-at-risk and final infarct size by cardiac magnetic resonance imaging (CMRI) have been increasingly used in studies of potential cardioprotective interventions. The late gadolinium enhancement technique is validated in numerous experimental and clinical studies and has established CMRI as the reference method for quantifying infarct size, and is even superior to SPECT for detecting subendocardial infarcts due to a higher spatial resolution. In contrast, quantification of area-at-risk by CMRI remains challenging, not only because the optimal protocol to quantify the edema that is thought to represent area-at-risk, remains to be defined [53] but also because any cardioprotective intervention that reduces final infarct size also seems to reduce edema, hence potentially underestimating salvage [54]. On the other hand, CMRI may add pathophysiological insight, as this modality allows differentiation of acute from chronic infarction since only recent infarcts contain edema. Moreover, CMRI characterizes different infarct components such as intramyocardial hemorrhage because different relaxation times, characterized as T1 and T2, and use of gadolinium contrast allow characterization of tissue morphology (Figure 15.4) [55].

Effect of Remote Ischemic Conditioning in Acute Myocardial Infarction

The option of initiating cardioprotective treatment after the onset of myocardial ischemia has simplified translation of RIC into the clinical setting. In the first proof-of-concept study demonstrating that RIC can increase myocardial salvage in patients with ST-elevation myocardial infarction [26], RIC was initiated in the ambulance during transportation to primary PCI.

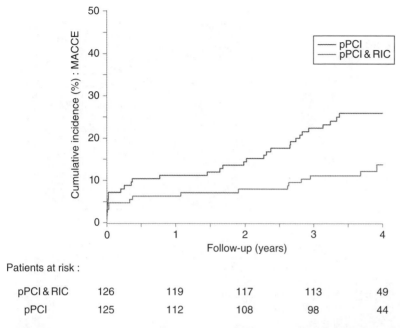

Figure 15.4 Cumulative incidence (%) of major adverse cardiovascular events (MACCE) by year since randomization (per-protocol analysis). $P = 0.010$ (source: Sloth et al. *European Heart Journal*, 2014; 35: 168–7557 with permission). PPCI, primary percutaneous coronary intervention; RIC, remote ischemic conditioning.

RIC increased salvage by 36%. In patients with left anterior descending (LAD) infarcts and patients with occluded culprit artery (thrombolysis in myocardial infarction, TIMI, 0–1) on admission, infarct size reduction, measured by SPECT, was 44% and 31%, indicating that patients at highest risk seem to have the largest benefit by RIC as an adjunctive therapy to primary PCI. The findings translated into an increment of left ventricular ejection fraction in LAD infarcts [56]. Although not powered to evaluate clinical outcome, a follow-up study of the total cohort showed that the beneficial effect of RIC translated into a reduction of major cardiovascular events by RIC up to 4 years after the index event (Figure 15.5) [57]. A simultaneous study demonstrated that RIC increases the number of patients achieving complete ST-segment resolution and a statistically borderline reduction of troponin-T release [58]. Most recently, RIC was shown to reduce myocardial biomarker release in patients undergoing thrombolytic reperfusion (Table 15.1) [59].

Remote ischemic postconditioning also reduces infarct size as assessed by the area under the curve of CK-MB release [60]. Consistently, infarct size was reduced by CMRI-delayed gadolinium enhancement volume; T2-weighted edema volume and ST-segment resolution greater than 50% was observed in twice as many patients in the treatment group as in the control group. At vital-status assessment after 1-year follow-up, one patient died in the control group (from refractory heart failure) and none in the remote postconditioning group. Cardiovascular events were lower in the treatment group. Combining RIC with local postconditioning does not reduce infarct size further in either experimental or in clinical settings [61,62].

Present reperfusion therapy is effective in the majority of patients undergoing primary PCI. Demonstrating additional clinical benefit beyond current reperfusion therapy may be challenging, owing to difficulties in demonstrating further reduction in small myocardial infarcts

(a)   (b)

(c)   (d)

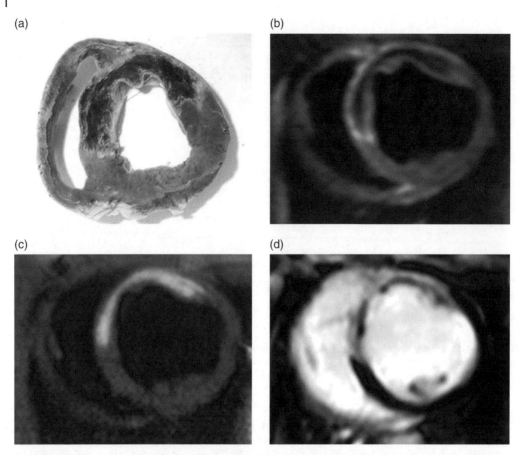

Figure 15.5 Short axis cardiac magnetic resonance images and corresponding pathology four days after ischemia/reperfusion injury in a porcine heart. Pathology shows intramural hemorrhage in the anteroseptal myocardium (a), which corresponds to a hypointense region on a T2-weighted area-at-risk (b). On the T1-weighted image, intramyocardial hemorrhage is depicted by a hyper-intense region (c). The late gadolinium image, which reflects the final infarct size, shows that microvascular obstruction is present within the infarct core (d) (source: Botker et al. *Cardiovascular Research*, 2012; 94: 266–7555, with permission).

and translating a minor reduction into a clinical benefit in low-risk patients. Some patients, predominantly those with large anterior infarcts, develop heart failure due to myocardial injury and subsequent remodeling of the left ventricle months or years after the infarct, despite optimal medical treatment according to guidelines. Because RIC reduces final tissue necrosis, improved clinical outcome may be assessed by reducing postinfarction left ventricular dysfunction and heart failure in combination with mortality reduction [63]. To achieve widespread acceptance of RIC in the clinical world, focus should be kept on patients at risk of extensive myocardial injury and global tissue damage. An emerging concept, known as chronic conditioning, is the extended use of RIC on a daily basis for weeks. In a study of rats, RIC demonstrated a dose-dependent effect on cardiac remodeling, heart failure and even death rate in the absence of a significant reduction of infarct size by administration daily for the first 28 days after the myocardial infarction [64]. This effect demonstrates beneficial effects beyond modification of acute ischemic effects, whereas a 2014 pilot study demonstrated no immediate translation into an improved exercise capacity in stable heart failure patients [65].

Table 15.1 Clinical studies of remote ischemic conditioning in acute myocardial infarction.

Study	Patients: Control/RIC (*n*)	RIC Regimen	Endpoint	Outcome
Botker et al. 2010 [26]	69/73	Upper limb 4 cycles I/R (5/5 minutes)	Salvage index (SPECT)	20% increase in salvage index
Munk et al. 2010 [56]	110/108	Upper limb 4 cycles I/R (5/5 minutes)	LVEF at 30 days	5% increase in LVEF in anterior infarcts
Rentoukas et al. 2010 [58]	30/33	Upper limb 3 cycles I/R (5/5 minutes)	STRes	20% increase in proportion of patients achieving full STRes
Crimi et al. 2013 [60]	50/50	Lower limb 3 cycles I/R (5/5 minutes)	CK-MB (AUC 72 hours after PCI)	20% reduction of CK-MB release
Prunier et al. 2014 [61]	17/18	Upper limb 4 cycles I/R (5/5 minutes)	CK-MB (AUC 72 hours after PCI)	31% reduction of CK-MB release
Sloth et al. 2014 [57]	167/166	Upper limb 4 cycles I/R (5/5 minutes)	MACCE at 4 years	12% reduction in MACCE
Yellon et al. 2015 [59]	260/260	Upper limb 4 cycles I/R (5/5 minutes)	TnT (AUC 24 hours after PCI)	17% reduction of TnT release
White et al. 2015 [101]	40/43	Upper limb 4 cycles I/R (5/5 minutes)	CMR	27% reduction of infarct size

AUC, area under curve; CK, creatine kinase; CK-MB, creatine kinase-myocardial band; CMR, cardiac magnetic resonance; I/R, ischemia/reperfusion; LVEF, left ventricular ejection fraction; MACCE, major adverse cardiovascular and cerebral events; PCI, percutaneous coronary intervention; RIC, remote ischemic conditioning; SPECT, single photon emission computed tomography; STRes, ST-segment resolution; TnT, troponin T.

Confounding Factors in Remote Ischemic Conditioning

Experimental studies using diseased animal models suggest that the effect of local ischemic conditioning may be modulated by aging, gender and comorbidities. Although less investigated, some of these conditions may also affect the efficacy of RIC in patients.

Comorbidities and Cardiovascular Risk Factors

Preclinical studies suggest that age [66] and comorbid diseases [67] such as hyperlipidemia, diabetes, and hypertension, raise the threshold for protection such that the presence of comorbidity requires an intensified conditioning signal. The change of cardioprotective threshold is reflective of the fundamental molecular alterations within the heart that affect both the sensitivity to ischemia/reperfusion injury and the response to a particular cardioprotective strategy [66,68–70]. Most experimental models use healthy young animals free of any comorbid diseases [71]. Experimental studies using human atrial muscle from aged and diabetic patients and patients with heart failure [49,72–74] undergoing coronary artery bypass graft, seem to confirm that comorbidity may affect the conditioning threshold and induce resistance to various conditioning strategies. Although diabetes mellitus attenuates the effect of RIC in experimental studies [75], the degree of cardioprotection may depend on stimulus intensity [76] and diabetes duration [77]. In a 2015 study of patients undergoing primary PCI for STEMI, any attenuation was absent and no influence of the glycemic status was observed [78]. Hence, diabetic patients should not be precluded from RIC.

Comedication

Pharmacological therapy may impact the cardioprotective effect of RIC. Specific sulphonylureas for treatment of type 2 diabetes can attenuate the conditioning response [79,80]. Conversely, insulin, metformin, some statins, angiotensin converting enzyme inhibitors and – of specific importance in STEMI patients – platelet $P2Y_{12}$ receptor antagonists and opioids can themselves be cardioprotective and raise the threshold for an additional benefit [10,31,70,81–83]. Intravenous nitroglycerine and nitroprusside, each protective in experimental settings, may interfere with the efficacy of cardioprotective interventions [70,84,85].

Other Potential Confounders in STEMI Patients

Infarct location and patient selection are important as only a quarter of all patients with STEMI have infarcts of sufficient size to realize benefit from adjunctive therapy [86]. Patients presenting with right and/or circumflex coronary artery occlusion usually have minor left ventricular involvement and do not gain as much benefit from cardioprotective therapy as those presenting with proximal left anterior descending coronary artery occlusion where the infarct is significantly larger [26,87]. "All-comer" trials will inevitably recruit more patients with small infarcts and little additional myocardial salvage, and hence will dilute a beneficial effect elicited by any novel protective strategy. On the other hand, recruitment of only patients with large anterior infarcts is more challenging, since these are the most critically ill patients [88]. The benefit for proof-of-concept trials is that fewer patients need to be recruited to demonstrate a significant difference between treatment and placebo [89]. Large studies with clinical outcome endpoints must be adequately powered to allow stratification according to infarct location.

Influence of TIMI flow prior to RIC is of importance because some patients with acute myocardial infarction have already undergone spontaneous reperfusion, at least partially, prior to interventional reperfusion and may not achieve the full benefit from any cardioprotective therapy [90]. Although it seems appropriate to include only those patients with TIMI score less than 1 in such studies [26], it is impossible specifically for RIC because the intervention must be initiated before the coronary pathology is identified to avoid delay in reperfusion. Large studies are required to allow adequate power for stratification.

The importance of visible coronary collaterals is not straightforward. While substantial collateralization is intuitively thought to improve clinical outcome by reducing the size of the area at risk [91,92] studies have not confirmed this [93,94], so the impact on the size of the evolving infarct seems minor [93,94]. RIC increases coronary blood flow in an experimental pig model [18] but does not seem to modify baseline and hyperemic coronary flow velocity in patients undergoing elective PCI [95]. To what extent collateralization will modify the ability of new cardioprotective strategies needs to be specifically investigated in RIC, because its effect is dependent of the transport of a mediating humoral factor to the infarct zone.

Given the crucial events that occur in the first few minutes of reperfusion, any cardioprotective strategy must be applied prior to the opening of the infarct-related coronary artery. Accordingly, RIC given to patients in the ambulance while in transit to the interventional center demonstrated a beneficial effect [26]. The effect is instantaneous and lasts 2–3 hours. A continued RIC protocol for an extended period after the acute myocardial infarction may modulate post-infarction remodeling [64] but the clinical implications remain yet unknown.

Alternative Methods to Achieve Cardioprotection

Other approaches to achieve protection against myocardial ischemia-reperfusion injury have been investigated, including cooling and pharmacological conditioning. Moderate hypothermia (34–35 °C) induced prior to reperfusion may reduce infarct size in animal models [96]. The CHILL-MI study, using similar cooling showed that while cooling did not have a general cardio-protective effect, it seems to reduce infarct size in patients with anterior STEMI admitted for primary PCI within four hours of symptom onset [97]. In addition, cooling caused a significant reduction in heart failure events.

The increasing insight into the mechanisms involved in local and RIC has encouraged the search for potential targets for pharmacological intervention against ischemia-reperfusion injury. While a vast number of pharmacological agents have been shown to afford cardioprotection in experimental models, most of these drugs yielded ambiguous results when tested in clinical studies. To date, the most promising pharmacological approaches for cardioprotection include cyclosporine [87], exenatide [98], and metoprolol [99], all of which seem to provide cardioprotection consistently in the clinical setting. It still remains unknown whether the combination of pharmacological therapy and RIC yields an additional cardioprotective effect. In an experimental rat model, hypothermia (30–31 °C) extended cardioprotection by ischemic preconditioning to coronary artery occlusions of longer duration [100].

Introducing Remote Ischemic Conditioning as Standard Adjuvant Therapy in STEMI

RIC is one of the most promising methods to achieve cardioprotection in patients admitted with acute myocardial infarction. The evidence so far suggests significant clinical benefit from RIC in patients with larger infarcts, and no significant adverse effects have been reported. RIC is easily applicable, low cost and universally available. Thus, it may already seem attractive to introduce RIC as standard adjuvant therapy in STEMI patients. However, properly sized randomized clinical trials are still essential to clarify whether RIC affords clinically relevant prognostic benefits to the patients.

The full potential of RIC has not yet been explored. Because RIC appears to have multi-organ protective capability, patients with cardiogenic shock, severe arrhythmias, including cardiac arrest and threatening global ischemia of the brain, heart, liver and kidney during organ transplantation may benefit from this novel approach.

Optimally, RIC should be initiated during ambulance transport to the cardiac unit, which requires both efficient pre-hospital diagnosis and complete collaboration with involved ambulance services.

Conclusions

Remote ischemic conditioning is a low-cost, non-invasive and easily applicable adjunctive therapy to reperfusion therapy for STEMI. It has no apparent adverse effects and seems to confer prognostic benefit for patients undergoing acute percutaneous coronary interventions. Large-scale studies with clinical endpoints are needed to confirm the clinical effect before RIC should be applied as standard adjunctive therapy.

References

1 Sorensen JT, Terkelsen CJ, Norgaard BL, et al. Urban and rural implementation of pre-hospital diagnosis and direct referral for primary percutaneous coronary intervention in patients with acute ST-elevation myocardial infarction. *Eur Heart J*, 2011; 32(4): 430–436.

2 Yellon DM, Hausenloy DJ. Myocardial reperfusion injury. *N Engl J Med*, 2007; 357(11): 1121–1135.

3 Ibanez B, Heusch G, Ovize M, et al. Evolving therapies for myocardial ischemia/reperfusion injury. *J Am Coll Cardiol*, 2015; 65(14): 1454–1471.

4 Carden DL, Granger DN. Pathophysiology of ischaemia-reperfusion injury. *J Pathol*, 2000; 190(3): 255–266.

5 Moran AE, Forouzanfar MH, Roth GA, et al. The global burden of ischemic heart disease in 1990 and 2010: the Global Burden of Disease 2010 study. *Circulation*, 2014; 129(14): 1493–1501.

6 Schmidt M, Jacobsen JB, Lash TL, et al. 25 year trends in first time hospitalisation for acute myocardial infarction, subsequent short and long term mortality, and the prognostic impact of sex and comorbidity: a Danish nationwide cohort study. *BMJ*, 2012; 344: e356.

7 Chen J, Hsieh AF, Dharmarajan K, et al. National trends in heart failure hospitalization after acute myocardial infarction for Medicare beneficiaries: 1998-2010. *Circulation*, 2013; 128(24): 2577–2584.

8 Murry CE, Jennings RB, Reimer KA. Preconditioning with ischemia: a delay of lethal cell injury in ischemic myocardium. *Circulation*, 1986; 74(5): 1124–1136.

9 Yellon DM, Alkhulaifi AM, Pugsley WB. Preconditioning the human myocardium. *Lancet*, 1993; 342(8866): 276–277.

10 Heusch G. Cardioprotection: chances and challenges of its translation to the clinic. *Lancet*, 2013; 381(9861): 166–175.

11 Lonborg J, Kelbaek H, Vejlstrup N, et al. Cardioprotective effects of ischemic postconditioning in patients treated with primary percutaneous coronary intervention, evaluated by magnetic resonance. *Circ Cardiovasc Interv*, 2010; 3(1): 34–41.

12 Heusch G. Treatment of Myocardial Ischemia/Reperfusion Injury by Ischemic and Pharmacological Postconditioning. *Compr Physiol*, 2015; 5(3): 1123–1145.

13 Przyklenk K, Bauer B, Ovize M, et al. Regional ischemic 'preconditioning' protects remote virgin myocardium from subsequent sustained coronary occlusion. *Circulation*, 1993; 87(3): 893–899.

14 Kharbanda RK, Mortensen UM, White PA, et al. Transient limb ischemia induces remote ischemic preconditioning in vivo. *Circulation*, 2002; 106(23): 2881–2883.

15 Pedersen CM, Cruden NL, Schmidt MR, et al. Remote ischemic preconditioning prevents systemic platelet activation associated with ischemia-reperfusion injury in humans. *J Thromb Haemost*, 2011; 9(2): 404–407.

16 Konstantinov IE, Arab S, Li J, et al. The remote ischemic preconditioning stimulus modifies gene expression in mouse myocardium. *J Thorac Cardiovasc Surg*, 2005; 130(5): 1326–1332.

17 Konstantinov IE, Li J, Cheung MM, et al. Remote ischemic preconditioning of the recipient reduces myocardial ischemia-reperfusion injury of the denervated donor heart via a Katp channel-dependent mechanism. *Transplantation*, 2005; 79(12): 1691–1695.

18 Shimizu M, Konstantinov IE, Kharbanda RK, et al. Effects of intermittent lower limb ischaemia on coronary blood flow and coronary resistance in pigs. *Acta Physiol (Oxf)*, 2007; 190(2): 103–109.

19 Shimizu M, Saxena P, Konstantinov IE, et al. Remote ischemic preconditioning decreases adhesion and selectively modifies functional responses of human neutrophils. *J Surg Res*, 2010; 158(1): 155–1561.

20 Shimizu M, Tropak M, Diaz RJ, et al. Transient limb ischaemia remotely preconditions through a humoral mechanism acting directly on the myocardium: evidence suggesting cross-species protection. *Clin Sci (Lond)*, 2009; 117(5): 191–200.

21 Vinten-Johansen J, Shi W. Perconditioning and postconditioning: current knowledge, knowledge gaps, barriers to adoption, and future directions. *J Cardiovasc Pharmacol Ther*, 2011; 16(3-4): 260–266.

22 Schmidt MR, Smerup M, Konstantinov IE, et al. Intermittent peripheral tissue ischemia during coronary ischemia reduces myocardial infarction through a KATP-dependent mechanism: first demonstration of remote ischemic perconditioning. *Am J Physiol Heart Circ Physiol*, 2007; 292(4): H1883–H1890.

23 Andreka G, Vertesaljai M, Szantho G, et al. Remote ischaemic postconditioning protects the heart during acute myocardial infarction in pigs. *Heart*, 2007; 93(6): 749–752.

24 Breivik L, Helgeland E, Aarnes EK, et al. Remote postconditioning by humoral factors in effluent from ischemic preconditioned rat hearts is mediated via PI3K/Akt-dependent cell-survival signaling at reperfusion. *Basic Res Cardiol*, 2011; 106(1): 135–145.

25 Gritsopoulos G, Iliodromitis EK, Zoga A, et al. Remote postconditioning is more potent than classic postconditioning in reducing the infarct size in anesthetized rabbits. *Cardiovasc Drugs Ther*, 2009; 23(3): 193–198.

26 Botker HE, Kharbanda R, Schmidt MR, et al. Remote ischaemic conditioning before hospital admission, as a complement to angioplasty, and effect on myocardial salvage in patients with acute myocardial infarction: a randomised trial. *Lancet*, 2010; 375(9716): 727–7234.

27 Carroll R, Yellon DM. Myocardial adaptation to ischaemia--the preconditioning phenomenon. *Int J Cardiol* 1999; 68(Suppl 1): S93–S101.

28 Baxter GF. Ischaemic preconditioning of myocardium. *Ann Med*, 1997; 29(4): 345–352.

29 Zografos TA, Katritsis GD, Tsiafoutis I, et al. Effect of one-cycle remote ischemic preconditioning to reduce myocardial injury during percutaneous coronary intervention. *Am J Cardiol*, 2014; 113(12): 2013–2017.

30 Johnsen JP, Salman K, Kristiansen R, et al. Optimizing the cardioprotective effects of remote ischemic preconditioning. *Eur Heart J*, 2014; 35: (Suppl 1): 444.

31 Michelsen MM, Stottrup NB, Schmidt MR, et al. Exercise-induced cardioprotection is mediated by a bloodborne, transferable factor. *Basic Res Cardiol*, 2012; 107(3): 260.

32 Gross ER, Hsu AK, Urban TJ, et al. Nociceptive-induced myocardial remote conditioning is mediated by neuronal gamma protein kinase C. *Basic Res Cardiol*, 2013; 108(5): 381.

33 Redington KL, Disenhouse T, Strantzas SC, et al. Remote cardioprotection by direct peripheral nerve stimulation and topical capsaicin is mediated by circulating humoral factors. *Basic Res Cardiol*, 2012; 107(2): 241.

34 Merlocco AC, Redington KL, Disenhouse T, et al. Transcutaneous electrical nerve stimulation as a novel method of remote preconditioning: in vitro validation in an animal model and first human observations. *Basic Res Cardiol*, 2014; 109(3): 406.

35 Redington KL, Disenhouse T, Li J, et al. Electroacupuncture reduces myocardial infarct size and improves post-ischemic recovery by invoking release of humoral, dialyzable, cardioprotective factors. *J Physiol Sci*, 2013; 63(3): 219–223.

36 Jones WK, Fan GC, Liao S, et al. Peripheral nociception associated with surgical incision elicits remote nonischemic cardioprotection via neurogenic activation of protein kinase C signaling. *Circulation*, 2009; 120(11 Suppl): S1–S9.

37 Basalay M, Barsukevich V, Mastitskaya S, et al. Remote ischaemic pre- and delayed postconditioning: Similar degree of cardioprotection but distinct mechanisms. *Exp Physiol*, 2012; 97(8): 908–917.

38 Steensrud T, Li J, Dai X, et al. Pretreatment with the nitric oxide donor SNAP or nerve transection blocks humoral preconditioning by remote limb ischemia or intra-arterial adenosine. *Am J Physiol Heart Circ Physiol*, 2010; 299(5): H1598–H603.

39 Donato M, Buchholz B, Rodriguez M, et al. Role of the parasympathetic nervous system in cardioprotection by remote hindlimb ischaemic preconditioning. *Exp Physiol*, 2013; 98(2): 425–434.

40 Dickson EW, Lorbar M, Porcaro WA, et al. Rabbit heart can be "preconditioned" via transfer of coronary effluent. *Am J Physiol*, 1999; 277(6 Pt 2): H2451–H2457.

41 Skyschally A, Gent S, Amanakis G, et al. Across-species transfer of protection by remote ischemic preconditioning with species-specific myocardial signal transduction by RISK and SAFE pathways. *Circ Res*, 2015; 117(3):279–288.

42 Rassaf T, Totzeck M, Hendgen-Cotta UB, et al. Circulating nitrite contributes to cardioprotection by remote ischemic preconditioning. *Circ Res*, 2014; 114(10): 1601–1610.

43 Leung CH, Wang L, Nielsen JM, et al. Remote cardioprotection by transfer of coronary effluent from ischemic preconditioned rabbit heart preserves mitochondrial integrity and function via adenosine receptor activation. *Cardiovasc Drugs Ther*, 2014; 28(1): 7–17.

44 Giricz Z, Varga ZV, Baranyai T, et al. Cardioprotection by remote ischemic preconditioning of the rat heart is mediated by extracellular vesicles. *J Mol Cell Cardiol*, 2014; 68: 75–78.

45 Sahoo S, Losordo DW. Exosomes and cardiac repair after myocardial infarction. *Circ Res*, 2014; 114(2): 333–344.

46 Yellon DM, Davidson SM. Exosomes: nanoparticles involved in cardioprotection? *Circ Res*, 2014; 114(2): 325–332.

47 Arroyo JD, Chevillet JR, Kroh EM, et al. Argonaute2 complexes carry a population of circulating microRNAs independent of vesicles in human plasma. *Proc Natl Acad Sci USA*, 2011; 108(12): 5003–5008.

48 Li J, Rohailla S, Gelber N, et al. MicroRNA-144 is a circulating effector of remote ischemic preconditioning. *Basic Res Cardiol*, 2014; 109(5): 423.

49 Jensen RV, Zachara NE, Nielsen PH, et al. Impact of O-GlcNAc on cardioprotection by remote ischaemic preconditioning in non-diabetic and diabetic patients. *Cardiovasc Res*, 2013; 97(2): 369–378.

50 Kharbanda RK, Nielsen TT, Redington AN. Translation of remote ischaemic preconditioning into clinical practice. *Lancet*, 2009; 374(9700): 1557–1565.

51 Hausenloy DJ, Botker HE, Condorelli G, et al. Translating cardioprotection for patient benefit: Position paper from the Working Group of Cellular Biology of the Heart of the European Society of Cardiology. *Cardiovasc Res*, 2013; 98(1): 7–27.

52 Schmidt MR, Redington A, Botker HE. Remote conditioning the heart overview - translatability and mechanism. *Br J Pharmacol*, 2015; 172(8): 1947–1960.

53 Fernandez-Jimenez R, Sanchez-Gonzalez J, Aguero J, et al. Myocardial edema after ischemia/ reperfusion is not stable and follows a bimodal pattern: imaging and histological tissue characterization. *J Am Coll Cardiol*, 2015; 65(4): 315–323.

54 Thuny F, Lairez O, Roubille F, et al. Post-conditioning reduces infarct size and edema in patients with ST-segment elevation myocardial infarction. *J Am Coll Cardiol*, 2012; 59(24): 2175–2181.

55 Botker HE, Kaltoft AK, Pedersen SF, et al. Measuring myocardial salvage. *Cardiovasc Res*, 2012; 94(2): 266–275.

56 Munk K, Andersen NH, Schmidt MR, et al. Remote ischemic conditioning in patients with myocardial infarction treated with primary angioplasty: impact on left ventricular function assessed by comprehensive echocardiography and gated single-photon emission CT. *Circ Cardiovasc Imaging*, 2010; 3(6): 656–662.

57 Sloth AD, Schmidt MR, Munk K, et al. Improved long-term clinical outcomes in patients with ST-elevation myocardial infarction undergoing remote ischaemic conditioning as an adjunct to primary percutaneous coronary intervention. *Eur Heart J*, 2014; 35(3): 168–175.

58 Rentoukas I, Giannopoulos G, Kaoukis A, et al. Cardioprotective role of remote ischemic periconditioning in primary percutaneous coronary intervention: enhancement by opioid action. *JACC Cardiovasc Interv*, 2010; 3(1): 49–55.

59 Yellon DM, Ackbarkhan AK, Balgobin V, et al. Remote Ischemic Conditioning Reduces Myocardial Infarct Size in STEMI Patients Treated by Thrombolysis. *J Am Coll Cardiol*, 2015; 65(25): 2764–2765.

60 Crimi G, Pica S, Raineri C, et al. Remote ischemic post-conditioning of the lower limb during primary percutaneous coronary intervention safely reduces enzymatic infarct size in anterior myocardial infarction: a randomized controlled trial. *JACC Cardiovasc Interv*, 2013; 6(10): 1055–1063.

61 Prunier F, Angoulvant D, Saint Etienne C, et al. The RIPOST-MI study, assessing remote ischemic perconditioning alone or in combination with local ischemic postconditioning in ST-segment elevation myocardial infarction. *Basic Res Cardio,l* 2014; 109(2): 400.

62 Xin P, Zhu W, Li J, et al. Combined local ischemic postconditioning and remote perconditioning recapitulate cardioprotective effects of local ischemic preconditioning. *Am J Physiol Heart Circ Physiol*, 2010; 298(6): H1819–H1831.

63 Hausenloy DJ, Baxter G, Bell R, et al. Translating novel strategies for cardioprotection: the Hatter Workshop Recommendations. *Basic Res Cardiol*, 2010; 105(6): 677–686.

64 Wei M, Xin P, Li S, et al. Repeated remote ischemic postconditioning protects against adverse left ventricular remodeling and improves survival in a rat model of myocardial infarction. *Circ Res* 2011; 108(10): 1220–1225.

65 McDonald MA, Braga JR, Li J, et al. A randomized pilot trial of remote ischemic preconditioning in heart failure with reduced ejection fraction. *PLoS One*, 2014; 9(9): e105361.

66 Boengler K, Schulz R, Heusch G. Loss of cardioprotection with ageing. *Cardiovasc Res*, 2009; 83(2): 247–261.

67 Ferdinandy P, Hausenloy DJ, Heusch G, et al. Interaction of risk factors, comorbidities, and comedications with ischemia/reperfusion injury and cardioprotection by preconditioning, postconditioning, and remote conditioning. *Pharmacol Rev*, 2014; 66(4): 1142–1174.

68 Ferdinandy P, Schulz R, Baxter GF. Interaction of cardiovascular risk factors with myocardial ischemia/reperfusion injury, preconditioning, and postconditioning. *Pharmacol Rev*, 2007; 59(4): 418–458.

69 Whittington HJ, Babu GG, Mocanu MM, et al. The diabetic heart: Too sweet for its own good? *Cardiol Res Pract*, 2012; 2012: 845–698.

70 Ferdinandy P, Szilvassy Z, Baxter GF. Adaptation to myocardial stress in disease states: is preconditioning a healthy heart phenomenon? *Trends Pharmacol Sci*, 1998; 19(6): 223–299.

71 Ludman AJ, Yellon DM, Hausenloy DJ. Cardiac preconditioning for ischaemia: lost in translation. *Dis Model Mech*, 2010; 3(1–2): 35–38.

72 Loubani M, Ghosh S, Galinanes M. The aging human myocardium: tolerance to ischemia and responsiveness to ischemic preconditioning. *J Thorac Cardiovasc Surg*, 2003; 126(1): 143–147.

73 Hassouna A, Loubani M, Matata BM, et al. Mitochondrial dysfunction as the cause of the failure to precondition the diabetic human myocardium. *Cardiovasc Res*, 2006; 69(2): 450–458.

74 Sivaraman V, Hausenloy DJ, Wynne AM, et al. Preconditioning the diabetic human myocardium. *J Cell Mol Med*, 2010; 14(6B): 1740–1746.

75 Kristiansen SB, Lofgren B, Stottrup NB, et al. Ischaemic preconditioning does not protect the heart in obese and lean animal models of type 2 diabetes. *Diabetologia*, 2004; 47(10): 1716–1721.

76 Tsang A, Hausenloy DJ, Mocanu MM, et al. Preconditioning the diabetic heart: the importance of Akt phosphorylation. *Diabetes*, 2005; 54(8): 2360–2364.

77 Povlsen JA, Lofgren B, Dalgas C, et al. Protection against myocardial ischemia-reperfusion injury at onset of type 2 diabetes in Zucker diabetic fatty rats is associated with altered glucose oxidation. *PLoS One*, 2013; 8(5): e64093.

78 Sloth AD, Schmidt MR, Munk K, et al. Impact of cardiovascular risk factors and medication use on the efficacy of remote ischaemic conditioning: post hoc subgroup analysis of a randomised controlled trial. *BMJ Open*, 2015; 5(4): e006923.

79 Kottenberg E, Thielmann M, Kleinbongard P, et al. Myocardial protection by remote ischaemic pre-conditioning is abolished in sulphonylurea-treated diabetics undergoing coronary revascularisation. *Acta Anaesthesiol Scand*, 2014; 58(4): 453–462.

80 Kristiansen SB, Lofgren B, Nielsen JM, et al. Comparison of two sulfonylureas with high and low myocardial K(ATP) channel affinity on myocardial infarct size and metabolism in a rat model of type 2 diabetes. *Diabetologia*, 2011; 54(2): 451–458.

81 Roubille F, Lairez O, Mewton N, et al. Cardioprotection by clopidogrel in acute ST-elevated myocardial infarction patients: a retrospective analysis. *Basic Res Cardiol*, 2012; 107(4): 275.

82 Przyklenk K. Efficacy of cardioprotective 'conditioning' strategies in aging and diabetic cohorts: the co-morbidity conundrum. *Drugs Aging*, 2011; 28(5): 331–343.

83 Cohen MV, Downey JM. Combined cardioprotectant and antithrombotic actions of platelet P2Y12 receptor antagonists in acute coronary syndrome: just what the doctor ordered. *J Cardiovasc Pharmacol Ther*, 2014; 19(2): 179–190.

84 Heusch G, Botker HE, Przyklenk K, et al. Remote ischemic conditioning. *J Am Coll Cardiol*, 2015; 65(2): 177–195.

85 Kleinbongard P, Thielmann M, Jakob H, et al. Nitroglycerin does not interfere with protection by remote ischemic preconditioning in patients with surgical coronary revascularization under isoflurane anesthesia. *Cardiovasc Drugs Ther*, 2013; 27(4): 359–361.

86 Miura T, Miki T. Limitation of myocardial infarct size in the clinical setting: current status and challenges in translating animal experiments into clinical therapy. *Basic Res Cardiol*, 2008; 103(6): 501–513.

87 Piot C, Croisille P, Staat P, et al. Effect of cyclosporine on reperfusion injury in acute myocardial infarction. *N Engl J Med*, 2008; 359(5): 473–481.

88 Hausenloy DJ, Erik Botker H, Condorelli G, et al. Translating cardioprotection for patient benefit: position paper from the Working Group of Cellular Biology of the Heart of the European Society of Cardiology. *Cardiovasc Res*, 2013; 98(1): 7–27.

89 Ovize M, Baxter GF, Di Lisa F, et al, Working Group of Cellular Biology of Heart of European Society of C. Postconditioning and protection from reperfusion injury: where do we stand? Position paper from the Working Group of Cellular Biology of the Heart of the European Society of Cardiology. *Cardiovasc Res*, 2010; 87(3): 406–423.

90 Roubille F, Mewton N, Elbaz M, et al. No post-conditioning in the human heart with thrombolysis in myocardial infarction flow 2–3 on admission. *Eur Heart J*, 2014; 35(25): 1675–1682.

91 Desch S, de Waha S, Eitel I, et al. Effect of coronary collaterals on long-term prognosis in patients undergoing primary angioplasty for acute ST-elevation myocardial infarction. *Am J Cardiol*, 2010; 106(5): 605–611.

92 Hoole SP, White PA, Heck PM, et al. Primary coronary microvascular dysfunction and poor coronary collaterals predict post-percutaneous coronary intervention cardiac necrosis. *Coron Artery Dis*, 2009; 20(4): 253–259.

93 Lonborg J, Kelbaek H, Vejlstrup N, et al. Influence of pre-infarction angina, collateral flow, and pre-procedural TIMI flow on myocardial salvage index by cardiac magnetic resonance in patients with ST-segment elevation myocardial infarction. *Eur Heart J Cardiovasc Imaging,* 2012; 13(5): 433–443.

94 Ortiz-Perez JT, Lee DC, Meyers SN, et al. Determinants of myocardial salvage during acute myocardial infarction: evaluation with a combined angiographic and CMR myocardial salvage index. *JACC Cardiovasc Imaging,* 2010; 3(5): 491–500.

95 Hoole SP, Heck PM, White PA, et al. Remote ischemic preconditioning stimulus does not reduce microvascular resistance or improve myocardial blood flow in patients undergoing elective percutaneous coronary intervention. *Angiology,* 2009; 60(4): 403–411.

96 Tissier R, Ghaleh B, Cohen MV, et al. Myocardial protection with mild hypothermia. *Cardiovasc Res,* 2012; 94(2): 217–225.

97 Erlinge D, Gotberg M, Lang I, et al. Rapid endovascular catheter core cooling combined with cold saline as an adjunct to percutaneous coronary intervention for the treatment of acute myocardial infarction. The CHILL-MI trial: a randomized controlled study of the use of central venous catheter core cooling combined with cold saline as an adjunct to percutaneous coronary intervention for the treatment of acute myocardial infarction. *J Am Coll Cardiol,* 2014; 63(18): 1857–1865.

98 Lonborg J, Vejlstrup N, Kelbaek H, et al. Exenatide reduces reperfusion injury in patients with ST-segment elevation myocardial infarction. *Eur Heart J,* 2012; 33(12): 1491–149.

99 Ibanez B, Macaya C, Sanchez-Brunete V, et al. Effect of early metoprolol on infarct size in ST-segment-elevation myocardial infarction patients undergoing primary percutaneous coronary intervention: the Effect of Metoprolol in Cardioprotection During an Acute Myocardial Infarction (METOCARD-CNIC) trial. *Circulation,* 2013; 128(14): 1495–1503.

100 van den Doel MA, Gho BC, Duval SY, et al. Hypothermia extends the cardioprotection by ischaemic preconditioning to coronary artery occlusions of longer duration. *Cardiovasc Res,* 1998; 37(1): 76–81.

101 White SK, Frohlich GM, Sado DM, et al. Remote ischemic conditioning reduces myocardial infarct size and edema in patients with ST-segment elevation myocardial infarction. *JACC Cardiovasc Interv,* 2015; 8(1 Pt B): 178–88.

Part III

The STEMI Process

16

Reducing Door-to-Balloon Times

Michel Le May MD, Joshua PY Loh MD

Introduction

Time is a key prognosticator of morbidity and mortality in ST-segment elevation myocardial infarction (STEMI), and a modulator of the efficacy and safety of reperfusion therapies [1–3]. The onset of symptoms in STEMI patients marks the start of the total ischemic time interval, a period during which thrombotic occlusion of a coronary artery will lead to progressive myocardial necrosis in the territory it supplies [4]. Although the rate of myocardial necrosis in STEMI depends on multiple factors (Box 16.1), the infarction is generally completed within hours of the coronary occlusion [5,6]. If perfusion in the infarct-related artery is not promptly reestablished, the ischemic myocardium will become irreversibly injured, leading to significant morbidity and mortality.

Primary percutaneous coronary intervention (PPCI) has become the gold standard reperfusion strategy for STEMI [7–9]. When provided in a timely manner, PPCI provides a mechanical means of bringing the total ischemic time to a halt, by establishing rapid, complete, and sustained reperfusion in the infarct-related artery. However, as in fibrinolysis, the efficacy of PPCI is highly time dependent, as the fraction of the ischemic myocardium available for salvage will invariably decrease with time [1,2,10]. Early data from the Global Use of Strategies to Open Occluded Coronary Arteries (GUSTO)-IIb substudy demonstrated an inverse relationship between the time to angioplasty and mortality, with optimal outcomes achieved when PPCI was provided within 60 minutes of study enrollment (1.0% vs. 6.4% mortality when time to angioplasty was ≤ 60 minutes vs. ≥ 91 minutes, respectively) [11]. This notion of the "golden hour" of PPCI led to a growing emphasis on reducing delays in the provision of PPCI, and highlighted the importance of considering PCI-related delays when choosing an optimal reperfusion strategy.

Door-to-balloon time, defined as the time between the arrival of a STEMI patient to a hospital and first balloon inflation (or device used) during PPCI, is a valid, reliable, and widely used metric of the timeliness of PPCI for STEMI patients.12 Door-to-balloon time has been shown to be a predictor of morbidity and mortality in STEMI, and a strong modulator of the efficacy of PPCI [2,10,13]. Observational studies have demonstrated an inverse linear relationship between door-to-balloon time and mortality, with each 10-minute increase in door-to-balloon time resulting in a 9% increase in the odds of dying during the index hospitalization [14]. System delays during PPCI have also been correlated with increased long-term mortality, impaired left ventricular systolic function, and development of congestive heart failure [15–17]. Door-to-balloon time was adopted as a performance standard in American College of

---

Box 16.1   Factors That Affect the Rate of Necrosis in Myocardial Ischemia

- Availability of functioning collateral coronary arteries.
- Ischemic preconditioning.
- Duration of *sustained* ischemia.
- Myocardial oxygen demand.

Box 16.2   Non-System Based Delays in Door-to-Balloon Time Delays [8]

- Prolonged transport time due to geographic distance or weather.
- Uncertainty about STEMI diagnosis (e.g. suspected aortic dissection).
- Need to evaluation and treatment of potentially life threatening conditions (e.g. cardiac arrest).
- Delays while obtaining informed consent.

Cardiology/American Heart Association (ACC/AHA) STEMI guidelines in 1999 [18] and included in the European Society of Cardiology (ESC) STEMI guidelines in 2003 [19]. Although this recommendation was initially based on expert opinion, subsequent studies validated the use of door-to-balloon time as a quality of care measure, owing to its association with morbidity and mortality in STEMI [10,15,20]. Current STEMI guidelines recommend a door-to-balloon time of 90 minutes or less and 120 minutes or less for patients presenting to PCI-capable and non-PCI-capable hospitals, respectively [8,9]. Rather than benchmarks, door-to-balloon time limits are meant to represent the maximum acceptable time to reperfusion in STEMI patients without appropriate reasons for delay (Box 16.2) [8]. This is because, even within the recommended door-to-balloon time limits, there continues to be a linear association between further reductions in door-to-balloon time and decreased in-hospital mortality [14]. As a result, STEMI guidelines have adopted the notion that "every minute counts" during STEMI management [10].

During the early implementation of PPCI in healthcare systems, it became evident that the short door-to-balloon times achieved in large-volume centers participating in randomized controlled trials may not have been representative of those in smaller community hospitals [21–23]. In the Danish Trial in Acute Myocardial Infarction (DANAMI)-2, which compared on-site fibrinolysis to transfer for PPCI in STEMI patients presenting to non-PCI capable hospitals, PPCI was associated with a significant reduction in the composite of death, reinfarction, or stroke at 30 days [24]. However, in this study, 96% of patients in the invasive arm were transferred to a PCI-capable hospital within 2 hours. Although DANAMI-2 demonstrated the feasibility of a regional STEMI system, where patients presenting to non-PCI-capable hospitals with STEMI could be transferred for timely PPCI, early observational studies of STEMI management provided sobering data regarding door-to-balloon time during PPCI in a real-world setting. Data from the National Registry of Myocardial Infarction (NRMI) 2 registry showed that the median door-to-balloon time in the United States was nearly 2 hours, with only 29% of patients receiving PPCI within 90 minutes of presentation [1]. The results were concerning because of the increased mortality associated with prolonged door-to-balloon times, and the potential overreliance on PCI as a primary reperfusion strategy in centers with consistently prolonged PCI-related delays.

PPCI is a highly effective but resource intensive strategy, which requires infrastructure, technical expertise, and organizational schemes in order to be implemented with the timeliness and quality it requires. The superiority of PPCI over thrombolysis diminishes as PCI-related delays increase, with one observational study suggesting comparable mortality between reperfusion strategies when PCI related delay is greater than 114 minutes [25]. Hence, fibrinolysis should be considered as a primary reperfusion strategy in settings were PCI-related delays are consistently longer than 2 hours [9].

Large observational studies have identified several patient and institutional factors associated with prolonged door-to-balloon times. Similar to delays in thrombolysis, PCI-related delays are longer in STEMI patients who are older, female, and chest pain-free on presentation [26,27]. However, patients who require transfer for PPCI after presenting to a non-PCI-capable hospital, and those who present to hospital during off-hours or on weekends, are at highest risk of prolonged PCI related delays [26,27]. In a large observational study using data from NRMI 3/4, the median door to balloon time in patients requiring transfer for PPCI was 180 minutes, with only 4.2% achieving door-to-balloon times of 90 minutes or less [27]. Fortunately, during the 2000s, healthcare initiatives at institutional, regional, and national levels have led to significant reductions in door-to-balloon times, with a 2015 study demonstrating a decrease in the median door-to-balloon time in US hospitals from 86 minutes in 2005 to 63 minutes in 2011 [14,28]. The complexity of these initiatives ranges from quality improvement projects within hospital departments to complete redesigns of regional healthcare delivery systems [12,29–32].

Early Initiatives and Quality-of-Care Measures to Minimize Door-to-Balloon Time

STEMI systems can minimize system delays by addressing key door-to-balloon time subintervals: first medical contact to diagnosis time; diagnosis to catheterization laboratory time; and laboratory arrival to device time (Box 16.3) [33,34]. While all subintervals have not been independently correlated with mortality, they are important, as they allow the implementation of benchmarks and quality of care measures to systematically reduce door-to-balloon times. Current STEMI guidelines have targeted specific door-to-balloon time subintervals as quality of care measures in STEMI systems [8,9]. Both ACC/AHA and ESC guidelines use a door to electrocardiogram (EKG) time of 10 minutes or less as a quality of care measure. Although door to ECG time represents a small fraction (less than10%) of the door-to-balloon time in optimized STEMI systems, the value of a continuous focus on this quality of care measure cannot be overemphasized, as preventable delays in diagnosis do occur, and result in unnecessary morbidity and mortality [33]. Recent ACC/AHA guidelines have also adopted the use of the door in,door out time (DIDO), defined as the time between arrival of a STEMI patient to a non-PCI-capable hospital and departure from the same hospital for PPCI [8]. One of the objectives of the ACC/AHA door in,door out time target of 30 minutes or less is to reduce the EKG-to-catheterization laboratory interval, which accounts for approximately 60% of the door-to-balloon time interval in PPCI pathways [33]. Unlike the door-to-catheterization laboratory interval, the door in, door out time does not depend on transport time, which can vary widely and may not be entirely within an institution's control. In addition, in many modern STEMI systems, the door in, door out time will depend entirely on non-PCI-capable hospitals, as STEMI patients do not need to be accepted by a PCI-capable hospital prior to transfer [30]. As a result, the door in, door out time can serve as a robust quality of care measure in non-PCI-capable hospitals where an option of rapid transfer for timely PPCI is available.

Box 16.3 Strategies to Reduce Door-to-Balloon Time Based on Key Subintervals [12,30,33–35]

Reduction in first medical contact to diagnosis time

1) Rapid acquisition and interpretation of electrocardiogram (EKG) by paramedics.
2) Door-to-EKG time ≤ 10 minutes as a quality of care measure.

Reduction in diagnosis to catheterization laboratory time

1) Activation of the percutaneous coronary intervention (PCI) team by emergency physicians.
2) CODE STEMI protocol, including single call to a central operator activates the PCI team.
3) Arrival of PCI team to catheterization laboratory within 20 minutes of CODE STEMI deployment as quality of care measure.
4) Activation of PCI team while patient is en route to hospital.
5) Door in, door out time ≤ 30 minutes as a quality of care measure in non-PCI-capable hospitals transferring patients for primary PCI.

Reduction in catheterization laboratory to device time

1) Maximize staff experience:
   a) Primary PCI hospitals perform procedure 24 hours/day, 7 days/week; and
   b) STEMI regional systems designed to include a minimum catchment area (i.e. avoid small service areas which may have suboptimal experience).

General measures for all intervals above

1) Systematic feedback system to monitor progress and identify deficiencies.
2) A CODE STEMI protocol and organizational culture that fosters collaboration between interdisciplinary teams.

Regional STEMI Systems to Further Reduce Door-to-Balloon Time

One of the main barriers during the early implementation of STEMI pathways was achieving adequate door-to-balloon times in patients presenting to non-PCI-capable hospitals. NRMI data demonstrated that 96% of STEMI patients presenting to non-PCI-capable hospitals did not receive PPCI within the recommended door-to-balloon time of 90 minutes or less [27]. To circumvent these system delays, the initial STEMI pathway evolved from an institutional protocol to the modern STEMI system – a regional strategy encompassing neighboring hospitals, emergency medical services, and regional healthcare systems [30]. The design of the modern STEMI system relies on several basic tenets to minimize door-to-balloon-time, which include the use of EKG by paramedics before arrival to hospital, the option to bypass emergency department on route to a PCI-capable hospital, deployment of the PCI team by emergency department physicians without specialist consultation, and standardized protocols for pharmacotherapy, history taking, physical examination, and patient consent (Box 16.3) [12,30,34,35]. These measures reduce door-to-balloon times by streamlining the STEMI diagnosis, referral, and transfer process, and increasing the expertise and efficiency of PCI-capable hospitals by allowing them to safely and reliably serve larger catchment areas. This is of particular importance since center expertise with PPCI is associated with shorter door-to-balloon times and improved clinical outcomes [36,37]. Regional STEMI systems have been successfully implemented across North America and have resulted in significant, sizable reductions in door-to-balloon time, morbidity, and mortality [29,30,35].

Despite ongoing changes in patient demographics and advances in STEMI care, 2015 data from the National Cardiovascular Data Registry (NCDR) demonstrate that door-to-balloon time continues to be a robust prognosticator of morbidity and mortality in STEMI [14]. In a large prospective cohort of STEMI patients, there was a continuous association between door-to-balloon time and the odds of death during the index admission and at 6 months, which persisted across a wide spectrum of door-to-balloon times ranging from less than 60 minutes to greater than 120 minutes. This latter finding emphasizes the fact that, although a door-to-balloon time of 90 minutes or less is the standard quality of care measure, the institutional norm should be to treat all STEMI patients with the same rapidity, despite their place within the door-to-balloon time spectrum. This practice will maximize the benefits of PPCI for the individual patient and help improve and maintain the efficiency of the STEMI system.

Limitations of Door-to-Balloon Time

Despite its robustness as a predictor of morbidity and mortality in STEMI, the use of door-to-balloon times as a quality of care measure does have limitations. Several studies have demonstrated that the modulating effect of door-to-balloon time may be largely dependent on the duration of symptoms, patient demographics, and characteristics of the infarction [38]. Although clinically relevant, these factors do not negate the important of streamlining all STEMI patients through the PPCI pathway with the same rapidity to optimize outcomes for the individual patient and maintain the efficiency of the system. The current emphasis on reducing door-to-balloon time, rather than door-to-reperfusion time, has raised some valid concerns. In a real-world setting where fibrinolysis is widely available and PPCI is offered in a minority of hospitals, fixating on providing timely PPCI to all STEMI patients could lead to unjustifiable delays in door-to-reperfusion time and thereby worsen outcomes [39]. Previous studies have noted this issue in patients presenting to non-PCI-capable hospitals, in whom the median door-to-balloon time is as high as 180 minutes, with as many as 85% over the critical door-to-balloon time of less than 120 minutes, where fibrinolysis may have been preferred [27]. As a result, STEMI guidelines adopted the use of PCI-related delays, defined as the door-to-balloon time minus door-to-needle time, when addressing choice of reperfusion therapy for STEMI [8,9]. Although the modulating effect of PCI-related delays has been validated in post-hoc analyses of randomized controlled trials, estimates of the PCI-related delay that negates the benefits of PPCI have been quite variable, ranging from 60 minutes to 120 minutes [25,40]. Current STEMI guidelines have replaced an estimated PCI-related delay of 60 minutes by an estimated door-to-balloon time of 120 minutes or less as the critical period during which PPCI is preferred over fibrinolysis. Although this new recommendation is simple and based on more robust data, it does not address the fact that the mitigating effect of PCI-related delay on the efficacy of PPCI depends on multiple factors including duration of symptoms, patient characteristics, and the location of the infarct [25]. Despite this limitation, the standardization of STEMI care through prespecified pathways and regional systems, rather than a patient-specific approach, remains the most efficient strategy to achieve optimal and reliable reperfusion times during STEMI care.

A 2013 study questioned the appropriateness of the ongoing efforts to further reduce door-to-balloon times [41]. During the 2000s, public health initiatives to reduce door-to-balloon times have been highly effective. Despite their successes, some have noted that reductions in door-to-balloon time have not necessarily translated into reductions in mortality, and therefore question the validity of its predominance as a quality of care measure for PPCI. However, although reductions in door-to-balloon time may not correlate with mortality at the population level, door-to-balloon time continues to be a strong predictor of morbidity and mortality at the patient level in the current era [14]. The lack of correlation between reductions is door-to-balloon times and mortality at the population level should be interpreted with caution, as it will be confounded by the effect of the growing and changing demographics of STEMI patients on mortality.

Future Directions

The current digital era provides ample opportunities for improvement in door-to-balloon time. Electronic monitoring systems, which have been successfully implemented in emergency departments, can improve the efficiency of STEMI systems through live data display and automated data collection systems. Live data display can help practitioners identify and troubleshoot delays as they occur, and smooth transitions between the different stages of the STEMI pathway. Automated data collection systems can also provide accurate, current, and local data which could be used to identify areas for improvement and make optimal medical decisions (for example, choosing reperfusion therapy based on accurate estimates of door-to-balloon time). Lastly, the advent of intracardiac monitoring devices and the refinement of internet-based medical technologies may help to make palpable reductions in symptom-to-reperfusion time. Despite the significant reductions in door-to-balloon time, efforts in reducing total ischemic times are limited by the fact that the average STEMI patient presents later than 60 minutes after symptom onset, and a significant number die before medical contact. Ongoing public health efforts in patient education are needed to minimize patient-related delays in STEMI pathways.

References

1 Cannon CP, Gibson CM, Lambrew CT, et al. Relationship of symptom-onset-to-balloon time and door-to-balloon time with mortality in patients undergoing angioplasty for acute myocardial infarction. *JAMA*, 2000; 283: 2941–2947.

2 McNamara RL, Wang Y, Herrin J, et al. Effect of door-to-balloon time on mortality in patients with ST-segment elevation myocardial infarction. *J Am Coll Cardiol*, 47: 2180–2186.

3 Brodie BR, Hansen C, Stuckey TD, et al. Door-to-balloon time with primary percutaneous coronary intervention for acute myocardial infarction impacts late cardiac mortality in high-risk patients and patients presenting early after the onset of symptoms. *J Am Coll Cardiol*, 2006; 47: 289–295.

4 Reimer KA, Lowe JE, Rasmussen MM, et al. The wavefront phenomenon of ischemic cell death. 1. Myocardial infarct size vs duration of coronary occlusion in dogs. *Circulation*, 1977; 56: 786–794.

5 Maroko PR, Kjekshus JK, Sobel BE, et al. Factors influencing infarct size following experimental coronary artery occlusions. *Circulation*, 1971; 43: 67–82.

6 Braunwald E. Myocardial reperfusion, limitation of infarct size, reduction of left ventricular dysfunction, and improved survival. Should the paradigm be expanded? *Circulation*, 1989; 79: 441–444.

7 Keeley EC, Boura JA, Grines CL. Primary angioplasty versus intravenous thrombolytic therapy for acute myocardial infarction: A quantitative review of 23 randomised trials. *Lancet*, 2003; 361: 13–20.

8 O'Gara PT, Kushner FG, Ascheim DD, et al., American College of Cardiology Foundation/ American Heart Association Task Force on Practice G. 2013 ACCF/AHA guideline for the management of ST-elevation myocardial infarction: A report of the American College of Cardiology Foundation/American Heart Association Task Force on Practice Guidelines. *Circulation*, 2013; 127: e362–e425 (erratum appears in *Circulation*, 2013; 128(25): E481).

9 Steg PG, James SK, Atar D, et al. ESC guidelines for the management of acute myocardial infarction in patients presenting with ST-segment elevation. *Eur Heart J*, 2012; 33: 2569–2619.

10 De Luca G, Suryapranata H, Ottervanger JP, et al. Time delay to treatment and mortality in primary angioplasty for acute myocardial infarction: Every minute of delay counts. *Circulation*, 2004; 109: 1223–1225.

11 Berger PB, Ellis SG, Holmes DR Jr, et al. Relationship between delay in performing direct coronary angioplasty and early clinical outcome in patients with acute myocardial infarction: Results from the global use of strategies to open occluded arteries in acute coronary syndromes (GUSTO-IIB) trial. *Circulation*, 1999; 100: 14–20.

12 Bradley EH, Herrin J, Wang Y, et al. Strategies for reducing the door-to-balloon time in acute myocardial infarction. *N Engl J Med*, 2006; 355: 2308–2320.

13 Nallamothu BK, Bates ER. Percutaneous coronary intervention versus fibrinolytic therapy in acute myocardial infarction: Is timing (almost) everything? *Am J Cardiol*, 2003; 92: 824–826.

14 Nallamothu BK, Normand S-LT, Wang Y, et al. Relation between door-to-balloon times and mortality after primary percutaneous coronary intervention over time: A retrospective study. *Lancet*, 2015; 385: 1114–1122.

15 Terkelsen CJ, Sorensen JT, Maeng M, et al. System delay and mortality among patients with stemi treated with primary percutaneous coronary intervention. *JAMA*, 2010; 304: 763–771.

16 Terkelsen CJ, Jensen LO, Tilsted H-H, et al. Health care system delay and heart failure in patients with ST-segment elevation myocardial infarction treated with primary percutaneous coronary intervention: Follow-up of population-based medical registry data. *Ann Intern Med*, 2011; 155: 361–367.

17 Brodie BR, Stuckey TD, Wall TC, et al. Importance of time to reperfusion for 30-day and late survival and recovery of left ventricular function after primary angioplasty for acute myocardial infarction. *J Am Coll Cardiol*, 1998; 32: 1312–1319.

18 Ryan TJ, Antman EM, Brooks NH, et al. 1999 update: ACC/AHA guidelines for the management of patients with acute myocardial infarction. A report of the American College of Cardiology/American Heart Association Task Force on Practice Guidelines (committee on management of acute myocardial infarction). *J Am Coll Cardiol*, 1999; 34: 890–911.

19 Van de Werf F, Ardissino D, Betriu A, et al., Task Force on the Management of Acute Myocardial Infarction of the European Society of Cardiology. Management of acute myocardial infarction in patients presenting with ST-segment elevation. *Eur Heart J*, 2003; 24: 28–66.

20 Rathore SS, Curtis JP, Chen J, et al. Association of door-to-balloon time and mortality in patients admitted to hospital with ST elevation myocardial infarction: National cohort study. *BMJ*, 2009; 338: b1807.

21 McNamara RL, Herrin J, Bradley EH, et al. Hospital improvement in time to reperfusion in patients with acute myocardial infarction, 1999 to 2002. *J Am Coll Cardiol*, 2006; 47: 45–51.

22 Williams SC, Schmaltz SP, Morton DJ, et al. Quality of care in US hospitals as reflected by standardized measures, 2002–2004. *N Engl J Med*, 2005; 353: 255–264.

23 Rogers WJ, Canto JG, Barron HV, et al. Treatment and outcome of myocardial infarction in hospitals with and without invasive capability. Investigators in the national registry of myocardial infarction. *J Am Coll Cardiol*, 2000; 35: 371–379.

24 Andersen HR, Nielsen TT, Rasmussen K, et al. A comparison of coronary angioplasty with fibrinolytic therapy in acute myocardial infarction. *N Engl J Med*, 2003; 349: 733–742.

25 Pinto DS, Kirtane AJ, Nallamothu BK, et al. Hospital delays in reperfusion for st-elevation myocardial infarction: Implications when selecting a reperfusion strategy. *Circulation*, 2006; 114: 2019–2025.

26 Angeja BG, Gibson CM, Chin R, et al. Predictors of door-to-balloon delay in primary angioplasty. *Am J Cardiol*, 89: 1156–1161.

27 Nallamothu BK, Bates ER, Herrin J, et al. Times to treatment in transfer patients undergoing primary percutaneous coronary intervention in the united states: National Registry of Myocardial Infarction (NRMI)-3/4 analysis. *Circulation*, 2005; 111: 761–767.

28 Krumholz HM, Bradley EH, Nallamothu BK, et al. A campaign to improve the timeliness of primary percutaneous coronary intervention: Door-to-balloon: An alliance for quality. *JACC Cardiovasc Interv*, 2008; 1: 97–104.

29 Le May MR, Wells GA, So DY, et al. Reduction in mortality as a result of direct transport from the field to a receiving center for primary percutaneous coronary intervention. *J Am Coll Cardiol*, 2012; 60: 1223–1230.

30 Le May MR, So DY, Dionne R, et al. A citywide protocol for primary PCI in ST-segment elevation myocardial infarction. *N Engl J Med*, 2008; 358: 231–240.

31 Jollis JG, Granger CB, Henry TD, et al. Systems of care for ST-segment-elevation myocardial infarction: A report from the American Heart Association's Mission: Lifeline. *Circ Cardiovasc Qual Outcomes*, 2012; 5: 423–428.

32 Fosbol EL, Granger CB, Jollis JG, et al. The impact of a statewide pre-hospital STEMI strategy to bypass hospitals without percutaneous coronary intervention capability on treatment times. *Circulation*, 2013; 127: 604–612.

33 Bradley EH, Herrin J, Wang Y, et al. Door-to-drug and door-to-balloon times: Where can we improve? Time to reperfusion therapy in patients with ST-segment elevation myocardial infarction (STEMI). *Am Heart J*, 2006; 151: 1281–1287.

34 Bradley EH, Curry LA, Webster TR, et al. Achieving rapid door-to-balloon times: How top hospitals improve complex clinical systems. *Circulation*, 2006; 113: 1079–1085.

35 Le May MR, Davies RF, Dionne R, et al. Comparison of early mortality of paramedic-diagnosed ST-segment elevation myocardial infarction with immediate transport to a designated primary percutaneous coronary intervention center to that of similar patients transported to the nearest hospital. *Am J Cardiol*, 2006; 98: 1329–1333.

36 Nallamothu BK, Wang Y, Magid DJ, et al. Relation between hospital specialization with primary percutaneous coronary intervention and clinical outcomes in ST-segment elevation myocardial infarction: National Registry of Myocardial Infarction-4 analysis. *Circulation*, 2006; 113: 222–229.

37 Canto JG, Every NR, Magid DJ, et al. The volume of primary angioplasty procedures and survival after acute myocardial infarction. National Registry of Myocardial Infarction 2 investigators. *N Engl J Med*, 2000; 342: 1573–1580.

38 Brodie BR, Gersh BJ, Stuckey T, et al. When is door-to-balloon time critical? Analysis from the HORIZONS-AMI (harmonizing outcomes with revascularization and stents in acute myocardial infarction) and CADILLAC (controlled abciximab and device investigation to lower late angioplasty complications) trials. *J Am Coll Cardiol*, 2010; 56: 407–413 [erratum appears in *J Am Coll Cardiol*, 2010; 56(14): 1168].

39 Armstrong PW, Boden WE. Reperfusion paradox in ST-segment elevation myocardial infarction. *Ann Intern Med*, 2011; 155: 389–391.

40 Boersma E, Primary Coronary Angioplasty vs. Thrombolysis G. Does time matter? A pooled analysis of randomized clinical trials comparing primary percutaneous coronary intervention and in-hospital fibrinolysis in acute myocardial infarction patients. *Eur Heart J*, 2006; 27: 779–788.

41 Menees DS, Peterson ED, Wang Y, et al. Door-to-balloon time and mortality among patients undergoing primary PCI. *N Engl J Med*, 2013; 369: 901–909.

17

Pre-hospital Triage and Management

Ivan Rokas MD

Introduction

Over the last 30 years, a large body of clinical cardiology literature has consistently reinforced the "time is muscle" mantra. Accordingly, the primary therapeutic goal for acute ST-elevation myocardial infarction (STEMI) remains timely reperfusion with either fibrinolytics or primary percutaneous coronary intervention (PPCI). The current American College of Cardiology/ American Heart Association (ACC/AHA) [1] and European Society of Cardiology (ESC) guidelines [2] both prioritize PPCI as the preferred reperfusion strategy if performed in a timely manner by an expert interventional cardiologist. However, PPCI is the most complex, multidisciplinary, and time sensitive therapeutic intervention in the world of medicine today: The process is measured in minutes, the outcome in terms of short-term mortality, and teamwork and smooth transitions between various care provider units appear to be critically important [3]. Thus, the development of organized STEMI systems is essential for the consistent delivery of high quality PPCI.

Conceptually, the delivery of PPCI can be divided into the STEMI *process* and the STEMI *procedure* [4]. The STEMI procedure occurs within the cardiac catheterization laboratory (CCL) and is uniquely performed by interventional cardiologists supported by highly trained support staff. Occasionally, the STEMI procedure may also involve surgical revascularization. The technology and pharmacology of the STEMI procedure have advanced dramatically and are covered in detail by other chapters in this text.

In contrast, the STEMI process broadly defines all the events and personnel outside of the CCL procedure. It starts with a patient who recognizes the need to seek medical evaluation for chest discomfort or other angina-equivalent symptoms. This is followed by rapid and coordinated evaluation and/or treatment by various medical providers (9-1-1 dispatchers, first responders, paramedics, and emergency department physicians and nurses), frontline support staff (hospital registration clerks, laboratory personnel, security, chaplains, and page operators), and post-event administrators and quality-improvement personnel. Importantly, optimal patient-centered care should be the guiding principle driving the development of any STEMI system.

Critical to an efficient STEMI process is the actual 12-lead electrocardiogram (EKG) diagnosis of acute STEMI, which quickly stratifies the large group of general chest pain patients into two distinct groups: the small minority (less than 5%) of patients experiencing STEMI compared with the large majority (over 95%) with either a non-STEMI, unstable angina, or noncardiac chest pain. When STEMI is confirmed, an in-hospital "code STEMI" should activate a defined set of interventions in preparation for CCL angiography followed by PPCI as indicated.

This chapter describes pre-hospital triage and management, with a focus on key roles for emergency medical service (EMS) providers in the context of an organized STEMI receiving center (SRC) network. Topics include a description of three essential roles for EMS, three supplemental roles, EMS transport logistics, relevant quality improvement metrics, pre-hospital medications, and the overlap between resuscitation of out-of-hospital cardiac arrest (OHCA) and STEMI care.

The STEMI Receiving Center Network

At the core of any STEMI network is the SRC [3], which is a hospital that is capable of PPCI and meets additional criteria as summarized in Box 17.1. The basic framework for STEMI networks was first described in 2006–2007 [5,6] and includes two major parts: pre-hospital cardiac triage and inter-hospital transfer. The former is focused on EMS providers identifying and transporting all STEMI patients to the nearest appropriate SRC, whereas the latter is focused on transfer strategies for STEMI patients who initially arrive at the emergency department of a non-PCI-capable hospital. More recently, an advanced framework [7,8] for the planning and implementation of STEMI networks has evolved and provides a comprehensive picture of STEMI care for all four major points-of-entry for patients across any region. Figure 17.1 provides a schematic for this basic building block of any STEMI network. At the core is the SRC, which is PPCI-capable by definition. Four distinct "express lanes" into the receiving center are diagrammed and represent four unique points of entry, since each express lane has specific frontline providers, logistics, and guideline-based quality-improvement benchmarks.

Essential Roles for the Emergency Medical Services

Three essential roles [5] exist for EMS, as summarized in Table 17.1. First, frontline EMS providers (paramedics or emergency medical technicians) must be able to diagnose an acute STEMI using a 12-lead pre-hospital electrocardiogram (PH-EKG) device. This involves the correct application of 10 electrodes on each patient, the acquisition of the 12-lead PH-EKG tracing, and evaluation for the presence of EKG patterns consistent with acute STEMI or STEMI equivalent.

Second, EMS providers need to have destination protocols, such that any identified STEMI patient is transported directly to the nearest SRC. In fact, bypass of closer non-PCI-hospitals is specifically allowed in STEMI networks by local EMS regulations, so that all EMS-identified STEMI patients are always taken to a hospital that can provide PPCI at all times (24/7 year-round).

Box 17.1 Criteria for STEMI Receiving Center (SRC) Designation
1) Primary percutaneous coronary intervention capable hospital.
2) Accessible to the general public.
3) Operational 24/7 every day for 365 days a year.
4) Cardiac catheterization laboratory remains open for STEMI patients despite high inpatient hospital census or emergency department closure due to overcrowding.
5) Officially designated as part of a network by regional authorities.
6) Participation in a quality improvement registry, either regional or national.
7) Onsite surgical revascularization capable (usually).

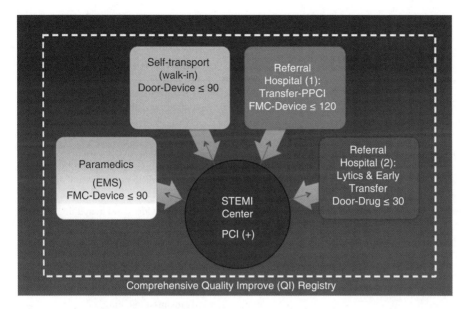

Figure 17.1 STEMI network: four express lanes (sources: *Critical Pathways in Cardiology*, 2013; 12: 43–44; *Circulation*, 2013; 128: 1799–1809). EMS, emergency medical services; FMC, first medical contact; PPCI, primary percutaneous coronary intervention.

Table 17.1 Emergency medical services roles.

Essential	Supplemental
Diagnose STEMI	Maximize appropriate CCL activation
Destination Protocols to SRC	Transmit the pre-hospital EKG
Defibrillation capable	Inter-hospital transport

CCL, cardiac catheterization laboratory; EKG, electrocardiogram;
SRC, STEMI receiving center; STEMI, ST-elevation myocardial infarction.

Consistent with standard EMS practice, all other chest-pain or angina-equivalent patients without STEMI on PH-EKG continue to be transported to the closest hospital emergency department.

Third, defibrillation capability is essential for all EMS providers. An acute coronary occlusion puts the STEMI patient at much higher risk for a malignant arrhythmia, such as ventricular fibrillation or ventricular tachycardia. Continuous EMS provider readiness to recognize sudden cardiac death and react with rapid defibrillation provides an important layer of safety for STEMI patients. In contrast, patients that self-transport forego access to immediate defibrillation while en route to the hospital and can die of untreated sudden cardiac arrest.

Supplemental Roles for the Emergency Medical Services

Beyond destination protocols and the ability to make an early STEMI diagnosis using the PH-EKG, EMS providers should strive to help maximize the rate of appropriate CCL activation [9]. Certainly, hospitals can save a significant amount of reperfusion time by pre-activating the

Table 17.2 Advantages and disadvantages of methods of interpreting pre-hospital electrocardiogram (adapted from the American Heart Association statement, *Circulation*, 2008; 118: 1066–1079) [10].

Method	Advantages	Disadvantages
Computer algorithm interpretation	Rapid, easy. No wireless network or technology requirements.	False positive and false negative rates higher than physician interpretation.
Paramedic interpretation	Rapid, easy. No wireless network or technology requirements.	Requires intensive education and quality assurance program More complex in communities with multiple EMS providers and agencies.
Wireless transmission and physician interpretation	Theoretically, lowest rate of false positives and false negatives. Medical oversight can provide guidance on destination hospital and treatment en route.	New technology requirement for EMS providers and hospital. Reliable wireless network transmission unit on ambulance. Receiver station unit at hospital Smartphones for physicians. Requires system to ensure immediate interpretation by physician. Transmission failures.

EMS, emergency medical services

CCL team prior to patient arrival in the emergency department, but run the risk of activating then cancelling the CCL team when hospital-based physicians are unable to review the index PH-EKG in real time. These CCL team cancellations cost hospitals money (overtime pay) and can be demoralizing to CCL staff.

As summarized in a 2008 American Heart Association Scientific Statement [10], three options exist for PH-EKG interpretation: Direct paramedic evaluation, computer algorithm reading, or wireless transmission for off-site interpretation. All three strategies rely on EMS providers initiating the PH-EKG interpretation process, so training and adherence to standardized protocols are important. Moreover, each option has its advantages and disadvantages (Table 17.2). Some STEMI systems exclusively use only one of these options, whereas many networks use a synergistic combination of all three PH-EKG interpretation strategies to optimize diagnostic accuracy.

Inappropriate CCL activations occur in almost all STEMI systems, but the frequency and root cause varies substantially across different regions [9,11–13]. However, as each STEMI network matures beyond the basic provision of fast reperfusion, it should strive to maximize efficiency and optimize resource use. The various concepts and strategies relevant to the pursuit of this goal are:

- Acute ST-elevation on any EKG is a very good (but imperfect) surrogate marker for an acute coronary occlusion that would benefit from PPCI.
- The adage "a picture is worth a thousand words" is very relevant to EKG interpretation.
- Transport and activation are indeed two separate steps in STEMI care: EMS can start driving to the SRC based upon their initial PH-EKG assessment, even if some uncertainty remains about whether or not the hospital will proceed with CCL team activation. Thus, a *pre-hospital* STEMI alert and an *in-hospital* code STEMI are distinct steps.
- The debate about which provider (EMS, emergency department, or cardiology) is the "best" at EKG interpretation is often counterproductive, when in fact collective and collegial

decision making in real time by all three on-duty providers is likely the most accurate. Advances in digital technology greatly facilitate this concurrent decision making.

- Pre-hospital EKG transmission is becoming more reliable and less expensive, and uses web-based receiving stations at each hospital, which automatically push the PH-EKG to a preset group of clinicians via email, text messaging or other smartphone applications. Immediate physician review of a transmitted PH-EKG (either on a desktop computer or a portable smartphone) builds into the STEMI process an instant "double-check" at a critical decision node. Parallel processing is encouraged, such that patient transport by EMS and CCL activation occur simultaneously.

- Each of the three major STEMI providers has a different clinical role, and thus expectations for each should be different:
  - EMS providers are the first point of contact for each patient, and thus EMS should strive for high sensitivity (minimizing false negatives) to detect acute STEMI across a wide spectrum of chief complaints and atypical presentations. A missed STEMI at this first stage of patient care may result in incorrect triage to a non-PCI-hospital and subsequent delays before the STEMI is finally recognized and the patient is transported to an SRC.
  - As the next downstream clinician, the emergency department physician should begin to focus on maximizing specificity (minimizing false positives) and look at each PH-EKG and patient with a critical eye before agreeing with the STEMI alert generated by the EMS. In particular, consideration should be given to the presence of both narrow- and wide-QRS complex ST-elevation mimics (Table 17.3), degree of comorbidities (dementia, advanced cancer, debility, frailty, etc.), and patient's advanced directives (do not resuscitate status or no heroic measures).
  - The on-duty interventionalist is the person who makes the final decision on whether to proceed with emergency angiography. Ideally, a lesion is identified and PPCI occurs. However, there are many reasonable scenarios in which an emergency angiogram is performed but subsequent PPCI is not indicated (Box 17.2). Despite their key role in a STEMI system, EKG interpretation by interventional cardiologists should not be the gold standard by which the rate of appropriate CCL activation is measured (see last point below).

- EMS and emergency department providers should confidently activate the CCL team in the cases of obvious STEMI in a patient who is clearly suitable for invasive revascularization. As the American College of Cardiology D2B Alliance initiative states, cardiology consultation is not needed in the majority of STEMI cases [14]. However, both EMS and emergency department providers need to be mindful of occasional "grey zone" or "challenging cases" that are best evaluated by a discussion with the on-duty interventionalist before activation of the entire CCL team. Real-time discussions about these equivocal cases prior to activation help preserve EMS and emergency department provider credibility with the cardiology department.

Table 17.3 Common QRS complex ST-elevation mimics.

Narrow	Tall/Wide
Benign early repolarization	Left ventricular hypertrophy
Pericarditis	Left bundle branch block
Left ventricular aneurysm	Paced rhythm
Normal variant "male pattern"	Hyperkalemia
Preexcitation	Brugada syndrome

Box 17.2   Catherization Laboratory Activation

Appropriate → Ideal
- Angiography and PPCI performed.

Appropriate → Reasonable
- Angiography *without* PPCI performed:
  - Surgical revascularization indicated.
  - Coronary anatomy is not amenable to PPCI intervention (i.e. medical therapy).
  - "Unavoidable angiogram" per index EKG and/or clinical scenario as documented by the real-time clinicians (e.g. Takotsubo cardiomyopathy, myocarditis).
  - No PPCI target lesion identified but cardiac markers become elevated.
- Before angiography, true STEMI per index EKG dies suddenly.
- Angiography ± PPCI for ROSC following witnessed out-of-hospital cardiac arrest from a shockable rhythm. Some ROSC patients may deteriorate and die before angiography.

Inappropriate → Goal is < 5% rate
- No angiography performed (catheterization laboratory activation cancelled by physician).
- Angiography without PPCI target-lesion being identified and normal cardiac markers:
  - "Avoidable angiogram" based upon erroneous EKG interpretation.
- Advanced comorbidities: patient is not a PPCI candidate.

Classification based on retrospective and multidisciplinary peer review of all index clinical data.
   Green zone represents the ideal scenario; orange zone events are all reasonable; red zone occurrences should be minimized.

EKG, electrocardiogram; PPCI, primary percutaneous coronary intervention; ROSC, return of spontaneous circulation; STEMI, ST-elevation myocardial infarction.

- Bypass of the emergency department within the SRC during regular CCL work hours is an emerging strategy. Following transmission and confirmation of true STEMI, frontline physicians at the hospital can plan for EMS to take these patients directly from the ambulance ramp to the CCL (with EMS stopping in the emergency department only for patient registration). This "ED bypass" strategy has been associated with a median 20-minute time saving in a 2013 Acute Coronary Treatment and Intervention Outcomes Network Registry–Get With The Guidelines (ACTION Registry–GWTG) analysis [15]. Patient safety remains paramount, so the emergency department bypass strategy should only occur at times when CCL staff are in the hospital and able to actively monitor the patient.
- Performance measurement of CCL activation requires correlation with subsequent clinical outcomes, angiogram findings, actual performance of PPCI, biomarker levels, imaging studies, and/or autopsy. This clinical gold standard is preferable to relying only on retrospective EKG interpretation by some designated "expert" and helps all stakeholders collaboratively identify sources of error that cause inappropriate CCL activations by the system. Advocates of STEMI system efficiency have proposed a target rate of 5% (or lower) for inappropriate CCL activation, such that 95 (or more) emergent angiograms are performed for every 100 CCL activations [9].

Inter-hospital transfer is another important supplemental role for EMS that is gradually gaining increased uptake across various regions. One of first published transfer networks using the 9-1-1 system (the national emergency response telephone number for the United States) came from Los Angeles County in California [16]. This strategy represents another paradigm shift, since traditionally, EMS providers only took patients to the closest hospital. However, in many regions, non-PCI-capable hospitals have no reliable method by which to rapidly get a newly diagnosed STEMI patient out of their emergency departments and into an SRC. A 9-1-1 call for assistance by clinicians at the non-PCI-capable emergency department represents a logical extension of current EMS practice: in the traditional model, the EMS provides both PH-EKG diagnosis and rapid transport for patients, whereas in this new transfer role, the EMS provides only transport between the emergency department of a referral hospital and the CCL of an SRC. Thus, the overarching goal for the EMS is to assist in getting all STEMI patients in their region to an SRC.

Emergency Medical Services Transport Logistics

Drive time (a combination of distance, geography, weather, and daily traffic patterns) between initial patient contact location and SRC location is a dominant issue for STEMI system authorities planning either pre-hospital cardiac triage or inter-hospital transfers. Drive time is usually a bigger issue for remote and rural regions, but can also be a problem during times of commuter gridlock in urban and suburban areas. A reasonable "rule of thumb" is a drive time of 30 minutes or less for two reasons. First, an EMS vehicle and crew are functionally taken out of service for at least 60 minutes (30 minutes one way is 60-minute round trip), often leaving the rest of the region understaffed and underserviced for at least 1 hour. Similarly, a 45-minute drive time becomes at least a 90-minute round trip, which can result in a serious coverage gap for rural regions that commonly have thin EMS staffing. Second, a 2015 ACTION Registry-GWTG analysis [17] found that only 43% of transfer patients with drive times exceeding 30 minutes achieved reperfusion within the guideline-based 120-minute first-door-to-balloon metric. This robust analysis spanned 5 years (2008–2012) and involved over 22,400 patients, 366 SRCs, and 1771 distinct referral hospitals in the United States. The report also stressed that clinicians should consider (if there are no contraindications) pre-transfer fibrinolytics for patients with drive times above 30 minutes, since guideline benchmarks for timely PPCI are not usually achievable.

Air transport is a potential solution to prolonged drive times by ground-based EMS. For example, the Minneapolis inter-hospital program successfully used helicopter transport for the vast majority (over 93%) of their zone 2 transfers (60–210 miles from the SRC) and reported a median first-door-to-device time of 120 minutes (interquartile range, IQR, 100–145 minutes) [18]. One-year mortality for these long-distance transfers was nearly identical to that of patients presenting directly to the SRC. Similarly, the Geisinger program (Pennsylvania) used helicopter transport in their regional inter-hospital transfer network (19 referral hospitals), with flight times ranging from 4 minutes to 32 minutes and demonstrated a significant reduction in first-door-to-balloon times from 189 minutes to 88 minutes over a 5-year study period (2004–2008) [19]. The emergency physician at the SRC served as the gatekeeper and first reviewed both a nine-item checklist and a faxed EKG with staff at the referral hospital before initiating helicopter dispatch and CCL activation.

Other analyses, however, highlight that challenges persist and that helicopters are not a universal panacea. A 2014 national ACTION Registry-GWTG database analysis compared over 10,700 ground and 6200 air-transport patients and found the median first-door-to-balloon to be 113 minutes compared with 124 minutes ($P < 0.001$) [20]. In the subanalysis restricted to patients with a transfer distance of over 40 miles, median first-door-to-balloon times for ground compared with air transport were 139 and 133 minutes ($P < 0.001$), respectively. Transport times were approximately 15 minutes faster in the air-transport cohort, but this gain was offset by a 10-minute (median) longer door-in, door-out time at the referral hospital. Additionally, a regional system in Texas first designed their system with helicopter transport but then switched to ground transport and found faster times [21]. Specifically, when comparing air with ground transport, transport time increased (as expected) from 20 minutes to 30 minutes, but door in, door out times at the referral hospital shortened from 70 minutes to 35 minutes and overall first-door-to-balloon was reduced from 123 minutes to 90 minutes ($P < 0.001$). This regional study highlights the impact of helicopter availability on the success of an air-transport program, as well as highlighting the importance of continually measuring key time points and making strategic adjustments in response to persistent delays.

Helicopters are the dominant form of air-transport for most STEMI networks, but exceptions do exist. For example, in Hawaii, current federal aviation regulations mandate the use of fixed-wing aircraft for the 100–150 miles trans-oceanic inter-island transport [7]. This adds additional complexity and delay, because the STEMI patient needs ground transport from the referral hospital to the airport, then the airplane flight, then a second ambulance drive from the destination airport to the nearest SRC. Again, pre-transfer fibrinolytic administration (unless contraindications exist) is a guideline-based strategy for those STEMI patients who are simply too far away from an SRC to receive timely PPCI.

Lastly, rural hybrid strategies have been described that combine the both ground and air transport into a seamless system. The Mayo network (Minnesota) has a number of key steps that are seamlessly coordinated [22]:

1) Rural EMS providers perform a PH-EKG.
2) Both Mayo and the local community hospital (non-PCI-capable) are notified if STEMI is identified on PH-EKG.
3) The EMS drives to the helipad of the local community hospital.
4) The Mayo (SRC) simultaneously launches a helicopter to meet the ambulance crew at the community hospital.
5) The Mayo activates their internal code STEMI so that CCL team is preactivated and ready to re-perfuse the patient upon arrival at the SRC.

In one extreme example, the Mayo team reported a first EMS contact to first device time of 82 minutes for a patient who was 5 miles from the non-PCI community hospital and 50 miles from the SRC.

Quality Improvement for Emergency Medical Services: Three Key Time Intervals

The delivery of pre-hospital patient care can be divided into three major intervals that should be followed by ongoing quality improvement surveillance: dispatch time, scene time, and transport time. Table 17.4 summarizes the four key time points that define these intervals. Both dispatch and transport time intervals are relatively fixed for any given patient, because they are a function of drive time (distance between EMS crew and patient location, modified by real-time weather and traffic conditions). In contrast, scene time represent the interval that is generally the most modifiable by efficient EMS providers using streamlined protocols and procedures.

The only guideline benchmark specifically pertaining to EMS timeliness is the recommendation of 10 minutes (or less) between first medical contact and EKG acquisition, representing a key subinterval of scene time [1,2]. Other universally agreed upon quality improvement

Table 17.4 Three scenarios for appropriate catheterization laboratory activation involving patients with out-of-hospital cardiac arrest.

First Event	Second Event	Action	Supplemental Action
Acute STEMI diagnosed by pre-hospital EKG	Cardiac arrest witnessed by EMS providers, followed by prompt defibrillation and ROSC	Catheterization laboratory team at SRC should have already been activated, based on original diagnosis of STEMI or STEMI equivalent	Initiate hypothermia protocol in post-resuscitation patients who remain unconscious
Bystander-witnessed out-of-hospital cardiac arrest, early activation of 9-1-1, and early chest compressions	Shockable rhythm and ROSC achieved, followed by EKG diagnostic of acute STEMI or STEMI equivalent	Activate catheterization laboratory team at cardiac resuscitation center	As above
As above	Shockable rhythm and ROSC achieved, but post-resuscitation EKG is not diagnostic of acute STEMI or STEMI equivalent	Consider activation of catheterization laboratory team at cardiac resuscitation center in patients whose clinical circumstance suggests acute ischemia and who are candidates for aggressive intervention	As above

EKG, electrocardiogram; EMS emergency medical services; ROSC, return of spontaneous circulation; STEMI, ST-elevation myocardial infarction.

benchmarks do not currently exist for the three major EMS time intervals, but the both the ACC/AHA and ESC guidelines stipulate an overarching goal of first medical contact to-device time of 90 minutes or less [1,2]. With time zero for first medical contact defined as arrival of the EMS at the patient, the combination of scene and transport times should ideally be less than 30 minutes to help the rest of the system (emergency department and CCL) achieve the 90-minute first medical contact to device benchmark. Perhaps, as previously proposed, first medical contact will be redefined by the guidelines as the time of the patient's first call for help to a 9-1-1 emergency operator [3]. This time is a more patient-centered definition of first medical contact, but using this earlier start time (reperfusion within 90 minutes from first call) would likely pose a significant challenge to many existing STEMI networks. For perspective, the United Kingdom's national Myocardial Ischaemia National Audit Project audit reports an 89% rate of call-to-balloon within 90 minutes in 2015 [23].

Experience from two regions in the United States further informs this discussion of what efficient STEMI systems can achieve. From San Diego, a quality improvement registry study of over 21,700 EMS runs for "chest pain" evaluated the impact of their PH-EKG implementation program on key time intervals [24]. The application of a PH-EKG did not effect scene times (approximately 19 minutes with or without PH-EKG). Moreover, the 303 patients identified with STEMI on PH-EKG had significantly shorter scene times (17 minutes 51 seconds vs. 19 minutes 31 seconds; $P < 0.0001$) and shorter scene and transport time (30 minuites 45 seconds vs. 33 minutes 29 seconds; $P < 0.001$). Similarly, from North Carolina, a contemporary study of almost 2700 patients transported directly to PPCI-hospitals by the EMS found the following time median intervals: dispatch, 10 minutes (approximately); scene, 14 minutes (IQR 10–18); and transport, 17 minutes (IQR 11–25) [25]. Overall, about 41 minutes elapsed in the pre-hospital setting.

Pre-hospital Medications

The generally accepted list of pre-hospital medications includes aspirin, nitrates, morphine, and oxygen. However, only aspirin has been proven to reduce mortality [1]. A one-time pre-hospital dose of aspirin is generally considered safe, except in the rare patient with a severe allergy. Additionally, there is the theoretical risk of inadvertently giving aspirin to a suspected STEMI patient who is actually suffering an acute aortic dissection, but the actual effect of this mistake on clinical outcomes in aortic dissection remains unknown.

With the evolution of dual antiplatelet therapy (DAPT) as the cornerstone of PPCI therapy, there has been interest in giving both aspirin and a second agent (clopidogrel, prasugrel, or ticagrelor) in the pre-hospital setting. The 2012 ESC guidelines state that this seems reasonable based upon pharmacokinetic data for oral antithrombotics, but also disclose that no clinical studies exist to definitively support this strategy [2]. In 2014, the ATLANTIC study began to address this issue and randomized 1862 STEMI patients to either pre-hospital or in-hospital ticagrelor [26]. Despite a 31-minute (median) earlier administration in the pre-hospital group, there was no effect on the co-primary endpoints (ST-segment resolution and pre-PCI thrombolysis in myocardial infarction flow grade 3) and no effect on major bleeding. The only potential benefit was a modest reduction in the secondary endpoint of definite stent thrombosis in the pre-hospital group (0% vs. 0.8% in the first 24 hours). A second contemporary single-center study used two platelet reactivity assays (VerifyNow and Multiplate Analyzer) to evaluate the 24-hour pharmacokinetics of both ticagrelor and prasugrel in 55 STEMI patients [27]. Prasugrel and ticagrelor performed similarly, as both took 2 hours to have the median pharmacokinetic level below the assay's standard benchmark for inhibition and 6 hours for the majority of patients to achieve this inhibitory benchmark.

Thus, at present, only aspirin appears to be worth the cost and effort by EMS to stock and administer to all suspected STEMI in the pre-hospital setting. DAPT in the pre-hospital setting appears to be safe (and common in parts of Europe [2]), but does not appear to have any major efficacy advantage over in-hospital administration.

STEMI Complicated by Out of Hospital Cardiac Arrest

Since 2000, there has been a focused effort by many organizations to build systems of care for OHCA on top of existing STEMI networks [9,28]. An acute coronary occlusion is a common cause of OHCA, especially when the patient initially suffers from a shockable rhythm (ventricular fibrillation or pulseless ventricular tachycardia). In other words, an OHCA patient is often an unfortunate STEMI patient whose chief complaint is sudden death.

Three major issues related to the merger of STEMI and OHCA systems deserve discussion. First, EMS providers should always strive to achieve return of spontaneous circulation (ROSC) in the pre-hospital setting by providing minimally interrupted chest compressions (push hard, push fast) and early defibrillation of shockable rhythms. Provider protocols should be focused on optimal pre-hospital resuscitation, because clinical outcomes are unlikely to improve with EMS transport of a persistently pulseless patient to the hospital. This focus also highlights the importance of termination of resuscitation protocols when ROSC by EMS providers cannot be achieved, such that deceased patients are kept on scene with adequate supplemental resources (chaplain, social worker, mortuary staff, coroner, etc.) to assist with the bereavement and funeral process [29].

The second issue relates to the identification of patients most likely to benefit from emergency angiography. The initial qualifier should be pre-hospital ROSC, as summarized above

Table 17.5 Three emergency medical services (EMS) time intervals.

Dispatch time	Scene time	Transport time
• EMS providers notified of patient's call[a] • EMS arrives at patient	• EMS arrives at patient • EMS vehicle departs scene • At scene, time to pre-hospital electrocardiogram should be 10 minutes or less, as guidelines	• EMS vehicle departs scene • EMS arrives at hospital door

[a] Date/time of dispatch should be recorded on the EMS care report. It provides a good surrogate for date/time of patient's actual call for help to a 9-1-1 emergency operator.

(unless extenuating circumstances exist). Based upon published results from two large datasets, only about 25% of all OHCA patients achieve ROSC [30,31]. The subsequent qualifier involves findings on the EKG. Importantly, because controversy still exists regarding the ability of a post-resuscitation EKG to reliably identify all patients with an acute coronary occlusion, emergent angiography (with PPCI as indicated) may be clinically prudent even when the post-resuscitation EKG is not diagnostic for a STEMI or STEMI-equivalent [9]. Table 17.5 shows three scenarios involving the EKG and clinical events in the setting of OHCA.

Third, the issue of anoxic encephalopathy remains a major concern for PPCI-focused STEMI systems that are expanding their entry criteria to include OHCA patients with ROSC. Specifically, interventional cardiologists have traditionally avoided treating unconscious OHCA patients because of perceived futility (i.e., the heart can be fixed but the brain remains dead). However, the more widespread dissemination of therapeutic hypothermia devices (surface or intravascular) and their potential to reduce hypoxic brain injury has recently changed the treatment paradigm (i.e., both the heart and brain can be saved) [28]. The overarching goal for OHCA care in the modern era is hospital discharge of neurologically intact patients with good cardiac function via a multidisciplinary team-based approach [28].

Conclusions

With the continued focus on creating regional SRC networks around the globe, pre-hospital triage and management of patients with acute STEMI (including the subset with OHCA) has evolved substantially in the 21st century. As frontline providers of clinical care, EMS staff need to be properly equipped and trained to perform optimally. Moreover, their pre-hospital efforts need to be seamlessly integrated with subsequent in-hospital care delivery to maximize efficiency and optimize patient outcomes.

References

1 O'Gara PT, Kushner FG, Ascheim DD, et al., American College of Cardiology Foundation/ American Heart Association Task Force on Practice G. 2013 ACCF/AHA guideline for the management of st-elevation myocardial infarction: A report of the american college of cardiology foundation/american heart association task force on practice guidelines. *Circulation*, 2013; 127: e362–e425.

2 Steg PG, James SK, Atar D, et al. ESC guidelines for the management of acute myocardial infarction in patients presenting with st-segment elevation. *Eur Heart J*, 2012; 33: 2569–2619.

3 Rokos IC, French WJ, Koenig WJ, et al. Integration of pre-hospital electrocardiograms and ST-elevation myocardial infarction receiving center (SRC) networks: Impact on door-to-balloon times across 10 independent regions. *JACC Cardiovasc Interv*, 2009; 2: 339–346.

4 Mehta S. The essence of stemi interventions – understanding the process and the procedure. *Cath Lab Digest*, 2008; 16: 14–16.

5 Rokos IC, Larson DM, Henry TD, et al. Rationale for establishing regional st-elevation myocardial infarction receiving center (SRC) networks. *Am Heart J*, 2006; 152: 661–667.

6 Jacobs AK, Antman EM, Faxon DP, et al. Development of systems of care for ST-elevation myocardial infarction patients: Executive summary. *Circulation*, 2007; 116: 217–230.

7 Rokos IC, Henry TD, Weittenhiller B, et al. Mission: Lifeline STEMI networks geospatial information systems (GIS) maps. *Crit Pathw Cardiol*, 2013; 12: 43–44.

8 Rokos IC, Schwamm LH, Konig M, et al. Variable impact of state legislative advocacy on registry participation and regional systems of care implementation: A policy statement from the american heart association. *Circulation*, 2013; 128: 1799–1809.

9 Rokos IC, French WJ, Mattu A, et al. Appropriate cardiac cath lab activation: Optimizing electrocardiogram interpretation and clinical decision-making for acute ST-elevation myocardial infarction. *Am Heart J*, 2010; 160: 995–1003.

10 Ting HH, Krumholz HM, Bradley EH, et al. Implementation and integration of prehospital ECGs into systems of care for acute coronary syndrome: A scientific statement from the American Heart Association. *Circulation*, 2008; 118: 1066–1079.

11 Larson DM, Menssen KM, Sharkey SW, et al. "False-positive" cardiac catheterization laboratory activation among patients with suspected ST-segment elevation myocardial infarction. *JAMA*, 2007; 298: 2754–2760.

12 Garvey JL, Monk L, Granger CB, et al. Rates of cardiac catheterization cancelation for ST-segment elevation myocardial infarction after activation by emergency medical services or emergency physicians: Results from the North Carolina Catheterization Laboratory Activation Registry. *Circulation*, 2012; 125: 308–313.

13 Mixon TA, Suhr E, Caldwell G, et al. Retrospective description and analysis of consecutive catheterization laboratory ST-segment elevation myocardial infarction activations with proposal, rationale, and use of a new classification scheme. *Circ Cardiovasc Qual Outcomes*, 2012; 5: 62–69.

14 Krumholz HM, Bradley EH, Nallamothu BK, et al. A campaign to improve the timeliness of primary percutaneous coronary intervention: Door-to-balloon: An alliance for quality. *JACC Cardiovasc Interv*, 2008; 1: 97–104.

15 Bagai A, Jollis JG, Dauerman HL, et al. Emergency department bypass for ST-segment-elevation myocardial infarction patients identified with a prehospital electrocardiogram: A report from the American Heart Association Mission: Lifeline program. *Circulation*, 2013; 128: 352–359.

16 Baruch T, Rock A, Koenig WJ, et al. "Call 911" STEMI protocol to reduce delays in transfer of patients from non primary percutaneous coronary intervention referral centers. *Crit Pathw Cardiol*, 2010; 9: 113–115.

17 Vora AN, Holmes DN, Rokos I, et al. Fibrinolysis use among patients requiring interhospital transfer for ST-segment elevation myocardial infarction care: A report from the US National Cardiovascular Data Registry. *JAMA Intern Med*, 2015; 175: 207–215.

18 Henry TD, Sharkey SW, Burke MN, et al. A regional system to provide timely access to percutaneous coronary intervention for st-elevation myocardial infarction. *Circulation*, 2007; 116: 721–728.

19 Blankenship JC, Scott TD, Skelding KA, et al. Door-to-balloon times under 90 min can be routinely achieved for patients transferred for ST-segment elevation myocardial infarction percutaneous coronary intervention in a rural setting. *J Am Coll Cardiol*, 2011; 57: 272–279.

20 Nicholson BD, Dhindsa HS, Roe MT, et al. Relationship of the distance between non-pci hospitals and primary pci centers, mode of transport, and reperfusion time among ground and air interhospital transfers using NCDR's Action Registry-GWTG: A report from the American Heart Association Mission: Lifeline program. *Circ Cardiovasc Interv*, 2014; 7: 797–805.

21 Mixon TA, Colato L. Impact of mode of transportation on time to treatment in patients transferred for primary percutaneous coronary intervention. *J Emerg Med*, 2014; 47: 247–253.

22 Pitta SR, Myers LA, Bjerke CM, et al. Using prehospital electrocardiograms to improve door-to-balloon time for transferred patients with ST-elevation myocardial infarction: A case of extreme performance. *Circ Cardiovasc Qual Outcomes*, 2010; 3: 93–97.

23 National Institute for Cardiovascular Outcomes Research. *Myocardial Ischaemia National Audit Project: How the NHS Cares for Patients with Heart Attack; Annual Public Report April 2014–March 2015*. London, UK: MINAP, University College London; 2015.

24 Patel M, Dunford JV, Aguilar S, et al. Pre-hospital electrocardiography by emergency medical personnel: Effects on scene and transport times for chest pain and ST-segment elevation myocardial infarction patients. *J Am Coll Cardiol*, 2012; 60: 806–811.

25 Fosbol EL, Granger CB, Peterson ED, et al. Prehospital system delay in ST-segment elevation myocardial infarction care: A novel linkage of emergency medicine services and in hospital registry data. *Am Heart J*, 2013; 165: 363–370.

26 Montalescot G1, van't Hof AW, Lapostolle F, et al. Prehospital ticagrelor in ST-segment elevation myocardial infarction. *N Engl J Med*, 2014; 371(11): 1016–1027.

27 Alexopoulos D, Xanthopoulou I, Gkizas V, et al. Randomized assessment of ticagrelor versus prasugrel antiplatelet effects in patients with ST-segment-elevation myocardial infarction. *Circ Cardiovasc Interv*, 2012; 5: 797–804.

28 Nichol G, Aufderheide TP, Eigel B, et al. Regional systems of care for out-of-hospital cardiac arrest: A policy statement from the American Heart Association. *Circulation*, 2010; 121: 709–729.

29 Sasson C, Forman J, Krass D, et al. A qualitative study to identify barriers to local implementation of prehospital termination of resuscitation protocols. *Circ Cardiovasc Qual Outcomes*, 2009; 2: 361–368.

30 Sasson C, Hegg AJ, Macy M, et al. Prehospital termination of resuscitation in cases of refractory out-of-hospital cardiac arrest. *JAMA*, 2008; 300: 1432–1438.

31 Stiell IG, Nichol G, Leroux BG, et al. Early versus later rhythm analysis in patients with out-of-hospital cardiac arrest. *N Engl J Med*, 2011; 365: 787–797.

18

Creating Networks for Optimal STEMI Management

David C. Lange MD, David M. Larson MD, David Hildebrandt RN,
Timothy D. Henry MD

Introduction

When performed in a timely manner by experienced operators, primary percutaneous coronary intervention (PPCI) is the preferred method of reperfusion for patients presenting with ST-segment elevation myocardial infarction (STEMI) [1,2]. However, only a minority (around 25%) of hospitals within the United States have the ability to perform PPCI [3]. Long delays in transferring STEMI patients to PPCI hospitals may offset the expected benefits of mechanical reperfusion, but not all delays are created equal [4–6]. One approach to expand the availability of PPCI for STEMI is integration of the pre-hospital electrocardiogram (PH-EKG) to determine patient triage. STEMI systems which integrate PH-EKG diagnosis of STEMI and immediate triage to the nearest PPCI-capable facility (bypassing non-PPCI-capable facilities) have consistently demonstrated reduced time delays in treatment, reduced infarct size, and improved survival among triaged patients compared with those who require subsequent inter-hospital transfer for PPCI [7–9]. However, as roughly 50% of STEMI patients do not present by ambulance and require ad hoc transfer for PPCI, this strategy may result in long transfer times prior to the initial medical assessment, definitive diagnosis and initiation of medical therapy [10]. An alternative approach is necessary to improve access to PPCI and improve STEMI care. Organized, integrated regional STEMI systems have drastically changed the method of healthcare delivery for STEMI, while providing access to PPCI for an ever-expanding population [11].

Transfer for PPCI Trials

The first randomized controlled trials to compare long-distance transport to PPCI centers with primary fibrinolysis performed at non-PCI community hospitals were performed in Europe in the early 2000s [12–15]. The PRAGUE study was a multicenter trial in which patients with STEMI were randomized to receive fibrinolysis at the presenting hospital without transfer for PPCI (group A, $n = 99$), fibrinolytic therapy during transport to a PPCI center (group B, $n = 100$), or immediate transfer to a PPCI center without fibrinolysis (group C, $n = 101$) [12]. The primary outcome was a combined endpoint of death, reinfarction or stroke at 30 days. Investigators found a significant reduction in the combined endpoint in group C compared with groups A or B (8% vs. 23% vs. 15%, respectively, $P < 0.02$) and concluded that transferring patients with STEMI to a PPCI facility was both safe and effective [12]. The PRAGUE-2 trial randomized

Manual of STEMI Interventions, First Edition. Edited by Sameer Mehta.

850 patients with STEMI who presented within 12 hours to fibrinolysis ($n = 421$) or immediate transfer for PPCI ($n = 429$). Intention to treat analysis showed a trend toward improved mortality in the PPCI group (6.8% in PPCI vs. 10.0% in the fibrinolysis group; $P = 0.12$) in spite of significantly longer times to randomization and revascularization. On-treatment analysis demonstrated a significant improvement in mortality (6.0% vs. 10.4%; $P < 0.05$) and the investigators noted that the mortality curves separated as time to randomization and revascularization grew longer, again favoring PPCI [13].

In the same year that PRAGUE-2 was published, investigators in Denmark published results of the DANAMI-2 trial. The trial design, similar to PRAGUE-2, was a randomized controlled trial of 1572 patients comparing primary angioplasty with fibrinolysis with alteplase. The primary composite endpoint of death, reinfarction, or disabling stroke at 30 days, occurred less in the angioplasty group compared with the fibrinolysis group (8.5% vs. 14.2% $P = 0.002$), driven by a lower incidence of reinfarction in the angioplasty group [14]. The only US STEMI trial to examine the issue of transfer for PPCI was the Air-PAMI trail [15]. This trial included high-risk STEMI patients and was terminated after only 138 patients were enrolled because of difficulties in recruitment. The authors reported major adverse cardiac event rates of 8.4% in the PPCI group compared with 13.6% in the fibrinolysis group, although this did not reach statistical significance due to the small sample size. Additionally, the median door-to-balloon time was 155 minutes, which may have mitigated the potential benefit of PPCI [15].

These four trials were included in a meta-analysis of six studies (3750 patients) comparing transfer for PPCI to fibrinolysis [16]. The authors demonstrated a significant reduction in the combination of death, reinfarction and stroke (Figure 18.1a,b). In spite of the convincing evidence, many remained pessimistic that such a system would work within the construct of the US healthcare system [17].

Growth and Success of STEMI Systems of Care Within the United States

In 2003, the Minneapolis Heart Institute (MHI) at Abbott Northwestern Hospital built one of the first regional STEMI systems in the United States. The system was modeled after successful regional trauma networks and built on the premise that an accelerated diagnosis, streamlined processes, and standardized care protocols were the keys to implementing and maintaining a successful STEMI system. The MHI system functioned as a "wheel-and-spoke" model with MHI at the center of the system. Referral hospitals and clinics within a 60-mile radius of MHI were included in zone 1, and used a standardized protocol which included evidence-based adjunctive medications (aspirin, clopidogrel, weight-based intravenous heparin loading dose and intravenous beta-blockers) and a prespecified transfer plan from each site. The regional STEMI system grew rapidly and expanded into a wider area (zone 2), which included referral hospitals within a 60–210-mile radius using a similar standardized protocol, with the addition of half-dose intravenous fibrinolytic and immediate transfer to MHI for pharmacoinvasive PCI (Figure 18.2a,b,c) [11]. In addition to the standardized protocol, the MHI group placed high priority on gathering data for quality assurance purposes and feedback. Over the next several years, MHI was able to demonstrate marked improvements in a variety of outcomes including death, reinfarction, stroke and length of hospital stay (Box 18.1) [11,18,19].

In the coming years, regional STEMI systems were developed throughout the United States (Figure 18.3) [20]. These systems were individually built and tailored to the unique political, geographical and socioeconomic landscapes of the various regions. Some were built in a

(a)

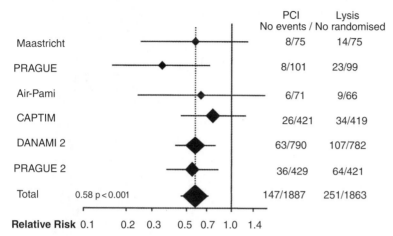

Death/Reinfarction/Stroke

	PCI	Lysis
	No events / No randomised	
Maastricht	8/75	14/75
PRAGUE	8/101	23/99
Air-Pami	6/71	9/66
CAPTIM	26/421	34/419
DANAMI 2	63/790	107/782
PRAGUE 2	36/429	64/421
Total 0.58 p < 0.001	147/1887	251/1863

Relative Risk 0.1   0.2 0.3   0.5 0.7 1.0 1.4

M. Dalby et al. Circulation. 2003;108:1809–1814

(b)

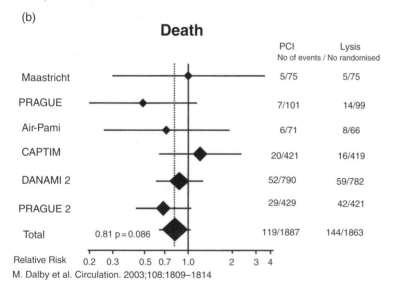

Death

	PCI	Lysis
	No of events / No randomised	
Maastricht	5/75	5/75
PRAGUE	7/101	14/99
Air-Pami	6/71	8/66
CAPTIM	20/421	16/419
DANAMI 2	52/790	59/782
PRAGUE 2	29/429	42/421
Total 0.81 p = 0.086	119/1887	144/1863

Relative Risk   0.2 0.3   0.5 0.7 1.0   2   3 4

M. Dalby et al. Circulation. 2003;108:1809–1814

Figure 18.1 Relative risks for the composite of death, reinfarction, and stroke (a) and Death (b) with thrombolysis and transfer for primary percutaneous cardiopulmonary support in individual trials and the combined analysis (Dalby M, et al., *Circulation*, 2003; 108: 1809–1814 [16]; reproduced with permission from American Heart Association).

wheel-and-spoke fashion similar to MHI, while others were built more as a "web-like" network, with multiple tertiary centers serving as hubs for PPCI in the area. In spite of their differences in structure, organization and providers, these systems demonstrated a combined rate of door-to-balloon time of 90 minutes or less in 86% of STEMI patients. Additionally, each region individually surpassed the American College of Cardiology's door-to-balloon benchmark of more than 75% of STEMI cases achieving a door-to-balloon time of 90 minutes or less [20]. These systems were able to demonstrate that, through a variety of models, regional STEMI systems provide diverse communities with timely access to quality STEMI care (Figure 18.4).

(a)

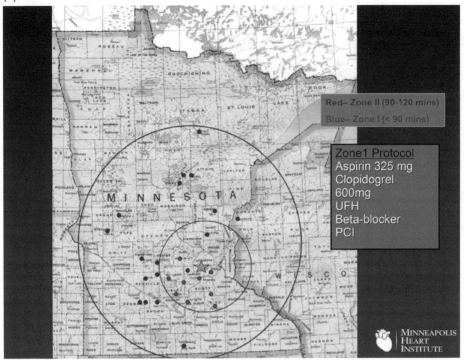

(b)

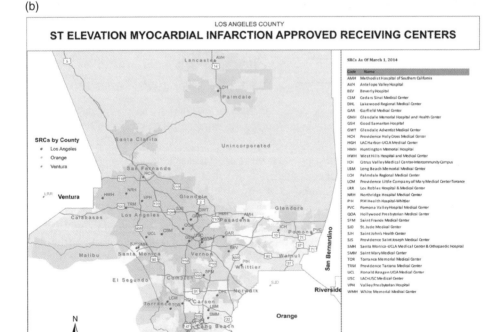

Figure 18.2 (a) Map of Minnesota with the percutaneous coronary intervention (PCI) center (Abbott Northwestern Hospital) in Minneapolis, zone 1 hospitals (≤60 miles from PCI hospital, and zone 2 hospitals (60–210 miles from PCI hospital. UFH, unfractionated heparin. (b) Map of Los Angeles County STEMI system of care. (c) Map of North Carolina state-wide Reperfusion of Acute Myocardial Infarction in Carolina Emergency Departments (RACE) STEMI system of care (source: Jollis J, et al. *JAMA*, 2007; 298(20): 2371–2380; reproduced with permission).

(c)

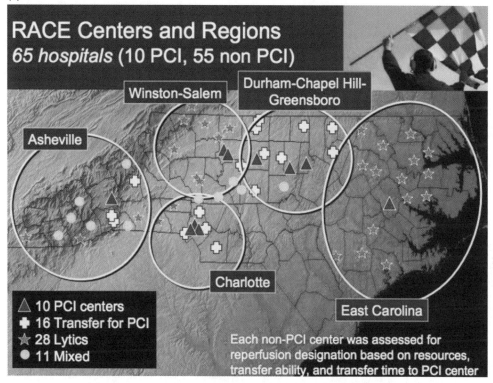

Figure 18.2 (Continued)

Box 18.1   Advantages and Successes of STEMI Systems of Care

- Improved access to tertiary care facilities and primary percutaneous coronary intervention.
- Decrease number of "eligible but untreated" patients.
- Shorter time to treatment through standardized protocols.
- Improved patient outcomes, including all-cause mortality, cardiovascular mortality, reinfarction, and length of hospitalization.

These were not necessarily preselected, high-performing centers. For example, in Los Angeles (LA) County, less than 50% of STEMI patients had a door-to-balloon time of 90 minutes or less prior to the implementation of the regional STEMI system. Within 1 month of implementing the system, more than 90% of the STEMI patients had a door-to-balloon time of 90 minutes or less [20]. To effectively triage patients to the appropriate STEMI receiving center (SRC) rather than to closest available hospital), LA County became one of the first STEMI systems to integrate PH-EKGs into the emergency medical service (EMS) care plan, with the computer readout determining the destination of patient triage. Meanwhile in North Carolina, collaborators built the first state-wide STEMI system, which included both PPCI and fibrinolytic-based strategies [21]. Through this integrated approach, the Reperfusion of Acute Myocardial Infarction in Carolina Emergency Departments (RACE) providers were able to demonstrate significant improvements in reperfusion rates and time-to-treatment metrics. Outcome data improved as well, but these measures did not reach statistical significance [21].

Mission: Lifeline STEMI Systems Coverage

As of 03/28/2015
(848 Systems - 83.13% Population Coverage)

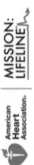
American Heart Association.

MISSION: LIFELINE

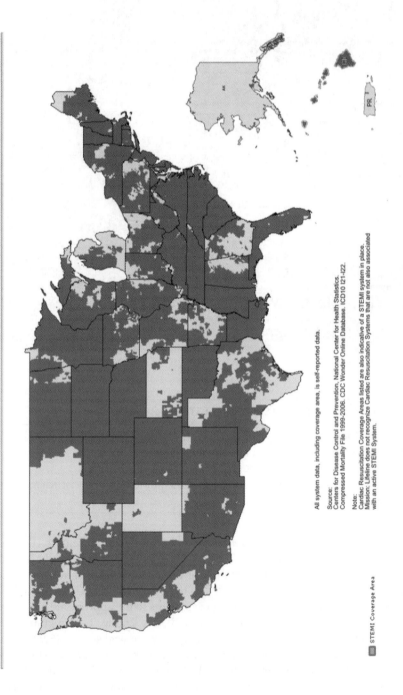

All system data, including coverage area, is self-reported data.

Source:
Centers for Disease Control and Prevention, National Center for Health Statistics.
Compressed Mortality File 1999-2006. CDC Wonder Online Database. ICD10 I21-I22.

Note:
Cardiac Resuscitation Coverage Areas listed are also indicative of a STEMI system in place.
Mission: Lifeline does not recognize Cardiac Resuscitation Systems that are not also associated with an active STEMI System.

STEMI Coverage Area

Figure 18.3 US STEMI systems of care from the Mission: Lifeline coverage Map (© American Heart Association); reproduced with permission.

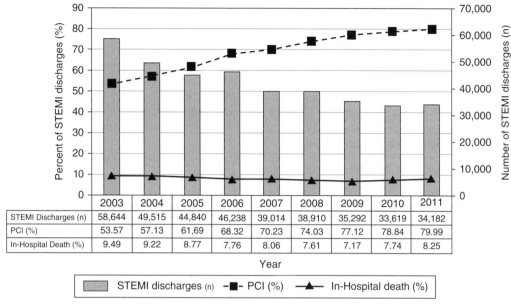

Number of STEMI Discharges and Rates of PCI and In-Hospital Death in the United States, 2003 to 2011
PCI = percutaneous coronary intervention; STEMI = ST-segment elevation myocardial infarction.

Figure 18.4 Trends in US STEMI Care 2003–2011. Increasing PCI to 80% with decreasing mortality (Shah RU, et al. *J Am Coll Cardiol Interv*, 2015; 8: 139–146); reproduced with permission. PCI, percutaneous coronary intervention; ST-segment elevation myocardial infarction.

The successes in Minnesota, North Carolina and California were replicated across the United States and contributed to a change in the American College of Cardiology/American Heart Association (ACC/HA) guidelines for STEMI patients. Current guidelines give a class I, level of evidence B recommendation that "all communities should create and maintain a regional system of STEMI care" [1].

Organizing A System for Inter-Hospital Transfer

An integrated, organized system with prespecified relationships and transfer agreements is needed to achieve the recommended door-to-balloon times for STEMI patients requiring transfer for PPCI. Such a system requires collaboration and buy-in from key stakeholders such as cardiologists, emergency medicine, nursing, EMS, and administration. The key components for organizing a regional system are addressed in the following section. Initially, transfer systems considered a "30-30-30 goal" (Box 18.2); however, after the ACC/AHA guidelines adopted the goal 120 minutes or less for patients transferred from a non-PCI center, a more realistic goal could be used:

- 30–45-minute door in, door out time at the referral hospital
- 30–45-minute inter-hospital transport time
- 30-minute door-to-balloon time at PPCI center.

Hospitals which cannot reasonably achieve a total door-to-balloon time of 120 minutes or less should consider alternative strategies such as pharmacoinvasive PCI [11,19].

Box 18.2   30-30-30 Goal

Door-in-door-out at referral hospital (30–45 minutes):

- Pre-hospital EKG and notification.
- Institution-specific STEMI protocol.
- STEMI team: emergency doctor, nurse, laboratory, radiology.
- STEMI kit with laboratory supplies, transfer forms, adjunctive medications.
- One call to activate STEMI transfer protocol.
- Dispatch transport team immediately.

Transport time (30–45 minutes):

- Highest priority for transfer (same as trauma).
- Rapid turnaround times (< 10 minutes).
- Air – hot loads.
- Ground – same crew, evaluation on gurney.
- Prearranged transfer agreements – no delays due to Emergency Medical Transport and Active Labor Act (EMTALA) restrictions.
- Community specific transfer plan.

EMTALA restrictions:

- Community-specific transfer plan.
- Door-to-balloon time at the percutaneous coronary intervention hospital (< 30 minutes).
- Cardiac catheterization laboratory team activated while the patient is en route.
- Direct admission to the cardiac catheterization laboratory: bypass emergency department and intensive care/coronary care unit.
- Preregistration based on demographic information from community hospital.
- Clinical and laboratory data faxed directly to cardiac catheterization laboratory from community hospital.

Key Components of a STEMI System of Care

The key components of a STEMI system of care are:

- standardized protocols
- empower the emergency department physician
- single telephone call activates the system
- individualize transfer agreements
- direct admission to the cardiac catheterization laboratory
- education and training
- feedback and quality improvement.

Standardized Protocols

In any STEMI system, the referral hospitals should have standardized "point-of-entry" protocols that clearly delineate which patients should be transferred to a referral center based on patient-specific risk criteria, indications and contraindications to alternative therapies and the proximity to the nearest receiving center. Standardized protocols and order sets that use guideline-based adjunctive therapy (antiplatelet and antithrombin medications) ensure the efficient delivery of evidenced-based therapies for all patients, while minimizing variability in the delivery of care. However, the same system needs to allow flexibility to address the individual needs of patients and physicians. These prespecified plans and arrangements should be agreed upon by the relevant stakeholders including the cardiologists, emergency department and primary care physicians within the system. Discussions between the emergency department physician and the treating cardiologist regarding the reperfusion strategy, which antithrombotic or antiplatelet regimen should be used, which tests to order, and so on, introduce unnecessary delays into the system. Each hospital should therefore have a written, institution-specific protocol for STEMI patients that includes appropriate laboratory studies, initial diagnostic tests, and adjunctive medications. Key details of the protocol should be available in checklists and standing orders in the emergency department. Tools such as laminated cards, posters, or prepopulated electronic order sets are helpful in streamlining this process (Figure 18.5).

Empower the Emergency Department Physician

The ACC/AHA STEMI guidelines recommend that an emergency department physician be responsible for making the initial diagnosis and treatment disposition for STEMI patients [1]. A single phone call from the emergency department physician should activate the entire system, mobilizing the interventional cardiologist and cardiac catheterization laboratory (CCL) staff to be available within 30 minutes. Non-diagnostic EKGs or diagnostic dilemmas can be discussed with the cardiologist, but these should be the exception, not the rule.

Individualize Transfer Agreements

As mentioned earlier, each referral center should have prespecified criteria for the transfer of patients and agreements which dictate where patients will be transferred and the mode of transportation (ground, air, etc.). Helicopter emergency medical services need to be instructed to use a trauma transfer approach that includes 10-minute turnaround times and "hot loads" (keeping the rotors running during patient loading). Furthermore, these centers should have integrated plans for the return of patients to their local community hospitals and care centers for post-discharge follow-up care.

Direct Admission to the Cardiac Catheterization Laboratory

Referral centers should have mechanisms that promote efficient transfer of data (medical records, study results, etc.) to the receiving centers for purposes of continuity of care and to avoid redundancies in the system. As transfer STEMI-patients have already been evaluated and diagnosed at the referral center, the patient should be taken directly to the CCL, bypassing the emergency department, intensive care or cardiac intensive care unit. Demographic data obtained from the referral center can be used to pre-admit the patient to the receiving center, and key clinical and laboratory data can be faxed directly to the CCL during patient transport (Figure 18.6).

Education and Training

Proper education and training are essential components to any successful STEMI system. This training should be directed at all parties, including transport personnel, nursing and ancillary staff, CCL staff, emergency department physicians, interventional cardiologists, cardiac intensive care staff, and primary care providers within the network. Each team member should understand their role and the roles of their colleagues in facilitating collaboration and mutual respect. Additionally, team members should understand the details of the critical

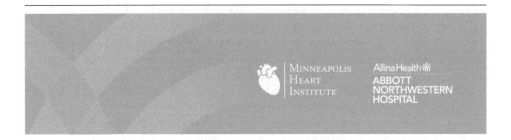

Level One Heart Attack Protocol

Criteria: ST Elevation Myocardial Infarction with
onset of symptoms less than 24 hours

- Activate emergency team and transport team (in-the-door to out-
  the-door goal is less than 30 minutes)
- Contact Minneapolis Heart Institute® at **612-863-3911** to page
  cardiologist for a Level One STEMI
- Monitor, minimum of 2 IVs, 12 Lead EKG, O2, draw blood for labs
- Aspirin: 324 mg orally (four 81 mg chewable tabs) **OR** 300 mg
  rectally
- Ticagrelor: 180 mg **OR** Plavix: 600 mg orally or via NG/OG
  if intubated
- Heparin IV Push: Loading dose of 50 units/kg (max 4,000 units IVP)
- Nitroglycerin 0.4 mg SL, repeat as needed
- Morphine Sulfate as needed for pain
- If expected transfer to the cath lab is greater than 90 minutes,
  Thrombolytic: ½ dose TNKase IVP
- Chest x-ray: consider if condition warrants (send film with patient)
- Attach hands-free defibrillator pads
- If awaiting transport, remove patient's clothing prior to transfer.
  Gown only. Do not delay transport.

*This information is intended only as a guideline.
Please use your best judgment in the treatment of patients.*

Figure 18.5 Example protocol from Minneapolis Heart Institute's Level 1 STEMI protocol. © Allina Health
System; reproduced with permission.

Level One Heart Attack
Data Sheet

Onset Chest Pain Time _____ ED Arrival Time _____ ECG Time _____

BP _____ HR _____ Rhythm _____ Sending Physician _____

ECG Findings: Inferior (II, III, aVF)   Anterior   Lateral (I, aVL, V5-V6)   Posterior   LBBB

Allergies _____

Allergy to IV Contrast? ☐ YES ☐ NO   If YES, pretreated for constrast allergy? List meds below.

Past Medical History _____

_____

Patient weight _____ Patient height _____

Lab Data

Na _____ K _____ Cr _____ Troponin I _____ Hgb _____

PT/INR _____ WBC _____ Platelets _____ Glucose _____

Is Patient Intubated? ☐ YES ☐ NO   **If yes, was patient given paralytics?** ☐ YES ☐ NO

MEDICATIONS	DOSE		TIME	GIVEN BY
Aspirin (check with patient if already taken today)	324 mg (four, 81 mg chewable tabs)			
Ticagrelor 180 mg **OR** Clopidogrel 600 mg	Drug:	Dose:		
Heparin (loading dose) 50 units/kg (Max 4000 units)		Units IVP		
Thrombolytics: Zone 2 patients (Zone 1 only if delayed transfer). TnKase ½ dose.	Was patient given thrombolytics? ☐ YES ☐ NO mg given			
Administer as needed for pain				
Nitroglycerin 0.4 mg sublingual				
Morphine Sulfate IVP; 2-4 mg prn				
Other medications administered	Name	Dose		
Other medications administered	Name	Dose		
Other medications administered	Name	Dose		

FAX THIS FORM AND 12 LEAD EKG TO 1-888-764-8218.

MINNEAPOLIS HEART INSTITUTE   Allina Health
ABBOTT NORTHWESTERN HOSPITAL   S413061A 20364 0614

PATIENT LABEL

Figure 18.6 Sample patient transfer datasheet from Minneapolis Heart Institute's Level 1 STEMI protocol; reproduced with permission.

pathway to facilitate rapid diagnosis, initial stabilization, and transfer. This training should be facilitated by the cardiovascular staff from the PCI hospital. All members of the system must share a sense of teamwork and singular common purpose – to provide the highest quality of care in the timeliest fashion possible. To do this, system members must share a mutual respect for each individual player and must understand that for the system to succeed, each member plays a critical role. Finally, local community education appears to decrease the time from symptom onset to arrival at the referral hospitals.

Feedback and Quality Improvement

Once a system is built, it is imperative that data are collected and feedback be provided to facilitate ongoing improvement. This includes the transport paramedics observing an angiogram, the interventional cardiologist calling the emergency department physician immediately following the procedure, and communication the following day between the system coordinators, emergency department managers, the primary cardiologist and the primary care physician. Monthly, quarterly, and yearly performance reports provide ongoing and system-wide quality improvement. A STEMI database will help to identify trends in time to treatment, protocol compliance, and clinical outcomes. A sample database has previously been published [22].

Leadership and Support

Financial and moral support from hospital administration is essential and, if missing, can create a major stumbling block. Perhaps the most important link in the chain is a passionate leader at every level. Dynamic leaders allow for ongoing improvements to be made in a rapid and efficient manner [23].

Challenges to Implementing and Maintaining a Regional STEMI System of Care

Each regional STEMI system faces its own political, socioeconomic and geographic hurdles. However, there are common challenges that most, if not all, STEMI system face (Box 18.3). One major challenge for STEMI systems is the total door-to-balloon time for patients who are transferred from a referral hospital. Door in, door out time at the referral hospitals appears to be a major system delay and a well-identified target for improvement [5,6,24]. PPCI centers must maintain adequate staffing to accept all patients, which requires manpower and financial overhead to operate. Reimbursement is a common challenge, as many different hospitals and providers may take care of a single patient during their stay within a STEMI system. Research and quality improvement measures take time, effort and financial backing. Incomplete data collection and inadequate exchange of information are ongoing issues, while under-reporting of outcomes and "scrubbing" data do little to enhance our understanding of patient outcomes [25]. Multiple isolated, incompatible medical record systems, both electronic and handwritten, are often forced to interact with one-another within a given STEMI system.

Public policy and oversight is another arena that provides unique challenges to each STEMI system. This is a particular problem given the large number and generally underfunded EMS agencies. Regional transportation systems still need to be developed in many areas of the country and ongoing discussions regarding the requirements for an acceptable "receiving" center and "referring" center is needed (Box 18.4). Public education and community outreach is necessary to teach patients and community members to recognize the signs and symptoms of a cardiac emergency and appropriately respond by activating EMS (via 9-1-1) immediately. Accurate mapping and denotation of receiving centers and referral centers is necessary to identify regions in need of more robust STEMI system. In-hospital STEMIs are a

---

Box 18.3   Challenges for STEMI Systems of Care

Pre-hospital:

- Availability of pre-hospital electrocardiogram.
- Use of 9-1-1 compared with self-transport.

Time to treatment for transfer patients:

- Door in, door out times.
- Weather.
- Transportation modality.
- Traffic.

Manpower and financial overhead to provide:

- Adequate staffing to care for all STEMI patients within the system.
- Research, data monitoring, and quality improvement.

Reimbursement for all members of the system.
Efficient exchange of information:

- Multiple incompatible medical record systems.
- Avoidance of duplication of diagnostic tests, laboratorys, studies, etc.

Public policy and oversight:

- Accurate mapping and denotation of percutaneous coronary intervention (PCI) centers and referral centers to identify regions in need.
- Minimal standards to define appropriate PCI centers and referral centers.

"In-hospital" STEMI.
"False positive" catheterization laboratory activation.
Reporting requirements, especially of out-of-hospital cardiac arrest and cardiogenic shock.

---

recently identified problem, associated with longer time to treatment and markedly worse clinical outcomes, which can be improved with standardized in-house STEMI protocols [26,27]. Finally, "false" or "inappropriate" activations are a challenging issue for some systems, particularly as we enter an era of performance-based reimbursement [28].

Conclusions

The past 30 years have seen great advances in the field of medicine, particular with regards to STEMI care. The advent of complex regional STEMI systems is one of many crowning achievements that has helped to improve the quality of cardiovascular care. Transfer from community and rural hospitals to a PCI center provides timely access to PPCI to an ever-increasing proportion of the US population, while decreasing the numbers of "eligible but untreated" patients. Randomized trials using this strategy have repeatedly demonstrated superiority to fibrinolytics if the transfer times are reasonable. Key components of the regional STEMI system include standardized protocols, empowering the emergency department physician, a single call to activate the system, community-specific prearranged transfer plans, direct transfer to the CCL and quality improvement programs.

Box 18.4   Requirements of a Primary Percutaneous Coronary Intervention STEMI Receiving Center

Institutional:

- Primary percutaneous coronary intervention (PPCI) available 24 hours a day, 365 days a year.
- PPCI performed as timely as possible (D2B Alliance for Quality™ goal of 75% door-to-balloon times less than 90 minutes).
- Able to provide supportive care on site for STEMI and complications.
  - Prespecified transfer agreement with tertiary care center for any PPCI center that does not have surgical back-up on site.
- Commitment by hospital administration in support of STEMI system program participation.
  - Mechanisms for monitoring performance.
  - Multidisciplinary team for quality improvement review.

Physician:

- Interventionalists should meet American College of Cardiology/American Heart Association guidelines for competency.
  - 11 PPCI per year for STEMI.
  - 75 total PCI per year.
- Formal on-call schedule.

References

1 O'Gara PT, Kushner FG, Ascheim DD, et al. 2013 ACCF/AHA guideline for the management of ST-elevation myocardial infarction: a report from the American College of Cardiology Foundation/American Heart Association Task Force on Practice Guidelines. *J Am Coll Cardiol*, 2013; 61(4): e78–e140.

2 Keeley E, Boura J, Grines CL. Primary angioplasty versus intravenous thrombolytic therapy for acute myocardial infarction: a quantitative review of 23 randomised trials. *Lancet*, 2003; 361: 13–20.

3 Nallamathu BK, Bates ER, Wang Y, et al. Driving times and distances to hospitals with percutaneous coronary intervention in the United States: implications for prehospital triage of patients with ST-elevation myocardial infarction. *Circulation*, 2006; 113: 1189–1195.

4 DeLuca G, Suryapranata H, Ottervanger JP, et al. Time delay to treatment and mortality in primary angioplasty for acute myocardial infarction: every minute of delay counts. *Circulation*, 2004; 109: 1223–1225.

5 Terkelsen CJ, Sørensen JT, Maeng M, et al. System delay and mortality among patients with STEMI treated with primary percutaneous coronary intervention. *JAMA*, 2010; 304(7): 763–771.

6 Miedema MD, Newell MC, Duval S, et al. Causes of delay and associated mortality in patients transferred with ST-elevation myocardial infarction. *Circulation*, 2011; 124(15): 1636–1644.

7 Diercks DB, Kontos MC, Chen AY, et al. Utilization and impact of pre-hospital electrocardiograms for patients with acute ST-segment elevation myocardial infarction: data from the NCDR (National Cardiovascular Data Registry) ACTION (Acute Coronary Treatment and Intervention Outcomes Network) Registry. *J Am Coll Cardiol*, 2009; 53: 161–166.

8 Pedersen SH, Galatius S, Hansen PR, et al. Field triage reduces treatment delay and improves long-term clinical outcome in patients with acute ST-segment elevation myocardial infarction treated with primary percutaneous coronary intervention. *J Am Coll Cardiol*, 2009; 54: 2296–2302.

9 Le May MR, So DY, Dionne R, et al. A citywide protocol for primary PCI in ST-segment elevation myocardial infarction. *N Engl J Med*, 2008; 358: 231–240.

10 Canto JG, Zalenski RJ, Ornato JP, et al. Use of emergency medical services in acute myocardial infarction and subsequent quality of CRE: observations from the National Registry of Myocardial Infarction 2. *Circulation*, 2002; 106: 3018–3023.

11 Henry TD, Sharkey SW, Burke N, et al. A regional system to provide timely access to percutaneous coronary intervention for ST-elevation myocardial infarction. *Circulation*, 2007; 116: 721–728.

12 Widimsky P, Groch L, Zelizko M, et al. Multicenter randomized trial comparing transport to primary angioplasty vs. immediate thrombolysis vs. combined strategy for patients with acute myocardial infarction presenting to a community hospital without a catheterization laboratory. The PRAGUE study. *Eur Heart J*, 2000; 21: 823–831.

13 Widimsky P, Budesinsky T, Vorac D, et al. Long distance transport for primary angioplasty vs. immediate thrombolysis in acute myocardial – PRAGUE-2. *Eur Heart J*, 2003; 24: 94–104.

14 Anderson HR, Nielsen TT, Rasmussen K, et al. A comparison of coronary angioplasty with fibrinolytic therapy in acute myocardial infarction – DANAMI-2. *N Engl J Med*, 2003;349(8): 733–742.

15 Grines CL, Browne KF, Marco J, Rothbaum D, Stone GW, O'Keefe J. Overlie P, Donohue B, Chelliah N, Timmis GC, Viletstra RE, Strzelecki M, Puchroqicz-Ochocki S, O'Neill WW, and the Primary Angioplasty in Myocardial Infarction Study Group. A Comparison of Immediate Angioplasty with Thrombolytic Therapy for Acute Myocardial Infarction. *N Engl J Med*, 1993; 328: 673–679.

16 Dalby M, Bouzamondo A, Lechat P, et al. Transfer for primary angioplasty versus immediate thrombolysis in acute myocardial infarction: a meta-analysis. *Circulation*, 2003; 108(15): 1809–1814.

17 Henry TD, Atkins JM, Cunningham MS, et al. ST-segment elevation myocardial infarction: recommendations on triage of patients to heart attack centers: is it time for a national policy for the treatment of ST-segment elevation myocardial infarction? *J Am Coll Cardiol*, 2006; 47: 1339–1345.

18 Miedema MD, Newell MC, Duval S, et al. Causes of delay and associated mortality in patients transferred with ST-elevation myocardial infarction. *Circulation*, 2011; 124(15): 1636–1644.

19 Larson DM, Duval S, Sharkey SW, et al. Safety and efficacy of a pharmaco-invasive reperfusion strategy in rural ST-elevation myocardial infarction patients with expected delays due to long distance transfers. *Eur Heart J*, 2012; 33: 1232–1240.

20 Rokos IC, French WJ, Koenig WJ, et al. Integration of pre-hospital electrocardiograms and ST-elevation myocardial infarction receiving (SRC) networks: Impact on door-to-balloon times across 10 independent regions. *J Am Coll Cardiol Cardiovasc Interv*, 2009; 2(4): 339–346.

21 Jollis J, Roettig M, Aluko A, et al. Implementation of a statewide system for coronaryreperfusion for ST-segment myocardial infarction. *JAMA*, 2007; 298(20): 2371–2380.

22 Henry TD, Unger BT, Sharkey SW, et al. Design of a standardized system for transfer of patients with ST-elevation myocardial infarction for percutaneous coronary intervention. *Am Heart J*, 2005; 150: 373–384.

23 Henry TD. From concept to reality: a decade of progress in regional ST-segment elevation myocardial infarction systems. *Circulation*, 2012; 126: 166–168.

24 Wang TY, Nallamothou BK, Krumholz HM, et al. Association of door-in door-out time with reperfusion delays and outcomes among patients transferred for primary percutaneous coronary intervention. *JAMA*, 2011; 305(24): 2540–2547.

25 Campbell AR, Satran D, Larson DM, et al. ST-elevation myocardial infarction: Which patients do quality assurance programs include? *Circ Cardiovasc Qual Outcomes*, 2009; 2: 648–655.

26 Kaul P, Federspeiel JJ, Dai X, et al. Association of inpatient vs. outpatient onset of ST-elevation myocardial infarction with treatment and clinical outcomes. *JAMA*, 2014; 312(19): 1999–2007.

27 Garberich RF, Traverse JH, Claussen MT, et al. ST-elevation myocardial infarction diagnosed after hospital admission. *Circulation*, 2014; 129(11): 1225–1232.

28 Larsen DM, Menssen KM, Sharkey SW, et al. False positive cardiac catheterization laboratory activation among patients with suspected ST-segment elevation myocardial infarction. *JAMA*, 2007; 298: 2754–2760.

19

Pharmacoinvasive Management of STEMI

Neeraj Bhalla MD

Introduction

The primary goal of STEMI management is early reperfusion to establish coronary blood flow to the ischemic myocardium. Currently, there are three main reperfusion strategies: Primary percutaneous coronary intervention (PPCI), fibrinolytic therapy, and fibrinolysis followed by PCI which includes facilitated PCI, rescue PCI and elective pharamacoinvasive strategies. Facilitated PCI, or thrombolysis followed mandatorily by immediate PCI, seemed to offer promise as a way of combining both strategies. It has been discarded as a strategy for managing STEMI following several clinical trials (ASSENT-4, FINESSE), which showed greater harm, in terms of stent thrombosis and/or greater bleeding rates when full dose thrombolytic was immediately followed by PCI [1,2]. This practice should be discouraged.

Rescue PCI is by definition a strategy for failed thrombolysis and can be viewed as a salvage procedure. PPCI, however, is currently the gold standard of STEMI care when offered in a timely fashion. It is often not available 24 hours a day, 7 days a week to all comers, even in PCI-capable hospitals, owing to practical limitations: 1) Applicability, which is limited by availability; 2) cost issues and reimbursement, which is relevant in those areas of the world where the payee is not the state or an insurance company.

Multiple randomized trials and registries have shown the benefit of PCI over thrombolysis only if performed in a timely manner. Early reperfusion is the key for decreasing mortality in STEMI patients and that mortality benefit is lost once there is delay in PCI, compared with immediate administration of a fibrin-specific thrombolytic agent [3].

Fibrinolytic Therapy

Fibrinolytic therapy for STEMI has been studied in numerous randomized trials involving more than 1,000,000 patients, and it has been found to be effective [4]. It is most widely available, can be easily administered, and is a relatively inexpensive modality for achieving reperfusion. Only approximately 50–60% of STEMI patients are eligible for fibrinolytic therapy, and only 50% of the patients treated with fibrinolytic therapy achieve complete reperfusion (thrombolysis in myocardial infarction, TIMI, III flow). Fibrinolytic therapy is most effective when given within 3 hours from the onset of chest pain [5]. The mortality rates and infarct size in patients treated with very early fibrinolytic therapy (within first 60–90 minutes of symptom onset) are extremely low, which suggests that fibrinolytic therapy still has an important role to play in patients presenting to hospital without PPCI capability [6,7].

Manual of STEMI Interventions, First Edition. Edited by Sameer Mehta.
© 2017 John Wiley & Sons Ltd. Published 2017 by John Wiley & Sons Ltd.

Pharmacoinvasive Therapy

Pharmacoinvasive therapy is best defined as the administration of early fibrinolysis and then promptly and systematically sending the patient for PCI, which is performed 3–24 hours after the start of fibrinolytic therapy, regardless of whether thrombolysis results in successful reperfusion.

Trials Comparing Routine Early PCI After Fibrinolysis With Standard Therapy and Primary PCI Alone

TRANSFER-AMI

TRANSFER-AMI is one of the largest trials to have evaluated routine early PCI compared with fibrinolysis [8]. In this study, 1059 STEMI patients who received small fibrinolytic therapy were randomized to either standard therapy (transfer for angiography no less than 24 hours after lytic therapy) or PCI of the infarct-related artery within 6 hours of fibrinolysis (early PCI). The primary endpoint was the 30-day composite of death, reinfarction, recurrent ischemia, heart failure, or cardiogenic shock. At 30 days, the primary endpoint occurred in 11% of early PCI group compared with 17.2% of the standard group ($P = 0.004$). The favorable results for the early PCI group were primarily driven by a decreased rate of reinfarction. There was no difference in incidence of bleeding between the two groups [8]. The results of four smaller studies investigating early PCI after fibrinolysis (CAPITAL-AMI, CARESS-IN-AMI, GRACIA-I, and SIAM-III) are consistent with findings of TRANSFER-AMI [9–12].

GRACIA-2

In the GRACIA-2 trial, a total of 212 STEMI patients were randomized to full-dose tenecteplase followed by stenting within 3–12 hours (early routine post-fibrinolysis angioplasty; 104 patients), or to undergo primary stenting with abciximab within 3 hours of randomization (primary angioplasty; 108 patients) [13]. The primary endpoints were epicardial and myocardial reperfusion, and the extent of left ventricular myocardial damage, determined by means of the infarct size and 6 week left ventricular function. The secondary endpoints were reinfarction, stroke, or revascularization. Early routine post-fibrinolysis angioplasty resulted in higher frequency (21% vs. 6%, $P = 0.003$) of complete epicardial and myocardial reperfusion (TIMI 3 epicardial flow, TIMI 3 myocardial perfusion, and resolution of the initial sum of ST-segment elevation $\geq 70\%$) following angioplasty. Both groups were similar regarding infarct size, 6-week left ventricular function, end systolic volume index, major bleeding and 6-month cumulative incidence of the clinical endpoint (10% vs. 12%). In conclusion, early routine post-fibrinolysis angioplasty safely results in better myocardial perfusion than primary angioplasty, and despite its later application, this approach seems to be equivalent to primary angioplasty in limiting infarct size and preserving left ventricular function [13].

FAST-MI

The purpose of the FAST-MI French registry, which included 223 centers and 1714 patients over a 1-month period at the end of 2005, with 1-year follow-up, was to assess contemporary outcomes in STEMI patients, with specific emphasis on comparing a pharmacoinvasive strategy (thrombolysis followed by routine angiography) with PPCI [14]. Some 60% of the patients underwent reperfusion therapy, 33% with PPCI, and 29% with intravenous thrombolysis (18% pre-hospital). After thrombolysis, 96% of patients had coronary angiography, and 84% had subsequent PCI (58% within 24 hours). The results from this registry clearly showed that when used early after the onset of symptoms, a pharmacoinvasive strategy that combines thrombolysis with a liberal use of PCI yields early and 1-year survival rates that are comparable to those of PPCI [14].

WEST

The WEST (Which Early ST-elevation myocardial infarction Therapy) study was a randomized trial of approximately 300 patients with STEMI, comparing three strategies: Pre-hospital lysis and usual care (group A), pre-hospital lysis and provisional rescue PCI in case of failure to achieve ST-segment resolution (group B), and mandatory invasive management within 24 hours (group C) in other cases. The composite of 30-day mortality was 25% (group A), 24% (group B), and 23% (group C), respectively. However, there was a higher frequency of the combination of death and recurrent myocardial infarction in group A compared with between group B (6.7%, P-log rank = 0.378) and group C. Data from this study reinforced the fact that a timely delivered pharmacologic therapy, coupled with routine coronary intervention within 24 hours of initial treatment, may be as effective as primary PCI [15].

NORDISTEMI

The primary objective of the NORDISTEMI (NORwegian study on DIstrict treatment of ST-elevation myocardial infarction) study was to compare a strategy of immediate transfer for PCI with an ischemia-guided approach after thrombolysis in patients with a very long transfer distance to PCI. In this trial, 266 patients with an estimated time delay for PPCI more than 90 minutes were randomized to immediate transfer for PCI or to standard management in the local hospitals with early transfer only if indicated for rescue or clinical deterioration. The data at 30 days showed that the primary endpoint of death, reinfarction, and stroke in the early invasive arm was 4.5% compared with 9.8% in the conservative arm. The 12-month data outcome were similarly in favor of pharmacoinvasive therapy (primary endpoint 6% vs. 15.9%). No significant differences in bleeding or infarct size were observed in either group [16].

STREAM Trial

The STREAM trail was an open-label, prospective, randomized, multicenter trial in which 1892 STEMI patients who presented within 3 hours of symptom onset and who were unable to undergo primary PCI within 1 hour, were randomly assigned to undergo either primary PCI or fibrinolytic therapy with bolus tenecteplase (amended to a half dose in patients ≥ 75 years of age), clopidogrel, and enoxaparin before transport to a PCI-capable hospital [17]. Emergency coronary angiography was performed in case of failed fibrinolysis; otherwise, angiography was performed 6–24 hours after randomization.

The primary endpoint was a composite of death, shock, congestive heart failure, or reinfarction up to 30 days. The primary endpoint occurred in 116 of 939 patients (12.4%) in the fibrinolysis group and in 135 of 943 patients (14.3%) in the PPCI group. Emergency angiography was required in 36.3% of patients in the fibrinolysis group, whereas the remainder of patients underwent angiography at a median of 17 hours after randomization. More intracranial hemorrhages occurred in the fibrinolysis group than in the PPCI group. The rates of non-intracranial bleeding were similar in the two groups. The results of this trial suggest that fibrinolysis with timely coronary angiography resulted in effective reperfusion in the patients with early STEMI who could not undergo primary PCI within 1 hour after the first medical contact. However, fibrinolysis was associated with slightly increase risk of intracranial bleeding [17].

Current Guidelines for Pharmacoinvasive Therapy

Present-day management of STEMI is aimed at reducing the "total ischemic time", which is the time from onset of ischemic symptoms to reperfusion of the infarct related artery [18]. PPCI of the infarct artery is preferred to fibrinolytic therapy when time-to-treatment delays are short and the patient presents to a high-volume, well-equipped center with experienced interventional cardiologists and skilled support staff. Compared with fibrinolytic therapy, PPCI produces higher rates of infarct artery patency, TIMI 3 flow, and access-site bleeding, and lower rates of recurrent ischemia, reinfarction, emergency repeat revascularization procedures, intracranial hemorrhage, and death [19–21]. The benefits of fibrinolytic therapy in patients with ST-elevation or new-onset left bundle branch block myocardial infarction are well established, with a time-dependent reduction in both mortality and morbidity rates during the initial 12 hours after symptom onset.

Guideline Recommendations

According to the American College of Cardiology/American Heart Association 2013 STEMI guidelines for reperfusion at a non-PCI-capable hospital, fibrinolytic therapy is a class IA indication when there is an anticipated delay to performing PPCI within 120 minutes of first medical contact (Figure 19.1). Fibrin-specific agents are preferred when a choice of fibrinolytic agents is available. Adjunctive antiplatelet and/or anticoagulant therapies are indicated, regardless of the choice of fibrinolytic therapy.

Delayed PCI of a significant stenosis in a patent infarct artery is reasonable in stable patients with STEMI after fibrinolytic therapy. PCI can be performed as soon as logistically feasible at the receiving hospital, and ideally within 24 hours, but should not be performed within the first 2–3 hours after administration of fibrinolytic therapy (class IIa recommendation) [22].

According to the 2012 European Society of Cardiology guidelines for the management of acute myocardial infarction in patients presenting with ST-segment elevation guidelines, fibrinolysis is a class I indication for STEMI management if there is delay in primary PCI for more than 120 minutes. The optimal timing for transfer to a PCI-capable center following successful thrombolysis is 3–24 hours for coronary angiography (class IIa recommendation) (Figure 19.2) [23].

Discussion

The primary aim of STEMI management in the current era is the early and complete restoration of coronary flow and myocardial tissue perfusion. For patients with a clinical presentation of STEMI within 12 hours of symptom onset and with persistent ST-segment elevation or new or presumed new left bundle branch block, early mechanical (PCI) or pharmacological reperfusion

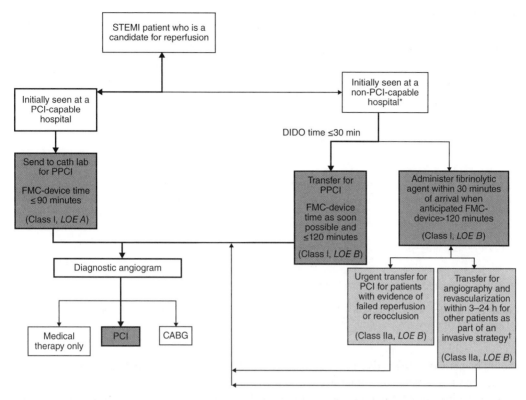

Figure 19.1 Reperfusion therapy for STEMI (adapted from ACC/AHA STEMI guidelines 2013). CABG, coronary artery bypass graft; DIDO, door in, door out; FMC, first medical contact; PPCI, primary percutaneous coronary intervention.

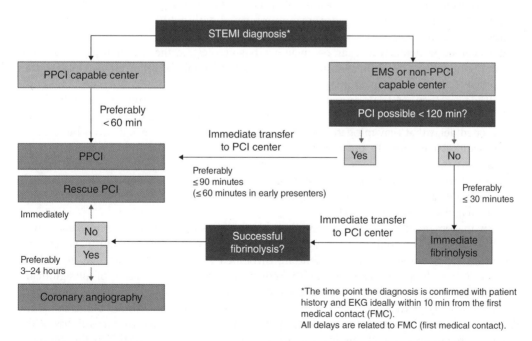

*The time point the diagnosis is confirmed with patient history and EKG ideally within 10 min from the first medical contact (FMC).
All delays are related to FMC (first medical contact).

Figure 19.2 Pre-hospital and in-hospital management, and reperfusion strategies within 24 hours of first medical contact (adapted from Wijns et al.) [24]. PPCI, primary percutaneous coronary intervention.

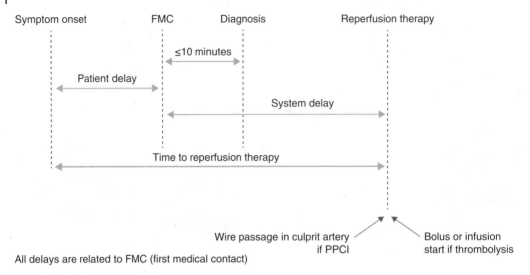

Figure 19.3 Components of delay in STEMI and ideal time intervals for intervention. EMS, emergency medical services; PPCI, primary percutaneous coronary intervention.

should be performed as early as possible. However, there are significant delays from the onset of chest pain to first medical contact to treatment, as shown in Figure 19.3.

PPCI (defined as an emergent percutaneous catheter intervention in the setting of STEMI, without previous fibrinolytic treatment) is the preferred reperfusion strategy in patients with STEMI, provided that it can be performed expeditiously (i.e. within guideline-mandated times), by an experienced team, and regardless of whether the patient presents to a PCI-capable hospital. In settings where PPCI cannot be performed within 120 minutes of first medical contact by an experienced team because of delays, as depicted in Figure 19.3, fibrinolysis should be considered, particularly if it can be given pre-hospital (e.g. in the ambulance) [25–27] and within the first 120 minutes of symptom onset [28,29]. It should be followed by consideration of rescue PCI or routine angiography.

Multiple randomized trials and registries have shown that significant delays to PPCI are associated with worse clinical outcomes. From randomized trials, it was calculated that the PCI-related delay that may mitigate the benefit of mechanical intervention varies between 60 minutes and 110 minutes. In another analysis of these trials, a benefit of PPCI over fibrinolytic therapy was calculated up to a PCI-related delay of 120 minutes [30]. In 192,509 patients included in the US National Registry of Myocardial Infarction 2–4 Registry, the mean PCI-related time delay, where mortality rates of the two reperfusion strategies were comparable, was calculated at 114 minutes [31].

The management of STEMI in contemporary times across the world is a complex and multi-variable situation. The gold standard is a timely PPCI, which offers the best coronary revascularization and addresses both the offending thrombus and the underlying culprit stenotic coronary lesion. It is now being debated whether simultaneous addressing of all significant coronary lesions offers a better outcome compared with only index or culprit-lesion PPCI. A 2013 trial suggests that the former is not only possible but possibly offers a better outcome. The limitations of this approach lies in its applicability, being dictated by accessibility of the STEMI population to a high-quality PCI center in a timely fashion [32]. On the contrary, fibrinolysis is available and applicable to a much larger STEMI population, and can be administered more easily and even in an emergency medical service or pre-hospital setting.

The syncretic and synergistic application of both these approaches underlies the philosophy of pharmacoinvasive management of STEMI.

Clinical trials to test this approach seem to suggest that when fibrinolysis is combined with a planned PCI approach (done within but not less than, 3–24 hours), the outcomes are salutary and equal PPCI with a suggestion of better coronary flow, albeit with a small increase in risk of bleeding. This offers the possibility of the best outcomes for a much larger STEMI population than does PPCI alone and serves a much larger socioeconomic purpose. It also reinforces the idea of developing local and regional STEMI networks and allows STEMI caregivers to organize functional systems with a clear plan for each patient who presents to them. Counter to this, once patient or system related delays dominate the presentation, due to lack of awareness, lack of emergency medical service systems and financial issues, current wisdom suggests that the benefit of fibrinolytic therapy would be lost. It would be worthwhile to perform a clinical trial with patients presenting beyond 4 hours to the first medical contact to assess whether pharmacoinvasive treatment still has equivalent outcomes to PPCI, as this would have worldwide implications.

References

1 ASSENT-4 PCI Investigators. Primary versus tenecteplase-facilitated percutaneous coronary intervention in patients with ST-segment elevation acute myocardial infarction (ASSENT-4 PCI): randomised trial. *Lancet*, 2006; 367: 569–578.
2 Ellis SG, Tendera M, de Belder MA, et al. FINESSE Investigators. Facilitated PCI in patients with ST-elevation myocardial infarction. *N Engl J Med*, 2008; 358: 2205–2217.
3 Van De Werf F, Baim DS. Reperfusion for ST segment elevation myocardial infarction: An overview of current treatment options. *Circulation*, 2002; 105: 2813–2816.
4 Gersch BJ, Stone GW, White HD, et al. Pharmacological facilitation of primary percutaneous coronary intervention for acute myocardial infarction: Is the slope of the curve the shape of the future? *JAMA*, 2005; 293: 979–986.
5 Rathore SS, Curtis JP, Chen J, et al. Association of door-to-balloon time and mortality in patients admitted to hospital with ST elevation myocardial infarction: national cohort study. *BMJ*, 2009; 338: b1807.
6 Antman EM, Anbe DT, Armstrong PW, et al. ACC/AHA guidelines for the management of patients with ST-elevation myocardial infarction--executive summary: A report of the American College of Cardiology/American Heart Association Task Force on Practice Guidelines (Writing Committee to Revise the 1999 Guidelines for the Management of Patients With Acute Myocardial Infarction). *Circulation*, 2004; 110(5): 588–636.
7 Nallamothu BK, Antman EM, Bates ER. Primary percutaneous coronary intervention versus fibrinolytic therapy in acute myocardial infarction: does the choice of fibrinolytic agent impact on the importance of time-to-treatment? *Am J Cardiol*, 2004; 94: 772–774.
8 Cantor WJ, Fitchett D, Borgundvaag B, et al. Routine early angioplasty after fibrinolysis for acute myocardial infarction. *N Engl J Med*, 2009; 360(26): 2705–2718.
9 Le May MR, Wells GA, Labinaz M, et al. Combined Angioplasty and Pharmacological Intervention Versus Thrombolysis Alone in Acute Myocardial Infarction (CAPITAL AMI Study). *J Am Coll Cardiol*, 2005; 46(3): 417–424.
10 Di Mario C, Dudek D, Piscione F, et al. Immediate angioplasty versus standard therapy with rescue angioplasty after thrombolysis in the Combined Abciximab REteplase Stent Study in Acute Myocardial Infarction (CARESS-in-AMI): An open, prospective, randomised, multicentre trial. *Lancet*, 2008; 371(9612): 559–568.

11 Fernandez-Aviles F, Alonso JJ, Castro-Beiras A, et al. Routine invasive strategy within 24 hours of thrombolysis versus ischaemia-guided conservative approach for acute myocardial infarction with ST-segment elevation (GRACIA-1): a randomised controlled trial. *Lancet,* 2004; 364(9439): 1045–1053.

12 Scheller B, Hennen B, Hammer B, et al. Beneficial effects of immediate stenting after thrombolysis in acute myocardial infarction. *J Am Coll Cardiol,* 2003; 142(4): 634–641.

13 Fernández-Avilés F, Alonso JJ, Peña G, et al. Primary angioplasty vs. early routine post-fibrinolysis angioplasty for acute myocardial infarction with ST-segment elevation: the GRACIA-2 non-inferiority, randomized, controlled trial. *Eur Heart J,* 2007; 28(8): 949–960.

14 Danchin N, Coste P, Ferrières J, et al. Comparison of thrombolysis followed by broad use of percutaneous coronary intervention with primary percutaneous coronary intervention for ST-segment-elevation acute myocardial infarction: data from the French registry on acute ST-elevation myocardial infarction (FAST-MI). *Circulation,* 2008; 118(3): 268–276.

15 Armstrong PW, WEST Steering Committee. A comparison of pharmacologic therapy with/without timely coronary intervention vs. primary percutaneous intervention early after ST-elevation myocardial infarction: the WEST (Which Early ST-elevation myocardial infarction Therapy) study. *Eur Heart J,* 2006; 27(13): 1530–1538.

16 Bohmer E, Hoffmann P, Abdelnoor M, et al. Efficacy and safety of immediate angioplasty versus ischemia-guided management after thrombolysis in acute myocardial infarction in areas with very long transfer distances results of the NORDISTEMI (NORwegian study on DIstrict treatment of ST-elevation myocardial infarction). *J Am Coll Cardiol,* 2010; 55: 102–111.

17 Armstrong PW, Gershlick AH, Goldstein P, et al. Fibrinolysis or primary PCI in ST-segment elevation myocardial infarction. *N Engl J Med,* 2013; 368: 1379–1387.

18 Denktas, H. Anderson V, McCarthy J, et al. Total ischemic time: The correct focus of attention for optimal ST-segment elevation myocardial infarction care. *JACC Cardiovasc Interv,* 2011; 4(6): 599–604.

19 Zijlstra F, Hoorntje JC, de Boer MJ, et al. Long-term benefit of primary angioplasty as compared with thrombolytic therapy for acute myocardial infarction. *N Engl J Med,* 1999; 341: 1413–1419.

20 Keeley EC, Boura JA, Grines CL, et al. Primary angioplasty vs. intravenous thrombolytic therapy for acute myocardial infarction: a quantitative review of 23 randomised trials. *Lancet,* 2003; 361(9351): 13–20.

21 Andersen HR, Nielsen TT, Rasmussen K, et al. comparison of coronary angioplasty with fibrinolytic therapy in acute myocardial infarction. *N Engl J Med,* 2003; 349: 733–742.

22 O'Gara PT, Kushner FG, Ascheim DD, et al. 2013 ACCF/AHA Guideline for the Management of ST-Elevation Myocardial Infarction A Report of the American College of Cardiology Foundation/American Heart Association Task Force on Practice. *Circulation,* 2013; 127: e362–e425.

23 Steg G, James SK, Atar D, et al. ESC Guidelines for the management of acute myocardial infarction in patients presenting with ST- segment elevation, The Task Force on the management of ST-segment elevation acute myocardial infarction of the European Society of Cardiology (ESC). *Eur Heart J,* 2012; 33: 2569–2619.

24 Wijns W, Kolh P, Danchin N, et al. Guidelines on myocardial revascularization: The Task Force on Myocardial Revascularization of the European Society of Cardiology (ESC) and the European Association for Cardio-Thoracic Surgery (EACTS). *Eur Heart J,* 2010; 31: 2501–2555.

25 Bonnefoy E, Steg PG, Boutitie F, et al. Comparison of primary angioplasty and pre-hospital fibrinolysis in acute myocardial infarction (CAPTIM) trial: a 5-year follow-up. *Eur Heart J,* 2009; 30: 1598–1606.

26 Morrison LJ, Verbeek PR, McDonald AC, et al. Mortality and pre-hospital thrombolysis for acute myocardial infarction: A meta-analysis. *JAMA*, 2000; 283: 2686–2692.

27 Bonnefoy E, Lapostolle F, Leizorovicz A et al. Primary angioplasty vs. pre-hospital fibrinolysis in acute myocardial infarction: a randomised study. *Lancet*, 2002; 360: 825–829.

28 Steg PG, Bonnefoy E, Chabaud S, et al. Impact of time to treatment on mortality after pre- hospital fibrinolysis or primary angioplasty: data from the CAPTIM randomized clinical trial. *Circulation*, 2003; 108: 2851–2856.

29 Pinto DS, Frederick PD, Chakrabarti AK, et al. Benefit of transferring ST-segment-elevation myocardial infarction patients for percutaneous coronary intervention compared with administration of onsite fibrinolytic declines as delays increase. *Circulation*, 2011; 124: 2512–2521.

30 Boersma E. Does time matter? A pooled analysis of randomized clinical trials comparing primary percutaneous coronary intervention and in-hospital fibrinolysis in acute myocardial infarction patients. *Eur Heart J*, 2006; 27: 779–788.

31 Pinto DS, Kirtane AJ, Nallamothu BK, et al. Hospital delays in reperfusion for ST-elevation myocardial infarction: implications when selecting a reperfusion strategy. *Circulation*, 2006; 114: 2019–2025.

32 Wald DS, Morris JK, Wald NJ, et al. Randomized Trial of Preventive Angioplasty in Myocardial Infarction. *N Engl J Med*, 2013; 369: 1115–1123.

Part IV

Global STEMI Initiatives

20

Stent for Life: The European Perspective on STEMI Interventions

Sasko Kedev MD PhD FESC FACC

Introduction

Percutaneous coronary intervention (PCI), thrombolytic treatment, or combinations of both are current strategies to treat patients with STEMI. Reperfusion therapy in STEMI patients is time dependent [1]. Survival rates after thrombolytic therapy are substantially higher if treatment commences within the first 2 hours after the onset of symptoms [2]. Mortality rates are also time dependent [3–5]. When applied in a timely fashion, primary PCI (PPCI) is able to reduce the risks of reinfarction and mortality compared with thrombolytic therapy [6]. PPCI, when performed in a timely fashion and by an experienced team, is thus the therapy of choice for patients with STEMI [7,8].

Several pharmacologic treatments, including antithrombotics, beta-blockers, angiotensin-converting enzyme inhibitors, angiotensin receptor blockers, and aldosterone blockade, have also proved to increase survival when administered to patients with STEMI. As a result, in-hospital and 30-day mortality rates for STEMI have decreased dramatically over the past 30 years [9–11].

Guidelines from the European Society of Cardiology (ESC) call for timely coronary artery reperfusion in patients with STEMI and stress that, if available, PPCI is the preferred strategy [12]. Despite its advantages, however, PPCI is not universally implemented and thrombolysis is still used in many patients, and a large group of patients presenting with STEMI are receiving no reperfusion therapy [13–15]. Certain clinical factors, financial concerns, obstacles, and organizational difficulties are key factors [6,16]. To overcome these types of barriers, systems of care have been developed, such as establishment of regional STEMI networks, with encouraging results [17,18].

In areas remote from PCI facilities, where PPCI cannot be delivered within the recommended time limit, the benefits of thrombolysis are well established and thrombolytic therapy remains an important reperfusion strategy [12,19]. Thrombolysis should preferably be administered in the pre-hospital setting and should be followed by transfer to a PCI center as soon as possible for urgent (rescue) or subacute coronary angiography [12,20]. The optimal timing for routine angiography following successful thrombolysis is not established, but trials have suggested a time window of 2–12 hours [12].

A well-organized system of care with clear treatment protocols and coordinated transfer systems is necessary for identifying treatment-eligible patients for on-site thrombolysis or transfer for PPCI, as treatment is highly dependent on time. Studies have shown that system delay (time from first medical contact to initiation of reperfusion) is strongly associated with mortality and the risk of readmission to hospital with congestive heart failure [21–24]. As stated in the 2012 STEMI guidelines from the ESC, the time from first medical contact to reperfusion with PPCI should not exceed 120 minutes, and indeed, even shorter time delays should be achieved [12].

STEMI patients who do not receive reperfusion therapy have a poor outcome [25]. A substantial proportion of STEMI patients are still not receiving any reperfusion therapy for a range of reasons, one of the most important being treatment delay. Delays in admission to the hospital, certain high-risk clinical features, and substantial comorbidity have all been shown to be associated with lower rates of reperfusion therapy [26,27]. The formation of STEMI networks involving the emergency medical services (EMS), non-PCI hospitals, and PPCI centers may be necessary to implement PPCI services effectively. These STEMI networks have been shown to reduce the number of patients who are not re-perfused [12,20,28].

Pre-hospital early diagnosis and immediate transport are of vital importance, and barriers to timely and appropriate intervention need to be identified and specifically targeted in order to impact on change. A prerequisite for effective STEMI management is education which aims to improve the quality of acute myocardial infarction (AMI) care, to improve the network of care to give more patients access to reperfusion therapy, and to decrease mortality from AMI. Several key issues should be addressed, including conducting public education and continuous physician training, setting up a local STEMI network focusing on pre-hospital alert by the EMS, inter-hospital transfer, bypassing the emergency department in hospital, and increasing the overall reperfusion ratio of STEMI.

Development of a system of care combining PPCI with the pharmacoinvasive strategy of reperfusion is required. Patients in rural or remote areas, with suspected long transportation time to PCI-capable hospitals, should employ the pharmacoinvasive strategy, with thrombolytic therapy followed by catheterization and PCI if indicated within 3–24 hours of thrombolysis [19]. Building partnerships between hospitals is critical in developing the pharmacoinvasive strategy and a mechanism for inter-hospital transfer of patients is needed. Patient awareness programs should be developed. Registries should be used by the health authorities for obtaining information about patients with acute coronary syndrome (ACS) that will help them improve the use of health resources to treat this patient group. A gross estimate of 600 PPCI procedures per one million inhabitants should serve as the recommended treatment goal in the development of optimal STEMI treatment strategy [29].

Stent for Life Initiative

Stent for Life (SFL), a coalition between the European Association of Percutaneous Cardiovascular Interventions and EuroPCR (the ESR official course in interventional cardiovascular medicine), was established in 2008 as a non-profit international network of national cardiac societies and partnering organizations to address inequalities in STEMI patients' access to a life-saving revascularization treatment [29–31]. SFL supports the implementation of European clinical practice guidelines at national and regional levels through the formulation of strategies, the creation and implementation of educational programs, and through advocacy activities and awareness campaigns. Currently, 18 national cardiac societies and partnering organizations are actively participating in the SFL initiative. The SFL model involves all stakeholders interested in the treatment of STEMI patients, from EMS providers to cardiologists, from STEMI-referral hospitals (non-PCI-capable) to STEMI-receiving hospitals (PCI-capable), from payers to policy makers, from patients to public.

The goal of the SFL initiative is to improve STEMI patients' timely access to appropriate treatment at a national level by establishing effective regional STEMI systems of care.

Geographic mapping and situational analyses of countries participating in SFL have shown that adherence to the ESC STEMI guidelines is influenced by many factors and varies from country to country, from region to region, and one model does not fit all. An in-depth understanding of system-level barriers and unique challenges in the regional context facilitates the development of more effective strategies for improving the quality of the STEMI system of care in a particular country.

Building regional STEMI systems of care and an EMS system infrastructure are critical success factors in the stepwise development of STEMI systems of care at a national level in Europe. An in-depth understanding of healthcare system-level barriers to timely and appropriate reperfusion therapy will facilitate the development of more effective strategies for improving the quality of STEMI care in each region and country. Participating countries already report striking rises in PPCI, reduction in mortality, and overall, a more effective management and organization of the STEMI treatment system, which strongly suggests the benefit of continuing a strategy of implementation and support for countries with low activity [30,32].

Summary

Early reperfusion of the occluded artery is the keystone of treatment for STEMI patients. The objective of STEMI networks is to coordinate the resources to deliver the best care as soon as possible and thereby diminish mortality among this group of patients. Despite strong evidence for the effectiveness of PPCI, not all STEMI patients are treated with PPCI. There is marked variation in treatment availability among countries.

SFL is a European platform for interventional cardiologists, government representatives, industry partners, and patient groups that aims to improve the delivery of care and patient access to PPCI. The main objectives of the SFL are defining the regions with an unmet medical need in the optimal treatment of ACS and implementing an action plan to increase patient access to PPCI. Its main targets are increasing the use of PPCI to more than 70% among all STEMI patients, offering 24/7 services for PPCI procedures at invasive facilities to cover a region's STEMI population at need, and achieving PPCI rates of more than 600 per million inhabitants per year. An action plan should adapt to specific national needs, since each country has different barriers for implementation of PPCI. Audit and quality control issues need to be addressed at every level. Inspired by the SFL model, by building STEMI systems of care region by region, a majority of patients will have access to a reperfusion therapy in remaining European countries in the near future. The model can be applied only by a close and enthusiastic collaboration between all stakeholders, respecting the local circumstances, and could be an example for other countries to follow [33].

References

1 Lambert L, Brown K, Segal E, et al. Association between timeliness of reperfusion therapy and clinical outcomes in ST-elevation myocardial infarction. *JAMA*, 2010; 303(21): 2148–2155.
2 Boersma E, Maas AC, Deckers JW, et al. Early thrombolytic treatment in acute myocardial infarction: reappraisal of the golden hour. *Lancet*, 1996; 348(9030): 771–775.
3 Pinto DS, Kirtane AJ, Nallamothu BK, et al. Hospital delays in reperfusion for ST-elevation myocardial infarction. *Circulation*, 2006; 114(19): 2019–2025.
4 McNamara RL, Wang Y, Herrin J, et al. Effect of door-to-balloon time on mortality in patients with ST-segment elevation myocardial infarction. *J Am Coll Cardiol*, 2006; 47(11): 2180–2186.

5 Rathore SS, Curtis JP, Chen J, et al. Association of door-to-balloon time and mortality in patients admitted to hospital with ST elevation myocardial infarction: national cohort study. *BMJ*, 2009; 338: b1807.

6 Keeley EC, Boura JA, Grines CL. Primary angioplasty versus intravenous thrombolytic therapy for acute myocardial infarction: a quantitative review of 23 randomized trials. *Lancet*, 2003; 361(9351): 13–20.

7 Van de Werf F, Bax J, Betriu A, et al. Management of acute myocardial infarction in patients presenting with persistent ST-segment elevation. *Eur Heart J* 2008; 29(23): 2909–2945.

8 Kushner FG, Hand M, Smith SC Jr, et al. 2009 focused updates: ACC/AHA guidelines for the management of patients with ST-elevation myocardial infarction (updating the 2004 guideline and 2007 focused update) and ACC/AHA/SCAI guidelines on percutaneous coronary intervention (updating the 2005 guideline and 2007 focused update) a report of the ACC Foundation/AHA Task Force on Practice Guidelines. *J Am Coll Cardiol*, 2009; 54(23): 2205–2241.

9 Gibson CM, Pride YB, Frederick PD, et al. Trends in reperfusion strategies, door-to-needle and door-to balloon times, and in-hospital mortality among patients with ST-segment elevation myocardial infarction enrolled in the National Registry of Myocardial Infarction from 1990 to 2006. *Am Heart J*, 2008; 156(6): 1035–1044.

10 Rosamond WD, Chambless LE, Heiss G, et al. Twenty-two year trends in incidence of myocardial infarction, CHD mortality, and case-fatality in four US communities, 1987 to 2008. *Circulation*, 2012; 125(15): 1848–1857.

11 Smolina K, Wright FL, Rayner M, et al. Determinants of the decline in mortality from acute myocardial infarction in England between 2002 and 2010: linked national database study. *BMJ*, 2012; 344: d8059.

12 Steg PG, James SK, Atar D, et al. ESC Guidelines for the management of acute myocardial infarction in patients presenting with ST-segment elevation: The Task Force on the management of ST-segment elevation acute myocardial infarction of the European Society of Cardiology (ESC). *Eur Heart J* 2012; 33: 2569–2619.

13 Goodman SG, Huang W, Yan AT, et al. The expanded Global Registry of Acute Coronary Events: baseline characteristics, management practices, and hospital outcomes of patients with acute coronary syndromes. *Am Heart J*, 2009; 158: 193–201.

14 Puymirat E, Simon T, Steg PG, et al. Association of changes in clinical characteristics and management with improvement in survival among patients with ST-elevation myocardial infarction. *JAMA*, 2012; 308(10): 998–1006.

15 Widimsky P, Wijns W, Fajadet J, et al. Reperfusion therapy for ST elevation acute myocardial infarction in Europe: description of the current situation in 30 countries. *Eur Heart J* 2010; 31(8): 943–957.

16 Laut KG, Pedersen AB, Lash TL, et al. Barriers to implementation of primary percutaneous coronary intervention in Europe. *Eur Cardiol*, 2011; 7: 108–112.

17 Labarere J, Belle L, Fourny M, et al. Regional system of care for ST-segment elevation myocardial infarction in the Northern Alps: a controlled pre- and postintervention study. *Arch Cardiovasc Dis*, 2012; 105(8–9): 414–423.

18 Huber K, Goldstein P, Danchin N, et al. Network models for large cities: the European experience. *Heart*, 2010; 96(2): 164–169.

19 Armstrong PW, Gershlick A, Goldstein P, et al. The Strategic Reperfusion Early After Myocardial Infarction (STREAM) study. *Am Heart J*, 2010; 160(1): 30–35.

20 Lassen JF, Botker HE, Terkelsen CJ. Timely and optimal treatment of patients with STEMI. *Nat Rev Cardiol*, 2013; 10(1): 41–48.

21 De Luca G, Biondi-Zoccai G, Marino P. Transferring patients with ST-segment elevation myocardial infarction for mechanical reperfusion: a meta-regression analysis of randomized trials. *Ann Emerg Med*, 2008; 52(6): 665–676.

22 De Luca G, Suryapranata H, Ottervanger JP, et al. Time delay to treatment and mortality in primary angioplasty for acute myocardial infarction: every minute of delay counts. *Circulation*, 2004; 109(10): 1223–1225.

23 Terkelsen CJ, Jensen LO, Tilsted HH, et al. Health care system delay and heart failure in patients with ST-segment elevation myocardial infarction treated with primary percutaneous coronary intervention: follow-up of population-based medical registry data. *Ann Intern Med*, 2011; 155(6): 361–367.

24 Terkelsen CJ, Sorensen JT, Maeng M, et al. System delay and mortality among patients with STEMI treated with primary percutaneous coronary intervention. *JAMA*, 2010; 304(7): 763–771.

25 Tunstall-Pedoe H, Vanuzzo D, Hobbs M, et al. Estimation of contribution of changes in coronary care to improving survival, event rates, and coronary heart disease mortality across the WHO MONICA Project populations. *Lancet*, 2000; 355(9205): 688–700.

26 Fox KA, Eagle KA, Gore JM, et al. The Global Registry of Acute Coronary Events, 1999 to 2009—GRACE. Heart. 2010;96(14):1095–1101.

27 Alter DA, Ko DT, Newman A, et al. Factors explaining the under-use of reperfusion therapy among ideal patients with ST-segment elevation myocardial infarction. *Eur Heart J*, 2006; 27(13): 1539–1549.

28 Huber K, Goldstein P, Danchin N, et al. Enhancing the efficacy of delivering reperfusion therapy: a European and North American experience with ST-segment elevation myocardial infarction networks. *Am Heart J*, 2013; 165(2): 123–132.

29 Widimsky P, Fajadet J, Danchin N, et al. 'Stent 4 Life' targeting PCI at all who will benefit the most. A joint project between EAPCI, Euro-PCR, EUCOMED and the ESC Working Group on Acute Cardiac Care. *EuroIntervention*, 2009; 4(5): 555–557.

30 Widimsky P, WijnsW, Kaifoszova Z. Stent for life: how this initiative began? *EuroIntervention*, 2012; 8(Pt): P8–P10.

31 Kaifoszova Z, Kala P, Alexander T, et al. Stent for Life Initiative: leading example in building STEMI systems of care in emerging countries. *Eurointervention*, 2014; 10: T87–T95.

32 Kristensen SD, Fajadet J, Di Mario C, et al. Implementation of primary angioplasty in Europe: stent for life initiative progress report. *EuroIntervention*, 2012; 8(1): 35–42.

33 Kristensen SD, Laut KG, Fajadet J, et al. Reperfusion therapy for ST elevation acute myocardial infarction 2010/2011: current status in 37 ESC countries. *Eur Heart J*, 2014; 35(29): 1957–1970.

21

Urban Combined Pharmacoinvasive Management of STEMI Patients as Antidote to Traffic in Large Metropolitan Cities

David G. Iosseliani MD FACC FESC

Introduction

Usually, when I present the experience of Moscow City Center of Interventional Cardioangiology with the treatment of acute myocardial infarction (AMI), the audience asks me if our methods of treatment correspond with the generally adopted guidelines of American College of Cardiology (ACC), American Heart Association (AHA), European Society of Cardiology, and so on. The audience is especially curious whether we respect all the steps and stages suggested by these guidelines in our daily practice. Let me say that, while I really respect most guidelines provided by highly professional organizations, I do not believe that we must take them for a dogma and cannot take a step aside. We should always leave a possibility for a certain improvisation and be ruled by an important postulate, namely "the simpler, the faster and the safer – the better".

In this connection, I would like to bring your attention to the letter of an eminent American cardiologist, the former ACC president Dr. David Holmes [1]. In this letter, David described his visit to the famous traditional Paris restaurant *"Tour d'Argent"*. When Holmes enquired whether they had wine, the waiter asked him to wait a little, then disappeared and came back with a velvet-colored book 10 inches thick. It was the wine list. David Holmes continues: "All I had asked was a simple question – *Do you have wine?* But instead of a direct answer I am given a wine bible – a veritable wine library". From this point on, Holmes draws an analogy with the everyday practice of physician–patient interaction. During the conversation, the patient can ask us many questions, and sometimes it is pretty difficult to give an unambiguous answer. In the words of Dr. Holmes, in attempting to support our answers "we try to rely on scientific evidence. Often we bring to the table the ACC and the AHA "guidelines bible". And then, the author asks: In what measure these reconditions may and should be used by our colleagues in their everyday practice? "They are luxurious documents, often with 150–200 pages full of wonderful details, including executive summaries, numerous references, tables, and graphs. Yet, how many of us have the luxury of sitting down and reading an entire textbook from front to back, particularly during a patient visit? All I want to know is the answer to a question about the patient I am asked to see". I agree with the author; the guidelines should simplify the process of diagnosis and the choice of adequate tactics of treatment, and not confuse and provide us with puzzles and conundrums. It seems that I am not alone in thinking so. Many physicians with whom I have talked on this subject believe that it is necessary to revise the process of guideline compilation to make them more condensed, compact, easier to read and comfortable for search; that is, to transform them into "living documents" that are so necessary to physicians and that will really be used in everyday practice.

Manual of STEMI Interventions, First Edition. Edited by Sameer Mehta.
© 2017 John Wiley & Sons Ltd. Published 2017 by John Wiley & Sons Ltd.

Such ample introduction before the presentation of our tactics of treatment of STEMI is not accidental; I wrote it so that the reader does not search for an absolute analogy, a blind copying of the existing guidelines on the treatment of STEMI. Our tactics can be described as a kind of improvisation on a given subject.

The Role of Coronary Thrombosis in Pathogenesis of STEMI

Before proceeding to the discussion of particular problems of the treatment of STEMI, namely, urban pharmacoinvasive management as an antidote to traffic in large, metropolitan cities, let me point out that while at present most clinical practitioners and researchers assign the leading role in the pathogenesis of STEMI to acute coronary thrombosis, this position has its opponents. The partisans base their position on the following reasons [2–8]:

1) There is a very high incidence of coronary occlusion associated with transmural (Q-wave) infarction.
2) There is a constant relationship between the location of the infarction and the obstruction in the infarct-related artery.
3) The severity of the underlying atherosclerotic plaques associated with coronary thrombosis seems not to be uniform.
4) The thrombosis is usually associated with local arterial lesions, such as plaque rupture and hemorrhage.
5) Radioactive fibrinogen studies demonstrating that a radio-negative central core exists in most human thrombi, which suggests that thrombosis occurs prior to deposition of radiolabeled fibrinogen.

The opponents of this position have their own reasons [9–12]:

1) The occurrence of coronary thrombi without the development of acute myocardial infarction and, vice versa, the occurrence of myocardial infarction without coronary thrombi.
2) The greater incidence of coronary thrombi with large infarctions, implying that larger infarct size predisposes to coronary thrombosis, cardiogenic shock and extensive congestive heart failure.
3) The low prevalence of coronary thrombi in cases of sudden death.
4) Implications from studies indicating that coronary thrombi incorporate radioactive tracers injected intravenously several hours after the onset of clinical infarction.

As one can see from these data, both sides have rather convincing arguments to justify their viewpoints. Today, however, the position of a large majority of clinical practitioners is that acute occlusive coronary thrombosis plays a leading trigger role in the pathogenesis of STEMI. This serves as a basis for the therapeutic principle of a maximally early myocardial reperfusion in such patients. Experimental and then clinical studies have provided convincing evidence that, in the presence of a totally occluded infarct-related artery (IRA), myocardial reperfusion limits the area of myocardial damage and improves left ventricular function, thus providing more favorable early and late prognosis in AMI patients. It is also proven that the earlier is reperfusion in STEMI, the lesser the apoptosis of cardiomyocytes in the myocardial infarction and the peri-infarction areas, and the necrotic focus within the myocardium, and hence, the more evident is the clinical effect. According to some authors, early blood flow restoration in the IRA is also favorable for long-term prognosis.

The Experience of Moscow

Today, few would contest the important role of early myocardial reperfusion in the prognosis of STEMI patients. Our studies also provide convincing evidence for this importance [13,14]. These studies have demonstrated that the longer the period of patient transportation and preparation for endovascular procedure, the less is the clinical effect of myocardial reperfusion and the worse the prognosis, especially in high-risk patients. It is also commonly accepted that if the patient can be transferred to the catheterization laboratory within the first 1–1.5 hours after the onset of angina pain, primary percutaneous coronary intervention (PCI) is the method of choice. In all probability, we can agree with this, but what is the real situation in the megalopolis with its crazy traffic, and in particular, in Moscow? Can the majority of STEMI patients reach the catheterization laboratory within this time interval?

In a large city such as Moscow, some STEMI patients arrive at the hospital far later than the "gold" time standard (the first 90 minutes from the onset of pain). Our study, performed in 2010, has shown that, on average, the patient with AMI is admitted to the hospital within 306.8 ± 46.4 minutes. Another 32.6 ± 13.5 minutes are spent in the clinics for patient transfer to the catheterization laboratory. There are several causes for late admission of patients, and most important among them are difficulties experienced by ambulances in heavy city traffic, and also the late ambulance call. Patients lose time in self-treatment, in seeking advice from acquainted physicians by telephone, and so on, and only after doing all this, do they dial the number for the ambulance. As a result, the majority of such patients arrive at the hospital at the earliest in 2–3 hours, and not infrequently within 5–6 hours after the onset of chest pain; that is, the precious time for the start of therapy is lost. Hence, the majority of Muscovites are deprived of the opportunity of receiving endovascular myocardial reperfusion within the first 90 minutes after the onset of angina status; that is, within the most optimal time interval. Such a situation is typical not only in Russia. In the United States, in barely 50% of patients with STEMI (51.3%) the door-to-balloon time is less than 120 minutes after the onset of angina status [15]. A significant time is spent in the transfer of patients from a non-PCI-capable community hospital to a clinic with around-the-clock PCI facilities. Among acute care hospitals in the United States, only about one-third deal with such procedures [15]. Naturally, in all such cases physicians face the question of the necessity of using an alternative for endovascular myocardial reperfusion, namely, pre-hospital systemic thrombolytic therapy (PH-TLT). According to some studies, thrombolytic therapy can be used in about 89–96% of STEMI patients [16,17].

It should be noted that, with this technique, myocardial reperfusion is obtained less frequently than with endovascular approach (according to our data, in about 70% of cases), and the recanalization of an IRA can be partial: after the dissolution of the thrombus, the IRA still contains the morphological substrate of the blood flow obstacle – a stenosing atherosclerotic plaque, which leads to the increased probability of re-thrombosis, recurrent ischemia, and other adverse events. Thus, in most cases, PH-TLT allows the restoration of the blood flow in the IRA at the earliest possible opportunity, but this restoration is incomplete, owing to persistent atherosclerotic plaque. On the other hand, endovascular myocardial reperfusion allows a significantly faster restoration of the blood flow in the IRA, but, because of the loss of time in patient transfer to a PCI-capable hospital and preparation for the procedure, the restoration of the blood flow in many occurs significantly later. This fact provided us with the basis for a clinical trial using a combination of two above-mentioned methods of STEMI management: a combination of PH-TLT with subsequent coronary angiography and, if indicated, percutaneous transluminal coronary angioplasty (PTCA) of the IRA. Such combined reperfusion therapy of STEMI allowed us to obtain the earliest and most complete correction of the blood flow in the IRA.

While conducting this trial, we paid special attention to the study of eventual complications (bleeding, hemorrhagic stroke, thrombus fragmentation and dislocation in the IRA, slow or no-reflow phenomenon and so on), which are used by the opponents of PH-TLT as a reason for not recommending its use in the treatment of STEMI patients during endovascular procedures on the coronary arteries performed after PH-TLT.

Before discussing our results, I should point out that, from 2001 through 2014, Moscow City Center of Interventional Cardioangiology accumulated experience with 12,350 cases of AMI; among these cases, 10,658 patients (86.2%) underwent selective coronary angiography. Endovascular myocardial reperfusion was performed in 8634 patients(81%), in 7856 (90.%) within the first 6 hours after the onset of angina; 1983 patients (16.4 %) received PH-TLT. Hospital mortality during these years was on average 3.44% (range 4.4–2.9%). Thus, from 2006 to 2013, we conducted a non-randomized study of clinical results of the treatment of STEMI in patients who received PH-TLT and subsequent in-hospital PTCA (*n* = 1252). A similar group of patients who received only primary PTCA was used for the comparison (*n* = 2062). The latter group also comprised patients with ineffective pre-hospital thrombolytic therapy. Another comparison group was formed from those STEMI patients who did not receive reperfusion therapy pre-hospital, or in hospital (*n* = 456). The reasons for non-performing reperfusion therapy included contraindications for thrombolytic therapy; the absence of non-stop coronary angiography at the time of admission; intolerance of iodine-containing contrast media; patient refusal of endovascular diagnostic and therapeutic procedures, and so on. As shown in the Table 21.1, the baseline history and demographic data were not significantly different between the groups.

PH-TLT was carried out with: Streptase® (streptokinase, 238 patients during the initial stage of the trial); Purolase® (prourokinase recombinant, 149 patients); Metalyse® (tenecteplase, 258 patients); Actilyse® (alteplase, 607 patients). While answering the question on the use of PH-TLT, we adopted the generally accepted indications and contraindications for this procedure. The effectiveness of the above agents (as evidenced by the data from coronary angiography) was, respectively: 70.7% for Streptase, 70% for Metalyse, 66.1% for Actilyse, 63.6% for Purolase. All procedures were performed by emergency teams, including cardiologists or specialists in intensive care and anesthesiology. The average interval between the onset of angina status and

Table 21.1 Main historical and demographic data in the studied groups of patients.

Index	Group			P value
	I (n = 1252)	II (n = 2062)	III (n = 456)	
Age (years)	58.2 ± 12.1	61.8 ± 10.5	59.1 ± 11.7	NS
Male *n* (%)	991 (79.2%)	1678 (81.,4%)	350 (76.7%)	NS
Smoker *n* (%)	893 (71.4%)	1406 (68.2%)	336 (73.7%)	NS
Arterial hypertension *n* (%)	660 (52.7%)	1198 (58.1%)	253 (55.5%)	NS
Hyperlipidemia *n* (%)	465 (37.1%)	740 (35.9%)	174 (38.1%)	NS
Diabetes mellitus *n* (%)	86 (6.9%)	151 (7.3%)	37 (8.2%)	NS
Duration of coronary heart disease (months)	4.6 ± 1.8	5.2 ± 2.3	5.7 ± 2.1	NS
History of myocardial infarction *n* (%)	206 (16.5%)	328 (15.9%)	82 (18%)	NS

Table 21.2 Complications in the pre-hospital thrombolysis group.

Complication	Occurrence (%)	
	Pre-hospital	In hospital
Allergic reactions	0.3	2.1
Bleeding:[a]	–	–
Gastrointestinal	–	1.2
Arterial puncture site	–	2.8
Other sites	–	3.5
Heart rupture	–	1.5
Hemorrhagic stroke	–	1.1
Hypotension[b]	21	–
Complex rhythm disturbances	2.8	2.1

[a] Transfusion necessary in 0.9% of in-hospital patients.
[b] Mainly after streptokinase administration.

the start of PH-TLT was 114.8 ± 25.8 minutes. Table 21.2 shows the main pre- and in-hospital complications seen in STEMI patients after PH-TLT.

Upon the admission to hospital and in the absence of contraindications, all patients underwent standard diagnostic coronary angiography. Then, in accordance with the tactics adopted in Moscow City Center of Interventional Cardioangiology, PTCA was performed immediately after pre-hospital thrombolysis in all cases, except for:

- residual stenosis of the IRA less than 50%;
- multiple coronary lesions with open IRA (given that there were indications for surgical myocardial revascularization);
- angiographic evidence of massive non-occlusive thrombosis of the IRA (if the team on duty could not perform thromboextraction);
- patient admission later than within 6 hours after the onset of angina attack (in the absence of angina pain).

As a rule, bare-metal stents were used. In the majority of cases only the IRA was stented, but in 8.6% of cases other coronary arteries were also stented. The indication for stenting of other vessels was the severe stenosis where the involved arteries perfused a significant region of the viable myocardium. The rates of endovascular diagnostic and therapeutic procedure-related complications and mortality did not reliably exceed those seen in patients with chronic coronary artery disease. Tables 21.3 and 21.4 present clinical and angiographic data from the studied groups of patients at the in-hospital stage.

The rates of no-reflow syndrome, heart rupture and bleeding in the group of patients after PH-TLT were not reliably higher than in the other studied groups. However, acute left ventricular failure was seen in this group significantly less often that in the two other groups. The rates of mortality and of second- to third-degree atrioventricular block were somewhat lower in the PH-TLT group compared with two other groups, but the difference with the endovascular reperfusion group was not statistically significant. Heart rhythm disturbances in the form of ventricular fibrillation in this group were significantly more common in comparison with two control groups: 8,1%, 5,4%, and 6.1%, respectively ($P < 0,05$). However, these rhythm

Table 21.3 In-hospital clinical and angiographic data in the studied groups of patients.

	Group I (N=1252)		Group II (N=2062)		Group III (N=456)		P values		
	n	%	n	%	n	%	I–II	I–III	II–III
Uncomplicated course	1085	86.6	1654	80.2	286	62.7	0.01	0.01	0.01
Acute left ventricular failure (Killip II–IV)	51	4.1	152	7.4	78	17.1	0.01	0.01	0.01
Acute and subacute stent thrombosis	–	–	–	–	–	–	0.01	0.01	0.01
Ventricular fibrillation	73	5.8	122	5.9	29	6.3	NS	NS	NS
Atrial fibrillation	53	4.2	161	7.8	55	12.2	0.01	0.01	0.01
AV block (II–III degree)	14	1.1	49	2.4	19	4.3	0.05	0.01	0.05
Total mortality	15	1.2	52	2.5	24	5.3	0.05	0.01	0.01
Slow or no-reflow		10.6		8.9	–	–	NS	–	–
Heart rupture		1		0.3		0.45	NS	NS	NS

Table 21.4 Frequency of ventricular fibrillation in the studied groups of patients.

	Group I (N=1252)		Group II (N=2062)		Group III (N=456)		P values		
Ventricular fibrillation	n	%	n	%	n	%	I–II	I–III	II–III
Total	73	5.8	122	5.9	29	6.3	NS	NS	NS
Primary	59	4.7	81	3.9	5	1.1	NS	0.01	0.05
Secondary	14	1.1	41	2	24	5.2	NS	0.01	0.01

disturbances developed mainly at pre-hospital stage during thrombolysis, so they had probably been triggered by so-called "reperfusion arrhythmia", and, importantly, all episodes of ventricular fibrillation were successfully stopped by cardioversion.

In accordance with the protocol adopted in the center, all STEMI patients who received myocardial reperfusion in the acute stage of the disease, were invited for control after 6 months of follow-up. Control examination has been performed on average at $7,2 \pm 0.6$ months, 6.9 ± 04 months, and 7.6 ± 0.5 months, respectively, after the procedure, the interval being not significantly different between the groups. Tables 21.5 and 21.6 show mid-term clinical and angiographic data in the studied groups of patients. Survival PH-TLT group was somewhat better than in two other groups, the difference being statistically significant. Functional capacity of the left ventricle and tolerance to physical exercise in this group also were better, but the differences were not significant.

Thus, according to our data, the lowest in-hospital mortality was seen among patients with STEMI after effective PH-TLT and successful PTCA. These patients also more often had an uncomplicated clinical course, better functional indices of the left ventricle, and physical tolerance during the in-hospital stage, as well as at mid-term. This was especially true for patients who received reperfusion within the first 3 hours after the onset of the angina attack. The analysis within this group gave a convincing evidence that these patients had the lowest mortality rate. Also, in the long term, this group had the largest increase in left ventricular ejection

Table 21.5 Long-term clinical and angiographic data in the studied groups of patients.

	Group I (N = 1252)		Group II (N = 2062)		Group III (N = 456)		P values		
	n	%	n	%	n	%	I–II	I–III	II–III
Information obtained	1158	92.5	1938	93.9	426	93.4	NS	NS	NS
Complete examination	935	74.7	1503	72.9	343	75.2	NS	NS	NS
Angina pectoris	227	19.5	411	21.2	102	23.9	NS	NS	NS
Re-stenosis/reocclusion of the IRA	210	16.8	385	18.7	82	17.9	NS	NS	NS
Reinfarction	27	2.3	43	2.2	14	3.3	NS	NS	NS
Heart failure (NYHA II–IV)	14	1.2	91	4.7	65	15.2	0.01	0.01	0.01
Mortality (8 months)	18	1.4	77	3.7	41	9	0.01	0.01	0.01

IRA, infarct-related artery.

Table 21.6 Long-term changes in left ventricular ejection fraction (LVEF) in the studied groups of patients.

LVEF	Group I (n = 935)	Group II (n = 1503)	Group III (n = 456)	P value I–III
Before PTCA (%)	53.6 ± 11.4	50.3 ± 9.7	46.6 ± 10.1	<0.05
Δ (%)	6.4 ± 2.9	2.1 ± 1.4	−2.6 ± 1.2	<0.05

PTCA, percutaneous transluminal coronary angioplasty.

fraction (6.4 ± 2.9%) and in exercise load during a stress test (78.9 ± 11.2 Вт). However, is should be noted that ventricular rhythm disturbances, including ventricular fibrillation, were seen significantly more often in PHP-TLT group compared with the other two groups. This observation coincides with the data from several studies where the rate of ventricular arrhythmia accompanying STEMI increased in the presence of fibrinolytic therapy, which, according to the authors, was related to reperfusion metabolic processes in the myocardium [18]. In all probability, it would be inappropriate to give an unambiguous prognostic evaluation of such reperfusion ventricular arrhythmia. If ventricular arrhythmia occurs at late stages of myocardial revascularization, it can have a negative impact on the prognosis, as a significant reperfusion injury caused by myocytolysis products develops simultaneously with ischemic necrosis. In other cases, also at early stages of myocardial reperfusion, the development of reperfusion arrhythmia, in our opinion, does not significantly influence the early and late prognosis in STEMI patients. Thus, our studies allow us to make certain conclusions about urban combined pharmacoinvasive management of STEMI patients:

- PH-TLT allows maximally early myocardial reperfusion in cases where endovascular myocardial reperfusion cannot be performed within the first 90 minutes after the onset of angina attack.
- Urgent selective coronary angiography and PCI allows:
  - evaluation of the state of the coronary arteries and verification of the results of PH-TLT;
  - restoration of the blood flow in the IRA in case of ineffective PH-TLT;
  - PTCA to be performed in successfully opened but still severely stenotic IRA and, if indicated, also in other narrowed coronary arteries.

- PH-TLT and PCI should be considered not as alternative, but as complementary methods of treatment of STEMI. This is related to the not uncommon situation when IRA stenosis persists after successful PH-TLT. This stenosis should be treated by PTCA at different stages of management. Thus, in most cases, PH-TLT should be considered as the first step towards more complete reperfusion therapy in STEMI patients; that is, a "bridge" to PCI.

Conclusions

Our study provides convincing evidence that, in megapolis with heavy traffic, PH-TLT allows for myocardial reperfusion significantly earlier than in-hospital PCI. In cases where the transfer of the patient to the hospital is delayed because of heavy traffic or other reasons, we consider it reasonable to perform PH-TLT (in the absence of contraindications) with subsequent in-hospital coronary angiography and eventual angioplasty of the IRA. And, finally:

1) It is desirable to perform PH-TLT in all STEMI patients excluding those with contraindications or those who are within walking distance from a hospital with 24-hour angiographic facilities.
2) Patients should be admitted urgently, by priority, to PCI-capable hospitals.
3) All STEMI patients admitted to hospital within the first 6 hours after the onset of angina attack should receive coronary angiography and PTCA (if indicated).
4) It is necessary to improve the ambulance service in terms of optimization of pre-hospital care of patients with STEMI, including the possibilities for performing PH-TLT in the absence of contraindications. Also, we consider it to be very important to develop mutual understanding and close contacts between the ambulance service and the hospitals dealing with emergency cardiology. Only such contact will allow us to maximally optimize the management of patients with STEMI and to minimize the time from the onset of angina status to the performance of necessary diagnostic and therapeutic procedures. Certainly, it is difficult to overestimate the role of ambulance service in terms of transportation of STEMI patients to the nearest hospitals with 24-hour emergency cardiologic and angiographic facilities.

References

1 Holmes DR. President's Page: Dining out in Paris: Wine and Guidelines. J *Am Coll Cardiol*, 2011; 58: 2015–2016.
2 Baroldi G. Coronary thrombosis: facts and beliefs. *Am Heart J*, 1976. 91: 683–688.
3 Davies MJ, Woolf N, Robertson WB. Pathology of acute myocardial infarction with particular reference to occlusive coronary thrombi. *Br Heart J*, 1976; 38: 659–664.
4 Horie T, Sekiguchi M, Hirosawa K. Coronary thrombosis in pathogenesis of acute myocardial infarction: Histopathological study of coronary arteries in 108 necropsied cases using serial section. *Br Heart J*, 1978: 40: 52–161.
5 Chandler AB, Chapman I, Erhardt LR, et al. Coronary thrombosis in myocardial infarction. Report of a workshop on the role of coronary thrombosis in the pathogenesis of acute myocardial infarction. *Am J Cardiol*, 1974; 34: 823–832.
6 Roberts WC, Buja LM. The frequency and significance of coronary arterial thrombi and other observations in fatal acute myocardial infarction: a study of 170 necroscopy patients. *Am J Med*, 1972; 52: 425–443.

7 Vlodaver Z, Freeh R, Van Tassel RA, et al. Correlation of the antemortem coronary arteriogram and the postmortem specimen. *Circulation*, 1973; 47: 162–169.

8 Chapman I. The cause–effect relationship between recent coronary artery occlusion and acute myocardial infarction. *Am Heart J*, 1974; 87: 267–271.

9 Ehrlich JC, Shinohara Y. Low incidence of coronary thrombosis in myocardial infarction: A restudy by the serial block technique. *Arch Pathol*, 1964; 78: 432–445.

10 Friedberg CK, Horn H. Acute myocardial infarction not due to coronary artery occlusion. *JAMA*, 1939; 112: 1675–1679.

11 Willerson JT, Campbell WB, Winniford MD, et al. Conversion from chronic to acute coronary artery disease: speculation regarding mechanisms. *Am J Cardiol*, 1984; 54: 1349–1359.

12 Baratashvili VL, Iosseliani DG, Koledinsky AG, et al. Early staged restoration of disturbed heart blood supply and improvement of early and mid-term prognosis in patients with acute myocardial infarction. Collection of articles (ed. DG Iosseliani, AP Seltsovsky) Moscow, 2009 (in Russian).

13 Iosseliani DG, Filatov AA, Rogan SV, et al. Restoration of the blood flow in the infarct-related coronary artery in acute myocardial infarction: is it effective or just spectacular? *Int J Interv Cardioangiol*, 2003; 1: 27–30.

14 Iosseliani DG, Semitko AP, Koledinsky AG, et al. Combined use of pre-hospital systemic thrombolytic therapy (TLT) and in-hospital PTCA of the infarct-related artery (IRA) in the treatment of acute myocardial infarction (AMI). *Int J Interv Cardioangiol*, 2005; 7: 20.

15 Vora AM, Holmes DN, Rokos I, et al. Fibrinolysis use among patients requiring interhospital transfer for ST-segment elevation myocardial infarction care: A report from the US National Cardiovascular Data Registry. *JAMA Intern Med*, 2015; 175(2): 207–215.

16 AIMS Trial Study Group. Effect of intravenous APSAC on mortality after acute myocardial infarction: Preliminary report of a placebo-controlled clinical trial. *Lancet* 1988; 1: 545.

17 Fibrinolytic Therapy Trialists (FTT) Collaborative Group. Indication for fibrinolytic therapy in suspected acute myocardial infarction: collaborative overview of early mortality and major morbidity results from all randomized trials of more than 1000 patients. *Lancet* 1994; 343: 311.

18 Gibson S, Pride Y, Buros J, et al. Association of impaired thrombolysis in myocardial infarction myocardial perfusion grade with ventricular tachycardia and ventricular fibrillation following fibrinolytic therapy for ST-segment elevation myocardial infarction. *J Am Coll Cardiol* 2008; 51: 546-551.

22

Lessons from the Puerto Rico Infarction National Collaborative Experience Initiative

Orlando Rodríguez-Vilá MD MMS FACC FSCAI, Jose Escabi-Mendoza MD FACC, Fernando Lapetina-Irizarry MD FACC, Miguel A. Campos-Esteve MD FACC

> *Coming together is a beginning; keeping together is progress; working together is success.*
>
> Henry Ford

Introduction and Background

The accumulation of knowledge in the 21st century has confirmed the benefit of ST-segment elevation myocardial infarction (STEMI) percutaneous coronary intervention (PCI) as a superior reperfusion strategy when performed in a timely manner [1–3]. Large-scale initiatives, such as those from the American College of Cardiology (ACC) Door-to-Balloon (D2B) Alliance, American Heart Association (AHA) Mission Lifeline, and the Stent for Life European Initiative, together with academic leaders in the field, have provided extensive guidance, rationale, and tools to help to develop primary PCI programs and STEMI-PCI systems of care [4–6]. As a result, geographic STEMI-PCI systems of care have arisen in the United States, Canada, and Europe. However, most of the world does not have access to STEMI-PCI and much less an integrated system of care. Other regions still face considerable variability in access and timeliness of STEMI-PCI protocols [7,8]. Although some countries simply do not have the resources or infrastructure to support PCI, many have the basic capabilities but have yet to align their assets into a working model of STEMI-PCI. In this chapter, we share the challenges faced, the lessons learned, and the success achieved in the journey to establish a nationwide STEMI-PCI network. We encourage other countries or regions to accept the challenge and commit to improving STEMI care in their communities.

The US territory of Puerto Rico is under the jurisdiction of the Food and Drug Administration (FDA) and other US agencies, and thus shares healthcare regulations with the United States. However, compared with the United States, the Commonwealth of Puerto Rico has unique social and economic circumstances that influences its potential to become "a good place to have a heart attack". On the positive side, its small geography and dense population allows 1-hour driving time access to a primary PCI (PPCI) hospital (Figure 22.1). The high eligibility for Medicare and Medicaid benefits also results in most of the population being insured. Nonetheless, Puerto Rico's healthcare industry has faced financial challenges that partly explain the struggle to keep up with quality improvement programs such as the STEMI-PCI care system. The territory's healthcare budget depends largely on allocations from the US federal government, but in comparison to the United States, Puerto Rico suffers from disparate allocation from the Medicaid

Manual of STEMI Interventions, First Edition. Edited by Sameer Mehta.
© 2017 John Wiley & Sons Ltd. Published 2017 by John Wiley & Sons Ltd.

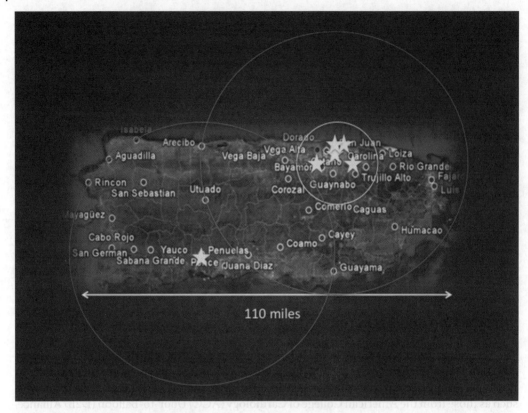

Figure 22.1 Map of Puerto Rico; stars represent Puerto Rico Infarction National Collaborative Experience ST-segment elevation myocardial infarction percutaneous coronary intervention centers, surrounded by bigger circles representing an approximate 1-hour driving time radius. The smaller circle represents the denser San Juan metro area.

and Medicare programs [9]. The 2006 economic crisis, as well as the ongoing working class exodus since that time, has made financing healthcare resources even more challenging. Limited healthcare funds have resulted in fewer resources being available for infrastructure, staff, education, and implementation of programs, which in turn can impact the quality of care. In fact, a study of Medicare beneficiaries showed that Puerto Rico ranked last among the 50 states and Washington DC in its adherence to quality indicators [10].

A study comparing US territories (where Puerto Rico accounted for almost 80% of the population studied) with the US mainland, within the Medicare population, showed worse outcomes in myocardial infarction, heart failure, and pneumonia in the US territories [11]. Within those suffering from myocardial infarction, studies showed that the rate of use of any reperfusion therapy or PCI for STEMI was low in Puerto Rico [12,13]. In spite of the rapid growth of clinical registries in the United States, such as the Society of Thoracic Surgeons (STS) and the National Cardiovascular Data Registry (NCDR) registries, the penetration of either registry in Puerto Rico is scant, lagging behind largely due to limited resources. With lower funding, worse quality, and scarce outcome data, Puerto Rico faced deep challenges at the time when the D2B Alliance was launched in 2006. Tackling this situation was urgent, as NCDR data began to show dramatic improvements in door-to-balloon times in the United States since 2005 [14].

Inspired to Make Changes

By 2010, 4 years after the launch of the ACC's D2B Alliance, only one of Puerto Rico's six major PCI hospitals had a 24/7 on-call roster and team for STEMI-PCI interventions. Other hospitals performed STEMI-PCI episodically. Scant data on door-to-balloon times estimated a less than 20% compliance with the 90-minute threshold and no concerted alignment between the emergency department and the cardiac catheterization laboratory (CCL). Data regarding better practices had been available for several years, but these did not percolate into the county's healthcare system.

Late in 2010, the Puerto Rican team had a lectureship visit from Dr. Sameer Mehta. Conversations began about the STEMI-PCI capabilities of Puerto Rico's hospitals and the geographic advantage that would make the country an excellent candidate to pursue the development of a nationwide STEMI-PCI network. This prospect led to a pivotal meeting in the fall of 2010, where local leaders from both academic centers and major private hospitals, together with Dr. Mehta, discussed the possibilities. The need was urgent and the direction was clear. This meeting lead to the constitution of what was later denominated the Puerto Rico Infarction National Collaborative Experience (PRINCE) Working Group.

The first issue addressed was that of governance. A chair and co-chairs were designated, together with an executive committee composed of at least one physician champion per participating institution. This team chose to operate within the umbrella of the Puerto Rico Chapter of the ACC. It was agreed that the mission was to "leave a legacy of improved care and survival from myocardial infarction in Puerto Rico". Also, for the designated physician champions of the six formerly competing institutions, it became a guiding principle that their endeavor would be characterized by collaboration, hence the use of "Collaborative Experience" when referring to the working group. When reflecting back on today's success, it can be determined that this commitment to collaborate was instrumental.

Second, a qualitative assessment of the strengths and weaknesses within each of Puerto Rico's PCI hospitals as candidates to become state of the art STEMI-PCI centers was conducted. Common flaws arose, including a lack of 24/7 on-call teams; no designated STEMI-PCI on-call interventional cardiologist; no specific pathway for the agile emergency department evaluation of suspected STEMI patients; slow, non-standardized processes to acquire and interpret electrocardiograms (EKG); and disorganized and variable processes for the early management and transport of patients to the CCL, among others. Notably, most hospitals had not made a commitment to use PPCI as the preferred method of reperfusion therapy, regardless of the time of day. This self-assessment helped to give structure to the execution plan.

The third step of the "coming together" stage was to agree with and standardize the target processes in the context of local realities. This would be done by drafting a quality improvement protocol that was ultimately called the PRINCE Initiative. Four pillars were designed for this concerted, sequential, collaborative effort to implement a staged renovation of STEMI care processes:

1) Establish standardized prospective data collection on STEMI-PCI cases.
2) Implement institutional processes to lower door-to-balloon times.
3) Integrate local emergency medical services (EMS) systems and referring hospitals to develop pre-hospital diagnosis and triage.
4) Public awareness campaign on symptom recognition and use of 911 to reduce total ischemia time.

Executing the Plan

Pillar 1: Data Collection

Any quality improvement intervention must begin with a process to measure variables and outcomes. In the absence of formal clinical databases at any hospital or lack of participation in the ACC NCDR, a data collection tool that relied on ACC data standards was designed (Figure 22.2). Without a data collection "culture", this initially proved to be a challenge, especially regarding door-to-balloon time intervals.

Processes promoted included the use of atomic clocks in the emergency room and CCL, monitoring correct hour programming of EKG machines, and training the nursing and interventional cardiology staff on the importance of documenting key time notations in their flow sheet for future reference. Monthly meetings of a quality improvement group consisting of the physician champion, STEMI coordinator, and representatives from the CCL and the emergency department were promoted. A quality department was also included to conduct case reviews and provide formal feedback. In addition, a 3-year prospective registry was designed. It consists on STEMI-PCI cases that meet prespecified criteria: Suspected STEMI within 12 hours of onset of sustained symptoms that were referred for emergency cardiac catheterization with the intention to perform primary (not rescue) PCI. Data collection is still ongoing. The objective is to examine trends in door-to-balloon times during the implementation and maintenance phases of the initiative.

Pillar 2: Hospital Door-to-Balloon Time Reducing Processes

Concurrently with setting up a data collection infrastructure, implementation of processes proven to help reduce door-to-balloon times became the rate-limiting step. Initially, each participating site was required to commit to:

- A 24/7/365 STEMI-PCI on call roster that included interventional cardiologist and a CCL team of at least one nurse and one cardiovascular technician.
- A designated institutional physician champion to serve as liaison between the PRINCE Working Group and their hospital.
- A designated STEMI coordinator to assist in the execution of the plan and data collection.
- Agreed for operators to incorporate evidence-based elements of STEMI-PCI procedures.

Having secured the aforementioned "core requirements", the implementation of the following "core quality elements", which included the seven success strategies known to reduce door-to-balloon times, was recommended [15]. For each strategy, specific means were encouraged to adapt them to their local realities, limitations and strengths, and to be creative about implementation:

- Early identification and triage of suspected STEMI: Most hospitals did not have a process to guide suspected STEMI patients through an accelerated pathway. Interventions included:
  - Signs in the emergency department alerting patients to proceed to the registration counter if they were having chest pain.
  - Immediate EKG and triage evaluation pathways for patients complaining of chest pain.
  - Availability of EKG machines at the triage station.
- Emergency room physician activates the team: This was a major shift in culture because it requires empowering the emergency department physician with "making the call". Following activation, the expectation was that the emergency department physician would directly contact the interventional cardiologists to provide a focused debriefing of the case and agree on the early management.

PRINCE Registry
Consenting adults with suspected STEMI within 12 hours of onset referred for PPCI

[82] □AUX □CCP □CMM □PAV □SLU □SPA □VAH [83]PCI Operator: □ | □□□□□□□
                                                                1st Initial   Last Name

□□□□ - □□□□ □□
[1] 4-Digit Year Cath Lab Case Number [2]Age

[3]Gender
□ Male
□ Female

[4]Race: □ Hispanic □ White □ Black □ Other
[5]Entry: □ ER from the field: [6]If yes, arrival mode: □ Self □ EMS

Pre-Cath therapy by:→	Patient	EMS	ED	None	Unk
[7]Aspirin	□	□	□	□	□
[8]Clopidogrel	□	□	□	□	□
[9]Prasugrel	□	□	□	□	□
[10]Ticagrelor	□	□	□	□	□
[11]Heparin IV	N/A □	□	□	□	□

OR □ Transferred from other HCF:[12]
  If yes, enter transfer facility arrival time & date in item 57-58:
OR □ In-hospital STEMI: use "trigger" ECG time as "door" time

STEMI trigger* ECG:	Origin of trigger ECG[13]	Dx criteria applied[14]
*This refers to the 1st ECG along the chain of care that "triggered" a STEMI alert Cath Lab Team activation.	□Ambulance/EMS □Transfer facility □1st PCI hospital ECG □Subsequent ECG	□ST elevation □New LBBB □True Posterior □Other

[15]12-lead ECG done & transmitted to ED? □Yes □No □Unknown
[16]Cath Team activated pre-hospital arrival? □Yes □No □Unknown

PRE-PCI CLINICAL ASSESSMENT: by Interventional Cardiologist

	Yes	No	Unk	
[17]ASA Allergy	□	□	□	Date of lytic start[27]
[18]Diabetes Mellitus	□	□	□	mm dd
[19]Prior CVA/TIA	□	□	□	
[20]ESRD/dialysis	□	□	□	
[21]Prior PCI	□	□	□	
[22]Prior CABG	□	□	□	Time of lytic start[28]
[23]Salvage PCI	□	□	□	24-hour : min
[24]Compassionate Use PCI	□	□	□	

[25]Pre-PCI Lytics (add 24:00 time)
[26]If Yes, PCI indication: □Rescue □Re-occlusion

PCI DATA: by Interventional Cardiologist

[29]Vascular access □Femoral □Radial □Brachial
[30]PCI attempted □Yes □No→**if no, go to item #51**
[31]If no, why: □Plan CABG □CAD/Med Tx □False (+)
[32]IRA Type □Native □SVG □IMA
[33]IRA Territory □LAD □CX □RCA □Left Main
[34]Stent Thrombosis □No □Yes, If Yes[35]: □A/SA □Late □VL
[36]#Vessel CAD (>50%) □0 □1 □2 □3 ±[37] □LM >50%
[38]Baseline TIMI Flow □0 □1 □2 □3
[39]Thrombus grade □No □Low grade □High grade
[40]Final TIMI Flow □0 □1 □2 □3
[41]Final TIMI MPG □0 □1 □2 □3 □Unknown
[42]Thrombectomy □Aspiration □Rheolytic □None
[43]Stent □BMS only □≥1 DES □None
[44]P₂Y₁₂ antagonist □clopidogrel □prasugrel □ticagrelor
[45]PCI Anticoagulant □UFH □LMWH □DTI
[46]IIb IIIa blocker (IV use) □No □Upstream □In-Lab
[47]IC microcirculation Rx: □No □Nip □Ade □CA □IIbIIIa
[48]Acute LV gram done: □No □Yes EF: ____%[49]
[50]Non-culprit vessel PCI done: □No □Yes □Planned staged

STEMI

Symptom Onset
24-hr : min

□□ : □□ [PCI Operator boxes top]

| mm | dd | yy[51] |

a) MI Symptom Onset[52]
Did the MI symptom include chest pain?[53]→ □Yes □No

EMS arrived at Scene[54] □N/A

1st EMS ECG[55] □N/A
STEMI trigger?[56] □Yes □No

Transfer site arrival[57] □N/A
Date[58]: □□□□

1st Transfer ECG[59] □N/A
STEMI trigger?[60] □Yes □No

b) PCI Hospital ED Arrival[61]
First recorded time of contact at ED

1st PCI Hospital ECG done[62]
STEMI trigger?[63] □Yes □No

Time of subsequent ECG only if STEMI trigger[64] □N/A

Interventional Cardiologist receives first contact[65]

Patient enters Cath Lab[66]
ED Bypassed?[67]: □Yes □No

Xylo applied / case start[68]
Date[69]: □□□□

c) 1st Device (if IRA has TIMI 3 flow at entry, use IRA angiogram time)[70]

Door to Balloon[71]
= c − b (minutes)

Total Ischemia time[72]
= c − a (hrs:minutes)

FOLLOW-UP: by STEMI coordinator

[73]D/H alive?
□ No→Death: □□□□ [74]
□ Yes→Date: □□□□ [75]
     mm   dd   yy

Discharge meds:	Yes	No	C/I	Unk
ASA[76]	□	□	□	□
P₂Y₁₂ antagonist [77]	□	□	□	□
Beta-Blocker[78]	□	□	□	□
ACE-inhibitor[79]	□	□	□	□
Statin[80]	□	□	□	□

[81]Formal feedback to ED: □Yes □No □Unk

Puerto **R**ico **I**nfarction **N**ational **C**ollaborative **E**xperience Working Group
Introduced December 2011
Revised September 2012

CONFIDENTIAL
PRINCEDB2010V4.0

Figure 22.2 Data collection sheet designed for the Puerto Rico Infarction National Collaborative Experience participating centers.

- Single call activation: Hospital operators were provided updated on-call rosters and were trained to call in each team member upon receiving a single call from the emergency department physician. They would also reply back with confirmatory response, to close the communication loop. In one site, the automated live process system was applied for simultaneous activation via email, text, and phone call with great success [16].

- Expectation for team to arrive within 20–30 minutes: Compliance with this expectation required monitoring of arrival times by the interventional cardiologist or by use of a clock to register arrival.
- CCL readiness from the emergency department: Delays were often encountered when transferring patients from the emergency department to the CCL, or by deferring the pre-procedure patient preparation to the CCL staff. Empowering emergency department nursing staff was encouraged. This helped to accelerate the pre-catheterization preparation, which involves preparing the access site, attaching the leads correctly out of the fluoroscopic field of view, administering per-protocol heparin and aspirin, having the patient on the monitor ready for transport on demand, transferring the patient and helping with the initial set-up. This immediately made the process agile and engaged emergency department nursing in a rewarding manner.
  - CCL "green light": At one center, a green light warning was installed at the emergency department. It was activated in the CCL. This signal indicated readiness for transfer to the emergency department. It sped up the process by obviating calling the emergency department.
  - Implementation of a STEMI briefing (expedited pre-procedure checklist): As soon as possible after the STEMI team activation, the emergency department physician was expected to contact the interventional cardiologist on call to provide a STEMI-PCI briefing to optimize physician to physician handoff at times of fast transit from the emergency department to the CCL. The briefing would include the following key information:
    Time of onset of sustained chest pain
    Initial assessment and management
    Medication allergies or contraindications
    EKG findings.
- Defined pathways for pre-hospital activation: Implementation of local hospital criteria for pre-hospital activation of the CCL and for "bypassing" the emergency department on the way to the CCL was promoted. This constituted a cultural shift. Recommended tools in this process included:
  - Standardized protocol and criteria for bypassing the emergency department.
  - A telephone that was used only for incoming call from paramedics or referring hospitals.
  - A computer that was used only for receiving EKG transmissions.
- Prompt feedback: The STEMI coordinator and physician champion were expected to hold monthly meetings to review the accumulated cases, giving special attention to those exceeding the 90-minute door-to-balloon performance goal. The use of a door-to-balloon time interval tool was encouraged. This would allow a closer examination of the time intervals that add up to the door-to-balloon time, as well as the role of the respective responsible member. This would be helpful in providing a focused feedback that would ultimately allow process improvement (Figure 22.3).
- Senior management support: A hospital administrator can facilitate the allocation of resources, quality officers may seek synergies with data collection efforts, nursing leadership can help redefine scopes of work of their staff, and the emergency department leadership may serve as key liaison between with the EMS system and the referring hospital community.
- Promote a culture of continuous improvement: Once it becomes clear that everyone involve in the door-to-balloon chain can make a difference, team members become engaged. Encouraging the involvement of emergency department nursing during the pre-procedure preparation and transport of the patient into the CCL led to favorable results. Similarly, paramedics were encouraged to follow-up on the case and receive immediate feedback of their performance as part of the chain.

Segmented STEMI Interval Feedback Form
STEMI-PCI case#:   Date:

Interval	Goal	Actual	Δ +/−	Possible Delay Sources	Yes	No	Comments
Door to ECG	10			No chest pain upon arrival			
Owner: Comments:				ECG machine unavailability			
				Clinical instability			
				Other:			
ECG to Activation	5			Absent or non-diagnostic ST segment elevation			
Owner: Comments:				Incorrect or delayed ECG diagnosis			
				Any activation process failure			
				Other:			
Activation to Cath Lab Entry	30			Any activation process failure			
Owner: Comments:				Delayed Cath-Lab readiness in ED			
				Clinical instability			
				Other:			
Cath Lab Entry to Xylo	25			Delayed arrival of Cath RN/MIT			
Owner: Comments:				Delayed arrival of Interv. Cardia			
				Equipment failure			
				Other:			
Xylo to Balloon	20			Clinical instability			
Owner: Comments:				Vascular access difficulty			
				Challenging coronary anatomy			
				Other:			
Door to Balloon	90			Comments or action items:			

Figure 22.3 Example of a ST-segment elevation myocardial infarction to percutaneous coronary intervention time interval form implemented as a tool to deliver focused feedback on case reviews to "interval owners".

Even before capitalizing on the pre-hospital strategies described below, simply implementing the aforementioned door-to-balloon reduction strategies at one of the PRINCE initiative PCI centers resulted in a measurable impact. The quality of performance was enhanced, and the measures of timeliness of reperfusion therapy improved (Figure 22.4).

Pillar 3: Pre-hospital Diagnosis and Triage

The EMS system has been shown to play a key role in the STEMI chain of survival [17]. Each link in this chain is crucial for reducing the time to reperfusion. An optimal EMS system may integrate the last three links of the STEMI chain into a single well-coordinated task, also known as a STEMI care system (Figure 22.5).

The most significant EMS contribution results from pre-hospital 12-lead EKG evaluation, which can significantly reduce the time to reperfusion by assisting with earlier STEMI diagnosis, advanced notification to the receiving hospital, triage directly to a PCI center, preactivation of the PCI

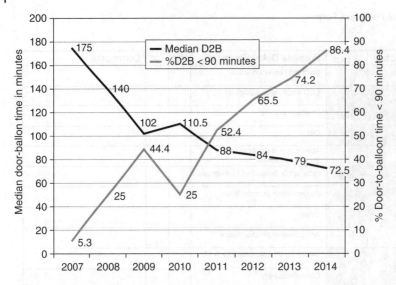

Figure 22.4 Reperfusion performance measures of median door-to-balloon times and percentage with door-to-balloon time of less than 90 minutes in one Puerto Rico Infarction National Collaborative Experience institution over an 8-year period.

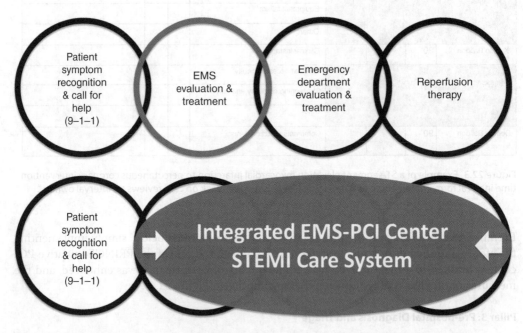

Figure 22.5 Schematic representation of integration in a ST-segment elevation myocardial infarction percutaneous coronary intervention system of care.

team and, in some cases, bypassing the emergency department directly into the CCL [18–20]. A meta-analysis from 2014 also found that this advance notification was associated with a reduction in short-term mortality [21]. One crucial aspect was acknowledging that, in Puerto Rico, only six (12%) acute-care hospitals had the capability to improve access to STEMI-PCI procedures. At the same time, records state that barely 5% of EMS activations for chest pain had an acute STEMI. Hence, the importance of pursuing a pre-hospital EKG diagnosis was crucial to most appropriately and optimally take advantage of the limited resources [22].

As with the hospitals' door-to-balloon reduction interventions, the first step was understanding and assessing the 9-1-1 and EMS systems. This consisted of a state (island wide) medical emergency system, municipal (town) systems, and private agencies. EMS activation proceeds via the 9-1-1 operators according to the scene location and service availability.

Recognizing the enormous challenge that restructuring a long-standing and dated response to 9-1-1 chest-pain calls posed, it was decided that organizing a PRINCE EMS Task Force was necessary. The initial objective was to gather key stakeholders to lead a coordinated, collaborative effort between independently operated municipal, private and state EMS systems, as well as PCI-capable institutions. This was done with the objective of establishing a national approach to STEMI response and triage (Box 22.1). This proposal was based on standardizing EMS unit capabilities for early STEMI diagnosis and therapeutic care, and also to facilitate a two-tiered triage algorithm for hospital destination selection according to lytic eligibility, clinical status, time from onset of symptoms, and transit time to assigned PCI-capable centers (Figure 22.6). Collaborative tasks led by the PRINCE EMS Task Force over the last 2 years have included the following actions:

- Holding meetings with EMS stakeholders and conducting site visits to the 9-1-1-dispatch centers.
- Encouraging EMS and other agencies to review protocols, equipment capabilities, and pre-hospital STEMI care issues. It was initially found that no EMS pre-hospital CCL activation processes were taking place within PCI centers, and that there was scarce access to 12-lead EKGs in the field.
- Seeking leadership integration between the state and municipal EMS, as well as integration of them both into the PRINCE working group meetings.
- Holding meetings with municipal and state health secretaries to raise awareness of this issue, as well as seeking their support.
- Holding periodic EMS task force meetings to discuss chest pain protocols, communication and equipment issues, processes, drill exercises, opportunities, and challenging cases.
- Implementing the use of telephones exclusively for STEMI cases in all PCI centers for EMS STEMI alerting.
- Advising on the implementation of new 12-lead EKG capability within the state and municipal EMS systems.
- Assisting in the development of transmission capability and processes within the state and municipal EMS systems.
- Establishing emergency department bypass protocols and agreements.
- Coordinating STEMI EKG workshops for EMS paramedics.
- Organizing monthly meetings with the state EMS, which addressed quality review of 9-1-1 calls for chest pain, 12-lead EKG performance, STEMI recognition, transmission and pre-hospital activation.
- Including quality metrics and benchmarking in EMS task force group meetings for process improvement.
- Assessing global EMS systems in Puerto Rico for the pre-hospital care of patients with suspected acute myocardial infarction through a survey adapted from the AHA (with their collaboration). This was done to assess gaps and barriers that needed to be improved and to review opportunities to assist with improvement.
- Seeking grants for 12-lead EKG equipment with transmission capability.

Box 22.1   Pre-hospital Strategies Focused on EMS Integration: PRINCE Recommended EMS Integration Goals and Processes

A Standardize EMS unit capabilities and protocols

1) 12-lead EKG acquisition with interpretation software in the field.
2) GPS recognition to allow for routing to nearest STEMI receiving center by the 9-1-1-dispatch center.
3) Wireless transmission of a 12-lead EKG to a designated STEMI-receiving center.
4) Paramedics trained in basic EKG interpretation and STEMI recognition.
5) Capability for and training to screen for and administer aspirin 325 mg according to a prespecified protocol.

B EMS triage algorithm for hospital destination selection

1) Immediate transfer for PCI and pre-hospital catheterization laboratory activation if:
   - cardiogenic shock
   - successful resuscitation from cardiac arrest
   - onset of symptoms < 2 hours and field to ED transit time < 60 minutes
   - onset of symptoms > 2 hours
   - any thrombolytic ineligible patient.
2) Immediate transfer to nearest lytic-capable hospital for thrombolysis for lytic-eligible patients may be considered if:
   - Onset of symptoms < 2 hours and field to emergency department transit time to PCI-capable hospital > 60 minutes (although the 1-hour radius to PCI centers covers all of Puerto Rico, an unexpected situation that may delay arrival would prompt the lytic pathway to the nearest center).
3) When the field to emergency department transit time is < 60 minutes to more than one PCI-capable hospital within the same distance radius, patient preference may be considered, as deemed appropriate by the paramedics and medical control.
4) Transportation to the nearest hospital (regardless of STEMI-PCI or lytic capability) should be considered if one or more of the following are present:
   - airway compromise that cannot be managed
   - refractory ventricular arrhythmias
   - ongoing cardiac arrest with no return of spontaneous circulation
   - determination by the paramedic that further transports delay may compromise the patient care.

- Exploring new or amended state legislation to improve the EMS activation process, such as assigning specific level 3 ambulance units to respond to all 9-1-1 calls (code alpha-10) with core capabilities.

The Ultimate Goal: Total Ischemia Time

The journey to improve access and quality of STEMI care in Puerto Rico goes on. Along the way, aims have been accumulated, challenges faced, and solutions have been found. Success has been achieved by implementing processes for reducing door-to-balloon time at major PCI centers in a sustainable manner. A culture of improvement has been instilled at those centers.

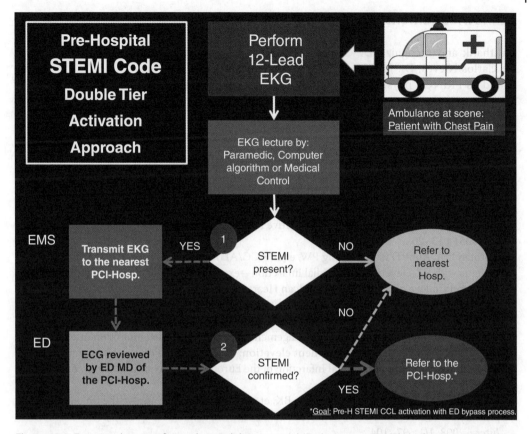

Figure 22.6 Two-tiered process for pre-hospital diagnosis and ST-elevation myocardial infarction (STEMI)-alert hospital activation in the Puerto Rico Infarction National Collaborative Experience initiative. CCL, cardiac catheterization laboratory; ED, emergency department; EKG, electrocardiogram; EMS, emergency medical services; PCI, percutaneous coronary intervention.

Disseminating education of this initiative across Puerto Rico through ACC Chapter live events and video-documentary on the PRINCE initiative is still ongoing [23]. Although these efforts have had an impact, they only begin to address the larger need for reducing overall STEMI morbidity and mortality by reducing the total ischemia time [24,25]. To this end, the final phase of the PRINCE initiative is the coordination of a public awareness campaign to educate the population to recognize symptoms of heart attack and to respond quickly by dialing 9-1-1. This would be done to increase entry into the system of care via EMS. As in other successful systems of care, being able to derive further benefits by incorporating the effective response to stroke and out of hospital arrest in Puerto Rico is desired.

Summary

In summary, any region or country with enough infrastructure, PCI capability, and an EMS system, can and should engage into putting the pieces to work together to improve the care of STEMI. Following the words of Henry Ford, after "coming together" in this ideal, and "keeping together" in this process, real progress will ensue from sustaining the will for "working together" in this pursuit.

Acknowledgements

We thank and recognize Dr. Sameer Mehta for his inspirational influence and guidance, Dr. Carlos Nieves, Dr. Jose Novoa, Dr. Efrain Feliciano, and Dr. Valentín del Rio, for having served as PRINCE physician champions, and emergency department physicians, cardiology fellows, nurses, cardiovascular technologists, and all who in one or more ways were part of this collaborative effort.

References

1 Keeley EC, Boura JA, Grines CL. Primary angioplasty versus intravenous thrombolytic therapy for acute myocardial infarction: a quantitative review of 23 randomized trials. *Lancet*, 2003; 361(9351): 13–20.

2 Antman EM, Anbe DT, Armstrong PW, et al. ACC/AHA guidelines for the management of patients with ST-Elevation myocardial infarction—executive summary: a report of the American College of Cardiology/American Heart Association Task Force on Practice Guidelines (writing committee to revise the 1999 guidelines for the management of patients with acute myocardial infarction). *J Am Coll Cardiol*, 2004; 44(3): 671–719.

3 Van deWerf F, Bax J, Betriu A, et al. Management of acute myocardial infarction in patients presenting with persistent ST-segment elevation: the Task Force on the Management of ST-Segment Elevation Myocardial Infarction of the European Society of Cardiology. *Eur Heart J*, 2008; 29(23): 2909–2945.

4 Krumholz HM, Bradley EH, Nallamothu BK, et al. A campaign to improve the timeliness of primary percutaneous intervention. Door-to-Balloon: an alliance for quality. *JACC Cardiovasc Interv*, 2008; 1(1): 97–104.

5 Rokos IC, Larson DM, Henry TD, et al. Rationale for establishing regional ST-elevation myocardial infarction receiving centre (SRC) networks. *Am Heart J*, 2006; 152(4): 661–667.

6 Jacobs AK, Antman EM, Faxon DP, et al. Development of systems of care for ST-elevation myocardial infarction patients. Executive summary. *Circulation*, 2007; 116(2): 217–230.

7 Widimsky P, Wijns W, Fajadet J, et al. Reperfusion therapy for ST elevation acute myocardial infarction in Europe: description of the current situation in 30 countries. *Eur Heart J*, 2010; 31(8): 943–957.

8 Huber K, Gersh BJ, Goldstein P, et al. The organization, function, and outcomes of ST-elevation myocardial infarction network worldwide: current state, unmet needs, and future directions. *Eur Heart J*, 2014; 35(23): 1526–1532.

9 Gutierrez N. Understanding health care disparities in the US territories. *Arch Intern Med*, 2011; 171(17): 1579–1581.

10 Jencks SF, Cuerdon T, Burwen DR, et al. Quality of medical care delivered to medicare beneficiaries: A profile at state and national levels. *JAMA*, 2000; 284(13): 1670–1676.

11 Nunez-Smith M, Bradley EH, Herrin J, et al. Quality of care in the us territories. *Arch Intern Med*, 2011;171(17):1528–40.

12 Sanchez M, Cox RA, Rodriguez JM, et al. Review of Clinical Characteristics and Management of Patients with ST Segment Elevation Myocardial Infarction at a Tertiary Center. *PR Health Sci J*, 2006;25(3):219–224.

13 Zevallos JC, Yarzebski J, Gonzalez JA, et al. Incidence, in-hospital case-fatality rates, and management practices in puerto ricans hospitalized with acute myocardial infarction. *PR Health Sci J*, 2013; 32(3): 138–145.

14 Krumholz HM, Herrin J, Miller LE, et al. Improvements in door-to-balloon time in the United States, 2005 to 2010. *Circulation*, 2011; 124(9): 1038–1045.

15 Bradley EH, Herrin J, Wang Y, et al. Strategies for reducing the door-to-balloon time in acute myocardial infarction. *N Engl J Med*, 2006; 355(22): 2308–2320.

16 Liveprocess. Available at http://www.liveprocess.com (accessed March 23, 2017).

17 Ornato J. The ST-segment-elevation myocardial infarction chain of survival. *Circulation*, 2007; 116(1): 6–9.

18 Ting H, Krumholz H, Bradley E, et al. Implementation and integration of prehospital ECGs into systems of care for acute coronary syndrome. *Circulation*, 2008; 118(10): 1066–1079.

19 Studnek JR, Garvey L, Blackwell T, et al. Association between prehospital time intervals and ST-elevation myocardial infarction system performance. *Circulation*, 2010; 122(15): 1464–1469.

20 Fosbol E, Granger C, Jollis J, et al. The impact of a statewide pre-hospital STEMI strategy to bypass hospitals without percutaneous coronary intervention capability on treatment times. *Circulation*, 2013; 127(5): 604–612.

21 Nam J, Caners K, Bowen J, et al. Systematic review and meta-analysis of the benefits of out-of-hospital 12-lead ECG and advance notification in ST-segment elevation myocardial infarction patients. *Ann Emerg Med*, 2014; 64(2): 176–186.

22 Weaver WD, Eisenberg MS, Martin JS, et al. Myocardial Infarction Triage and Intervention Project–phase I: patient characteristics and feasibility of prehospital initiation of thrombolytic therapy. *J Am Coll Cardiol*, 1990; 15(5): 925–931.

23 American College of Cardiology, Puerto Rico Chapter. Available at http://www.accpuertorico.org (accessed March 23, 2017).

24 De Luca G, Suryapranata H, Zijlstra F, et al. Symptom-onset-to-balloon time and mortality in patients with acute myocardial infarction treated by primary angioplasty. *J Am Coll Cardiol*, 2003; 42(6): 991–997.

25 Menees DS, Peterson ED, Wang Y, et al. Door-to-balloon time and mortality among patients undergoing primary PCI. N *Engl J Med*, 2013; 369(10): 901–909.

23

The STEMI Care Program in China

Yan Zhang MD, Yong Huo MD

Introduction

Ischemic heart disease was found to be the second leading cause of cardiovascular death in China in 2010 [1]. It is estimated that the number of patients with myocardial infarction in China will increase to 23 million by 2030 [2], mainly due to a worsening profile of cardiovascular risk factors and an increase in the aged population. Acute ST-segment elevation myocardial infarction (STEMI), a subtype of myocardial infarction as a result of sudden coronary artery occlusion, is one of the most life-threatening diseases and a worldwide public health issue.

It is well known that reperfusion is the key strategy to decrease mortality and major cardiovascular events of STEMI. Comparing the two major reperfusion methods, primary percutaneous coronary intervention (PPCI) is, overall, superior to thrombolysis [3]. Time is another key issue in the STEMI care as time means myocardium and life. Regardless of which reperfusion method is used, all patients benefit more from early treatment. Although extensive efforts have been taken to greatly improve the care of STEMI patients, a gap between demonstrated scientific evidence and actual practice still exists [4,5], especially in China.

Current Status of STEMI Reperfusion in China

Low Reperfusion Rate

Reperfusion is the most beneficial treatment for STEMI patients. The China PEACE-Retrospective Acute Myocardial Infarction Study [6] showed that the overall reperfusion rate is about 55% nationwide and had not significantly changed from 2001 to 2011, which means that the conservative strategy applied to candidate reperfusion patients had no improvement. However, the rate of PPCI increased from 10.2% to 27.6%, while the rate of thrombolysis concurrently decreased from 45.0% to 27.4% [6]. PCI was started in 1984 and has risen rapidly in China, especially since the year 2000. The national online PCI registry was set up by the Ministry of Health of China in 2009 to improve the quality of PCI, including the certification of institutions and individuals, and quality control of diagnostic and therapeutic interventions. Published data showed that, of the hundreds of thousands PCI procedures performed in China every year, PPCI accounted for only around 30% of all PCI procedures in hospitalized STEMI patients [7,8].

Manual of STEMI Interventions, First Edition. Edited by Sameer Mehta.
© 2017 John Wiley & Sons Ltd. Published 2017 by John Wiley & Sons Ltd.

Long Delays in Treatment

Many STEMI patients missed the window of reperfusion because of treatment delays, both within the healthcare system and from patients. The PEACE study showed that median time from symptom onset to hospital admission was 13–15 hours [6]. Around 50% of patients chose to self-transport to a PCI-capable hospital; 25% of them called the emergency medical service (EMS); the remainder were transferred from other hospital. Unfortunately, even patients who arrived at the hospital in a timely manner to receive reperfusion therapy did not reap the full benefit of the treatment. Results from a multiple-center registry conducted in Beijing showed median door-to-needle time to be 80 minutes and door-to-balloon time to be 135 minutes, much longer than the guideline recommendations [9].

Poor Prognosis

As a result of these less than ideal treatment times, average in-hospital mortality from STEMI was around 8.2% (7.0–9.4%) and had not changed in a decade. When survivors were discharged, only about 48.2% of patients with acute myocardial infarction (AMI) in level 2 hospitals and 49.1% of those in level 3 hospitals took all the recommended drug combinations, consisting of double antiplatelet agents, beta-blockers, statins, and angiotensin-converting enzyme inhibitor or angiotensin receptor blocker [10]. Thus, their long-term prognosis could hardly be favorable.

China STEMI Care Program

Shortening symptom to reperfusion time and choosing the optimal reperfusion strategy are both major challenges when treating STEMI patients in China. To narrow the gap between practice and evidence as well as decreasing the economic burden, a China STEMI care program was initiated in 2011. Supported by the former Ministry of Health, and organized by the Chinese Medical Doctor Association, this program is to be in implemented in three steps. The components and aims of the program are listed in detail in Table 23.1.

The pilot study, focusing on improving the in-hospital green channel, was carried out in 53 tertiary hospitals qualified for PPCI from 15 Chinese provinces in 2012. Based on the major findings of relative good medical care of top level hospitals and insufficient awareness of patients, a regional STEMI network with government support will then considered to be established. Since emergency medical services (EMS) and hospitals operate relatively independently in China, government support is especially important in enhancing the collaboration between the EMS and PCI-capable hospitals, as well as between non-PCI hospitals and PCI-capable hospitals.

The first aim of phase two is to increase the overall reperfusion rate of STEMI patients by prompting the use of PPCI and pharmacoinvasive strategy. Although PPCI is superior to thrombolysis under most conditions, it cannot replace thrombolysis in many areas in China, especially in rural areas. Thrombolytic therapy may be the only choice in those regions because of logistic constraints. Thus, the pharmacoinvasive strategy, known to improve patients' outcomes [11], should be methodically applied in conjunction with a well-established regional STEMI network.

The second aim of phase two is to shorten total ischemic time, as well as door-to-balloon time. As mentioned before, treatment delays result from both the healthcare system and patients. Delay attributed to patients accounts for up to two-thirds of the overall ischemic time, which is mostly due to their poor awareness regarding their symptoms and an inharmonious relationship (lack of trust) between doctors and patients. The inability to recognize symptoms

Table 23.1 Components and aims of the China STEMI care program.

Contents	Practices	Aims
Pre-hospital system	Public Health education	Transfer patients to the right hospital in time
	EMS training	
	Emergency network	
	EKG transmission	
In-hospital green channel	Chest pain center	Door-to-balloon time < 90 minutes
	Bypass to CCL	
	CCL 7/24	
Clinical pathway for PPCI	PCI training and certification	Implement standard operating procedure
Secondary prevention	Patient education	Improve prognosis
	Physician training	
	Guideline implementation	
Health economics evaluation	Cost effectiveness ratio	Health policy
Data collection and feedback	Database integration	Improve practice
	Measurement and feedback	

CCL, cardiac catheterization laboratory; EKG, electrocardiogram; EMS, emergency medical services; PPCI, primary percutaneous coronary intervention

of ischemia, failure to call an ambulance when symptoms occur, and prolonged discussions for obtaining reperfusion consent lead to major delays in medical treatment for suspected myocardial infarction. Improving patient knowledge through public education helps patients to seek medical assistant promptly in cases of suspected myocardial infarction, and to accept timely reperfusion without hesitations. Important aspects include recognizing the symptoms of ischemia, reducing transportation time to a PPCI-capable hospital via the EMS, and shorting discussion time for obtaining consent.

System-level barriers that affect the efficacy of STEMI treatment pathways include issues in leadership, capacity, ability, and lack of collaboration between EMS and hospitals [12]. An earlier study showed six in-hospital interventions that can significantly reduce door-to-balloon time [13]. Healthcare system delays could be further reduced by using pre-hospital 12-lead electrocardiograms (EKGs), activating PCI-capable centers early [14], and/or bypassing the emergency room [15]. Building chest pain centers dedicated to the efficient treatment of AMI is another option to optimize in-hospital green-channel process in order to reduce door-to-balloon time [16]. A notable problem in China has been the lack of any official criteria for accrediting chest pain centers, which has impeded the standardization of their establishment. Guidelines have now been created, based on observations of American chest pain centers, and a pilot accreditation process is in progress. Since then, 25 hospitals in 12 provinces have been accredited using Chinese standards.

The essence of phase 2 of our program is the improvement of the quality of medical care to reach levels similar to the US National Cardiovascular Data Registry (NCDR) model. With documents issued by the National Health and Family Planning Commission of the People's Republic of China, the program was initiated in a total of 200 PPCI-capable hospitals, together with hundreds of adjacent non-PPCI-capable hospitals across 15 provinces in March of 2015. STEMI patients with symptom onset within 30 days will be enrolled in three periods.

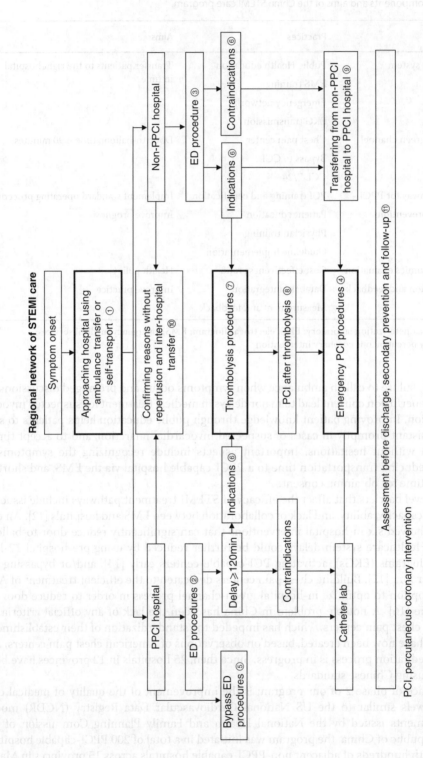

Figure 23.1 Regional network of STEMI care.

PCI, percutaneous coronary intervention

Regional network of STEMI care

- Symptom onset
- Approaching hospital using ambulance transfer or self-transport ①
- Confirming reasons without reperfusion and inter-hospital transfer ⑩

Non-PPCI hospital
- ED procedure ③
  - Indications ⑥
  - Contraindications ⑥
- Transferring from non-PPCI hospital to PPCI hospital ⑨

PPCI hospital
- ED procedures ②
  - Bypass ED procedures ⑤
  - Delay ≥ 120min
    - Indications ⑥
    - Contraindications
- Catheter lab
  - Thrombolysis procedures ⑦
  - PCI after thrombolysis ⑧
  - Emergency PCI procedures ④

Assessment before discharge, secondary prevention and follow-up ⑪

During each 6-month period, 30 patients will be enrolled consecutively from each PCI-capable center, leading to a total of 18,000 STEMI patients with follow-up period of 1 year. The entire system has been divided into 11 pathways in the STEMI process and procedure:

1) Approaching the hospital via ambulance transfer or self-transport.
2) Emergency department procedures in PPCI-capable hospitals.
3) Emergency department procedures in non-PPCI-capable hospitals.
4) Emergency PCI procedures such as PPCI and rescue PCI.
5) Emergency department bypass procedures.
6) Indications and contraindications of thrombolysis confirmation.
7) Thrombolysis procedures.
8) PCI after thrombolysis.
9) Transferring from non-PPCI-capable hospital to PPCI-capable hospital.
10) Reasons for no reperfusion and inter-hospital transfer.
11) Assessment before discharge, secondary prevention and follow-up.

STEMI patients with different conditions will follow the suitable clinical pathway to receive the optimal treatment (Figure 23.1).

Data collection, analysis, and feedback play a critical role in the cycle of devising a guideline, protocol, research, and evidence for improving medical services. Key performance indicators in STEMI care will be collected using both the national PCI online registry and a program STEMI online registry database for the purpose of improving medical care. Hospital performance indicators, rank report, and problem-based resolution will be shared with each participating hospital periodically after data analysis. Comparison of cross-sectional data will be used to evaluate whether there is improvement in the quality of medical services. Final reports will be released in 2019.

Conclusions

In conclusion, choosing the optimal reperfusion strategy for STEMI patients, and reducing the time from symptom onset to target vessel opening are great challenges in the real world. Improving the medical service system in accordance with guidelines for clinical practice will provide better insights and inspire us to move forward to eventually build a nationwide STEMI care network (phase 3).

References

1 Yang G, Wang Y, Zeng Y, et al. Rapid health transition in China, 1990–2010: findings from the Global Burden of Disease Study 2010. *Lancet*, 2013; 381: 1987–2015.
2 Human Development Unit East Asia and Pacific Region. *Toward a Healthy and Harmonious Life in China: Stemming the Rising Tide of Non-Communicable Diseases.* Washington, DC: World Bank.
3 Keeley EC, Boura JA, Grines CL. Primary angioplasty versus intravenous thrombolytic therapy for acute myocardial infarction: a quantitative review of 23 randomised trials. *Lancet*, 2003; 361: 13–20.
4 Widimsky P, Wijns W, Fajadet J, et al. European Association for Percutaneous Cardiovascular Interventions. Reperfusion therapy for ST elevation acute myocardial infarction in Europe: Description of the current situation in 30 countries. *Eur Heart J*, 2010; 31: 943–957.

5 Eagle KA, Nallamothu BK, Mehta RH, et al. Global Registry of Acute Coronary Events (GRACE) Investigators. Trends in acute reperfusion therapy for ST-segment elevation myocardial infarction from 1999 to 2006: we are getting better but we have got a long way to go. *Eur Heart J*, 2008; 29: 609–617.

6 Li J, Li X, Wang Q, et al., for the China PEACE Collaborative Group. ST-segment elevation myocardial infarction in China from 2001 to 2011 (the China PEACE-Retrospective AcuteMyocardial Infarction Study): a retrospective analysis of hospital data. *Lancet*, 2015; 385: 441–451.

7 Huo Y. Current status and development of percutaneous coronary intervention in China. *J Zhejiang Univ Sci B*, 2010; 11: 631–633.

8 Zhang Y, Huo Y. Early reperfusion strategy for acute myocardial infarction: a need for clinical implementation. *J Zhejiang Univ Sci B*, 2011; 12: 629–632.

9 Song L, Hu DY, Yan HB, et al. Influence of ambulance use on early reperfusion therapies for acute myocardial infarction. *Chin Med J (Engl)*, 2008; 121: 771–775.

10 Gao R, Patel A, Gao W, et al. CPACS Investigators. Prospective observational study of acute coronary syndromes in China: practice patterns and outcomes. *Heart*, 2008; 94: 554–560.

11 O'Gara PT, Kushner FG, Ascheim DD, et al. 2013 ACCF/AHA guideline for the management of ST-elevation myocardial infarction: a report of the American College of Cardiology Foundation/American Heart Association Task Force on Practice Guidelines. *J Am Coll Cardiol*, 2013; 61: e78–140.

12 Ranasinghe I, Rong Y, Du X, et al; CPACS Investigators. System barriers to the evidence-based care of acute coronary syndrome patients in china: qualitative analysis. *Circ Cardiovasc Qual Outcomes*, 2014; 7: 209–216.

13 Bradley EH, Herrin J, Wang Y, et al. Strategies for reducing the door-to-balloon time in acute myocardial infarction. *N Engl J Med*, 2006;355:2308–20.

14 Diercks DB, Kontos MC, Chen AY, et al. Utilization and impact of pre-hospital electrocardiograms for patients with acute ST-segment elevation myocardial infarction: data from the NCDR (National Cardiovascular Data Registry) ACTION (Acute Coronary Treatment and Intervention Outcomes Network) Registry. *J Am Coll Cardiol*, 2009; 53: 161–166.

15 Dorsch MF, Greenwood JP, Priestley C, et al. Direct ambulance admission to the cardiac catheterization laboratory significantly reduces door-to-balloon times in primary percutaneous coronary intervention. *Am Heart J*, 2008;155: 1054–1058.

16 Graff LG, Dallara J, Ross MA, et al. Impact on the care of the emergency department chest pain patient from the chest pain evaluation registry (CHEPER) study. *Am J Cardiol*, 1997; 80: 563–568.

24

STEMI INDIA

Thomas Alexander MD, Ajit S Mullasari MD

Introduction

The past few decades have seen a dramatic change in the pattern of disease in low and middle income countries, with a dramatic increase in non-communicable disease burden. This epidemiological transition has been magnified many times over in India, owing to its superimposition on a genetically predisposed population. This is reflected in the high burden of non-communicable diseases and the strain that this puts on scarce healthcare resources, which are already stretched to provide basic health care. Added to this, is the heterogeneity of the country. Large rural areas are grappling with infectious diseases while rapid urbanization exposes large populations to non-communicable diseases without going through a period of declining infections.

The rapid increase in cardiovascular disease is well documented, with an estimated 64 million cases by the year 2015 [1]. Although there are no accurate estimates of ST-elevation myocardial infarction (STEMI) in India, experts estimate a figure upwards of 3 million a year. The reduction in risk factors and the institution of systems of care in the United States and Europe for primary percutaneous coronary intervention (PPCI) have shown dramatic reductions in mortality and morbidity from STEMI. Developing systems of STEMI care in India is a challenge because of the complexities involved in allocating scarce healthcare resources, which should be effective and equitable, and the lack of adequate infrastructure and trained manpower. Finally, there is a disproportionately high prevalence of acute coronary syndrome in the lower socioeconomic classes. The consequent higher mortality caused through poor access to quality health care makes it imperative that any system devised should ensure equity, so that no patient falls through the system due to the unaffordability of care [2].

Current STEMI guidelines from the American College of Cardiology/American Heart Association and European Society of Cardiology emphasize the dominant role of PPCI as the reperfusion strategy to be followed in patients with STEMI. Unfortunately, data from the ACCESS registry from Africa, Latin America and the Middle East [3] and the CREATE registry data from India [2] show that a substantial proportion of patients do not receive any form of reperfusion. Furthermore, PPCI is seldom used as the means for reperfusion. Thrombolysis is the main mode for reperfusion and is almost always used as a stand-alone treatment. Data supporting the use of the pharmacoinvasive strategy as a reasonable option in this subset of patients has opened a window of opportunity for delivering a more practical and effective reperfusion treatment for the majority of patients in low and middle income countries [4,5].

Manual of STEMI Interventions, First Edition. Edited by Sameer Mehta.
© 2017 John Wiley & Sons Ltd. Published 2017 by John Wiley & Sons Ltd.

Beginnings

Focused STEMI meetings have been held in India in the past, but these have been sporadic and have mainly targeted cardiologists. The first real attempt to run a STEMI meeting and to train all the medical personnel involved in STEMI care was made when the first Kovai Lumen meeting was organized at Coimbatore in 2010. This meeting was modeled on the Lumen meeting run by Dr. Sameer Mehta in Miami. The Kovai Lumen meeting and was organized by Dr. Thomas Alexander and Dr. Sameer Mehta as course directors. Separate workshops were run to train paramedics, nurses, emergency room physicians, and cardiologists. While this meeting served the purpose of educating the medical teams in hospitals, it was considered that to impact the management of STEMI in the country, a national organization dedicated to all aspects of STEMI management was required. At the 2010 Cardiological Society of India (CSI) meeting at Calcutta, Dr. Thomas Alexander and Dr. Ajit Mullasari decided to set up a not for profit organization, STEMI INDIA, to pursue this goal. The organization was registered in February 2011.

Aims and Goals

STEMI INDIA is a not-for-profit national body dedicated to STEMI care in India. Its goals are:

- to impart and disseminate the latest information from across the world on STEMI management to all those involved in STEMI care in India;
- to help to organize and train "STEMI teams" in hospitals;
- to develop systems of care appropriate to STEMI care in India;
- to facilitate and contribute to developing a national STEMI guideline and to work towards a national STEMI program;
- public education to reduce delays in accessing appropriate STEMI care;
- to help organizations and individuals in research projects with expertise and, where feasible, funding.

Developing a STEMI System of Care: The STEMI INDIA Model

Data from the National Interventional Council shows that there is a steady increase in the numbers of PPCIs performed in India, although the percentage remains the same. However, only a small minority of STEMI patients receive this modality of reperfusion [2]. Data from the STREAM trial [4] and from the Indian data from the STEP-PAMI study [5] showed that the pharmacoinvasive strategy compared well with PPCI in overall morbidity and mortality. Based on this evidence, and on the success of the Pilot STEMI-Kovai Erodestudy [6], STEMI INDIA proposed that STEMI management in India adopt the dual strategy of combining PPCI with pharmacoinvasive reperfusion to develop a coherent framework for developing a system of care referred to as the STEMI-India Model (Table 24.1):

1) PPCI for patients located close to catheterization laboratories. Such an option would be available mostly for patients in urban areas with presumed short transportation time to the hospitals equipped with 24/7 PPCI capabilities.
2) Patients in rural areas, with a suspected long transportation time to PCI-capable hospitals would use the pharmacoinvasive strategy with thrombolysis therapy followed by catheterization and PCI, if indicated, within 3–24 hours of thrombolysis.

Table 24.1 STEMI INDIA model; two strategies, employing a) primary percutaneous coronary intervention (PCI) for patients with short transportation times, and b) pharmacoinvasive strategy for patients with long transportation times.

	Door to needle < 30 minutes			Pharmacoinvasive 3–24 hours
Variable	10 minutes		10 minutes	
Onset of patient symptoms	Arrival of patient at hospital/ambulance	EKG	Lysis	CCL to balloon
			Transport to PCI-capable hospital	
Variable	10 minutes		20–30 minutes	45–60 minutes
	Door to balloon < 90 minutes			
	Total ischemia time < 120 minutes			

CCL, cardiac catheterization laboratory; EKG, electrocardiogram

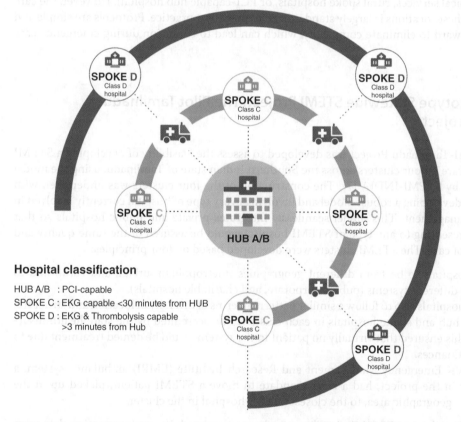

Hospital classification

HUB A/B : PCI-capable
SPOKE C : EKG capable <30 minutes from HUB
SPOKE D : EKG & Thrombolysis capable
>3 minutes from Hub

Figure 24.1 ST-elevation myocardial infarction cluster; hub and spoke model. EKG, electrocardiogram; PCI, percutaneous coronary intervention.

The system is based on a "hub and spoke" model, with each unit being termed a STEMI cluster (Figure 24.1). Each cluster is made up of two types of hub hospital (class A and class B), and two types of spoke hospital (class C and class D). The class A hospital is a hub hospital with a catheterization laboratory with 24-hour PPCI capability. The aim is to perform PPCI at class A hospitals with a door-to-balloon time of less than 90 minutes. Patients transferred from a linked spoke hospital would also have their catheterization and PCI performed within 3–24 hours of lysis. A class B hospital is also a hub hospital, but the catheterization laboratory does not function for 24 hours a day. Patients would have PPCI during regular hours but may be thrombolyzed during other times, with reperfusion management completed through the pharmacoinvasive approach and catheterization performed within 3–24 hours. Spoke hospitals linked to the class B hospital will thrombolyze patients and transfer them for further management. A class C hospital is a spoke hospital located within 30 minutes' transportation distance of the hub hospital. Patients presenting to these hospitals will have an EKG, will have STEMI confirmed, and will then be transferred to the hub hospital for PPCI. Finally, a class D hospital is a hospital located beyond 30 minutes' transportation time of a hub hospital, where a patient with STEMI is thrombolyzed, stabilized and then transported to the hub hospital within 3–24 hours for catheterization and PCI, if indicated.

Standardized protocols describing the expected care delivery for a STEMI patient have been designed. Different protocols have been implemented depending on the setting of care (emergency medical services, rural spoke hospitals, or PCI-capable hub hospital). However, the care at each of these locations is largely standardized to meet best practice. Protocols are simple and straightforward to eliminate complexity, which can lead to confusion during emergency care situations.

The Prototype Statewide STEMI Project: The Pilot Tamilnadu STEMI Project

The STEMI-Tamilnadu Project was developed to assess the feasibility of developing a STEMI system of care in four clusters across the Southern Indian state of Tamilnadu, using the model developed by STEMI-INDIA [7]. The construction of the four clusters was undertaken with the aim of developing a robust model and involving every type of hospital currently involved in STEMI management. This model seamlessly integrates private and public hospitals so that patients presenting to any type of STEMI hospital would be assured of the same quality and protocols of care. The STEMI clusters were developed based on four principles:

1) Hub hospitals to be from different geographies (metropolitan, urban, and rural) and to include different systems (public, corporate, and charitable hospitals).
2) Spoke hospitals also to follow a similar pattern in terms of diversity of location and structure.
3) All the hub and spoke hospitals in each cluster to be accredited by the state health insurance. This ensured that virtually no patient in the system would be denied treatment due to lack of finances.
4) The GVK Emergency Management and Research Institute (EMRI) ambulance system, a partner in the project, had a clear mandate to move a STEMI patient, picked up in the project's geographic area, to the closest STEMI hospital in the cluster.

The Pilot Tamilnadu STEMI Project has now been completed. Preimplementation data were collected on 927 patients and post-implementation data on 1742 patients. Preliminary analysis of the data has shown [8]:

- The feasibility of developing a STEMI system of care combining the two proven strategies of PPCI and the pharmacoinvasive strategy to manage patients with STEMI.
- Using technology to diagnose STEMI has helped in starting reperfusion treatment early, especially in rural and poorly served areas.

- The implementation of a system of care has increased access to pharmacoinvasive treatment, especially in patients from rural areas who traditionally have stand-alone thrombolysis as the only treatment for STEMI. Access to pharmacoinvasive treatment has increased from 3% to 30%.

Framework for a Statewide STEMI Program

Based on the success of the Pilot Tamilnadu Project, STEMI INDIA has developed a framework for establishing a statewide STEMI system of care. This model has now been endorsed by the CSI and the Association Physicians of India (API). For the STEMI program to be successful, the right infrastructure needs to be in place and a clear partnership needs to be developed among various key stakeholders.

The State Government

Any STEMI program requires the full support and involvement of the state government. Social insurance to cover the below-poverty population, ambulance services and participation of the state government hospitals in a STEMI program is crucial to its success, as all these are controlled and facilitated by the participation of the state government. Furthermore, funding for the program will come from the health budget of each state government. The other important areas where the state government, in consultation with the other stakeholders, such as STEMI-India, CSI and API, would be involved are:

- legislation to accredit STEMI hospitals and to prescribe minimum training requirements, infrastructure requirements, and manpower requirements to handle STEMI patients;
- legislation to enable the emergency medical services to bypass non-STEMI hospitals and transport patients to STEMI accredited hospitals for management;
- regulation of new STEMI hospitals, so that there is an even distribution of STEMI hospitals. This could be similar to the 'certificate of need' legislation in the United States. Such regulation would encourage newer centers in poorly served areas and would discourage the allocation of further resources in well-served areas.

Statewide Ambulance Network

The GVK EMRI ambulance service now exists in 15 states and union territories of India. It has a statewide presence and is an efficient and tested service. It is critical that an ambulance system similar to EMRI be available for primary collection and transfer of patients to STEMI hospitals and for inter-hospital transfer.

Cardiological Society of India

All the hub hospitals with CCLs and a significant number of thrombolytic spokes would have members of the CSI as the heads of the cardiology or medical departments. Each state has a state branch of the CSI and its involvement in the planning, development and running of the state program will be crucial for its success.

Association Physicians of India

A significant proportion of the thrombolytic spoke hospitals are managed by physicians and not by cardiologists. Involvement of the state branch of the API is also therefore important.

Involvement of STEMI INDIA

STEMI-India will lead the national program by setting the national strategy and facilitating its implementation in different states. The Tamilnadu Pilot STEMI project tools, such as the protocols and manuals, have already been developed and tested, technical knowledge and training programs are also available and can be used. However these may be modified when required, based on local needs, in consultation with the local state partners. STEMI-India also has the capability to map, develop and run the STEMI program in any state, in collaboration with the other partners.

Public Engagement

Engagement with the public to educate patients about symptoms of concern with STEMI and the availability of these services will need to be considered by states that begin to roll out these programs. Aside from this, technology and the telecommunication network will provide crucial input that will help to overcome many of the infrastructure and manpower deficiencies that exist in all low-and middle-income countries.

Other Important Activities of STEMI INDIA

"STEMI teams" are being developed in hospitals managing STEMI patients. The annual meeting of STEMI INDIA has been held in different regions of the country. Each meeting focuses on two or three states in that region. Hospitals that manage STEMI patients are encouraged to send "teams" to the meeting. These typically consist of a cardiologist or physician, emergency room physicians or intensivists and a senior nurse. Separate workshops to train each member of the team in their area of STEMI management helps to develop a core group in each hospital. This group would then help to develop a STEMI program in the hospital. Apart from the national meeting, many local meetings are run with STEMI INDIA partner organizations to promote this concept at local level.

Public education campaigns with partner organizations to improve early recognition of symptoms of heart attack are run periodically, focusing on areas where a STEMI system of care is planned.

STEMI INDIA has also been working with regional and national organizations in Africa and Asia to help them to develop STEMI systems of care based on the STEMI INDIA model. The prototype system of care model developed by STEMI INDIA and the use of technology to overcome manpower and infrastructure constraints will benefit many low and middle income countries that are in a similar position to India.

References

1 National Commission on Macroeconomics and Health. *Burden of Disease in India* (NCMH Background Papers). Delhi, India: Ministry of Health and Family Welfare, Government of India, 2005.

2 Xavier D, Pais P, Devereaux PJ, et al. Treatment and outcomes of acute coronary syndromes in India (CREATE): a prospective analysis of registry data. *Lancet*, 2008; 371: 1435–1442.

3 Schamroth C; ACCESS South Africa investigators. Management of acute coronary syndrome in South Africa: insights from the ACCESS (Acute Coronary Events- a Multinational Survey of Current Management Strategies) registry. *Cardiovasc J Africa*, 2012; 7: 365–370.

4 Armstrong PW, Gershlick AH, Goldstein P, et al. Fibrinolysis or primary PCI in ST-segment elevation myocardial infarction. *N Engl J Med*, 2013; 368: 1379–1387.

5 Victor SM, Subban V, Alexander T, et al. A Prospective, observational, multicentre study comparing tenectaplase facilitated PCI versus primary PCI in Indian patients with STEMI (STEPP-AMI). *Open Heart*, 2014: 1(1): e000133. doi:10.1136/openhrt-2014-000133.

6 Alexander T, Mehta S, Mullasari AS, et al. Systems of care for ST-elevation myocardial infarction in India. *Heart*, 2012; 98: 15–17.

7 Alexander T, Victor SM, Mullasari AS, et al. Protocol for a prospective, controlled study of assertive and timely reperfusion for patients with ST-segment elevation myocardial infarction in Tamil Nadu: the TN-STEMI programme. *BMJ Open*, 2013; 3(12): e003850. doi:10.1136/bmjopen-2013-003850.

8 Alexander T, Mullasari AS, Narula J. Developing a STEMI system of care for low- and middle-income countries. *Global Heart*, 2014; 9(4): 419–423.

25

The Role of Telemedicine in STEMI Interventions

Roberto Vieira Botelho MD PhD, Sameer Mehta MD FACC MBA, Julius Cezar Q. Ladeira DDS MSc,
Francisco Fernandéz MBA, Márcio Sanches MD, Denis Fabiano de Souza RN,
Wladimir Fernandes de Rezende MBA, Carlos Otávio Lara Pinheiro BSc

Definition of Telemedicine

Telemedicine is the practice of medicine at distance, by means of electronic communications, to improve a patient's clinical health status [1]. Once medical information can be digitized, a health professional can transmit it from one place to another. The telecommunication network simply needs to be adequate to transmit the particular file at a reasonable speed, provided that the file is protected for privacy, integrity and accessibility. The US Department of Health and Human Services issued the Privacy Rule to implement the requirement of the Health Insurance Portability and Accountability Act of 1996 to ensure that individuals' health information is properly protected while allowing the flow of health information needed to provide and promote high-quality health care and to protect public health and wellbeing [2].

Interesting applications have been developed for intervention in ST-elevation myocardial infarction (STEMI), which vary from the 12-lead tele-electrocardiogram [3–8], a near patient test for troponin or CKMB analysis [9] or even a complete picture archiving and communication system [10] to transmit an angiogram or any other image modality from one site to another. In this chapter, we discuss how technology is evolving towards singularity and how can it improve STEMI interventions.

Computer Power

Not only has the power of the computer increased, but also the way in which this power is delivered [11]. Decade by decade, progression can be seen (Box 25.1). Thus, instead of a single chip inside a computer, thousands of chips are scattered inside every artifact, all talking to one another and connected to the internet. When these chips are inserted into an appliance, it is dramatically transformed. In telephones, they became cell phones; cameras become digital cameras; into EKG machines, tele-EKG, and so on [12]. These devices can collect useful data with the help of Bluetooth, radio-frequency identification, near field communication and local wireless computer networking technologies, and then autonomously flow the data between other devices, giving a new approach to data exchange.

The superconvergence or ubiquity of "smart phones" (today the smart phone has more computer power than NASA had in 1969 when it placed two astronauts on the Moon), no limit

Manual of STEMI Interventions, First Edition. Edited by Sameer Mehta.
© 2017 John Wiley & Sons Ltd. Published 2017 by John Wiley & Sons Ltd.

Box 25.1   The Progression of Computing Power

1950s   Vacuum tube computers filling entire rooms. Only the United States military was rich enough to fund them.

1960s   Transistors replaced vacuum tube computers, and mainframe computers gradually entered the marketplace.

1970s   Integrated circuit boards, with hundred of transistors, created the minicomputer (the size of a large desk).

1980s   Chips, with tens of millions of transistors, allowed the creation of personal computers that can fit inside a briefcase.

1990s   The internet connected hundreds of millions of computers into a single, global computer network.

2000s   Ubiquitous computing freed the chip from the computer, when chips were dispersed into the environment.

---

for bandwidth, pervasive connectivity, social and health system networking, cloud computing, all lead to the concept of superconvergence, first described by Marshall McLuhan, who coined the word "surfing" nearly 30 years before the worldwide web existed. He also characterized media as extensions of human senses, bodies and minds.

Artificial Intelligence

Artificial intelligence is the science and engineering of making intelligent machines, according to John McCarthy, who coined the term in 1955 [13]. This science studies how to create computers and computer software that are capable of intelligent behavior; systems that perceive their environment and take actions that maximize their chances of success. A more specific tool is a decision support system; that is, a computer-based information system that supports organizational decision-making activities [14]. Decision support systems serve the management, operations, and planning levels of an organization and help to make decisions, which may be rapidly changing and not easily specified in advance. They can be either fully computerized, human-based or a combination of both.

A clinical decision support system is designed to assist physicians and other health professionals with clinical decision-making tasks [15]. Creating such systems is a major topic in artificial intelligence in medicine. A clinical decision support system is an active knowledge system that uses two or more items of patient data to generate case-specific advice. The main purpose of modern clinical decision support system is to assist clinicians at the point of care. The interaction between the physician and the support system helps the physician to analyze and reach a diagnosis or a therapeutic strategy based on the patient data. As a result, the interaction produces a better analysis of the patient data than either a human or clinical decision support system could make on their own. Knowledge-based systems contain the rules and associations of compiled data, which most often take the form of IF-THEN rules. In STEMI interventions, the rule might be that IF transfer time is shorter than 120 minutes, AND duration of chest pain is longer than 30 minutes, THEN transfer for primary percutaneous coronary intervention (PPCI) [16].

Non-knowledge-based systems use a form of artificial intelligence called machine learning, which allows computers to learn from past experiences and/or find patterns in clinical data.

Most clinicians do not use this system because no meaningful information about how they work can be discerned by human inspection, and reliability and accountability concerns may be raised. These systems can be used as post-diagnostic systems.

Pre-diagnosis clinical decision support system systems are used to help the physician to prepare the diagnosis. During-diagnosis clinical decision support systems help in filtering the diagnosis and improving it. Post-diagnosis clinical decision support systems are used to mine data to derive connections between patients and clinical research to predict future events.

Cloud Computing

Cloud computing refers to applications, hardware and systems software located in datacenters delivered as services over the internet (Figure 25.1). The National Institute of Standards and Technology's definition of cloud computing is "a model for enabling ubiquitous, convenient, on-demand network access to a shared pool of configurable computing resources that can be rapidly provisioned and released with minimal management effort or service provider interaction" [17] There are three "service models" (software, platform, and infrastructure) and four "deployment models" (private, community, public, and hybrid). We use the term "private cloud" to refer to internal data centers of an organization, not made available to the general public. It offers infinite computing resources available on demand, as well as wide geographical distribution of high-speed access to the servers. The global healthcare cloud computing market is estimated at US$4,216.5 million in 2014 and expected to reach US$12,653.4 million in 2020. However, factors such as the high cost involved in the implementation of clinical information systems, lack of security, and privacy of patient information and interoperability issues negatively impact its growth.

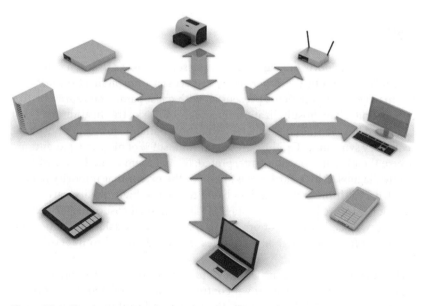

Figure 25.1 Cloud computing: Applications, hardware and systems software located in datacenters delivered as services over the internet.

Pervasive Computing, Ubiquitous Computing or the Internet of Things

Pervasive computing is the growing trend towards embedding microprocessors in everyday objects and things so they can communicate information. Pervasive computing devices are completely connected and constantly available. They rely on the convergence of wireless technologies, advanced electronics and the internet [18]. Smart devices communicate unobtrusively. They use the machine-to-machine concept, where a machine communicates with another machine, without human interference, and do all the talking [19]. They employ a device (sensor) to capture an event (heart rate, ST-elevation, arrhythmia), which is relayed through a network (wireless, wired, or hybrid) to an application (software program), translating the captured event into usable information (patient requires attention).

The pocket electrocardiogram (EKG) remote monitoring system [20] is a machine-to-machine enabled device which uses the secure, cloud-based, fully hosted platform that continuously receives data from the device. It transmits a two-lead EKG to a controlled and secure data center. Data can be viewed by physicians remotely. In cases of concern, the system can provide an alert to caregivers.

Socioeconomic Disparities

Lower socioeconomic status has been shown to be associated with a higher prevalence of cardiac risk factors, such as hypertension, cigarette smoking, obesity, diabetes, and prothrombotic factors such as elevated fibrinogen levels [21]. Thus, patients of lower socioeconomic status may have more extensive coronary disease, and they are certainly at greater risk for recurrent events. Occupational stress, social isolation, and depression are all more prevalent among persons with lower socioeconomic status and may contribute to higher mortality [22].

Healthcare Disparities

Healthcare disparities are costly. Poorly managed care or missed diagnoses result in expensive and avoidable complications [23]. On the other hand, unnecessary hospitalization plays an important role on the management of patients presenting with chest pain, who represent 10% of all visits to emergency units. The hospitalization for triage and risk stratification may cost $80,000 per quality adjusted life year [24]. Less than 30% of these patients do require hospitalization due to acute coronary syndrome. On the other hand, almost 9% of high-risk patients are not hospitalized because the EKG has been misinterpreted; 50% of them could have had their missed STEMI correctly diagnosed by a cardiologist [25]. To the extent that minority beneficiaries of publicly funded health programs are less likely to receive high-quality care, these beneficiaries may face higher future healthcare costs [26]. The personal cost of disparities can lead to significant morbidity, disability, and lost productivity at the individual level. At the societal level, distal costs follow from proximal opportunities that were missed to intervene and reduce burden of illness.

Although universal health insurance programs in developed countries have promoted greater equity in access to care, several studies have shown continuing income related differences in the rates of use of specific services [27]. Beyond that, there is a significant imbalance between supply and demand of physicians active in patient care, particularly cardiologists and emergency doctors. There is a linear correlation between distribution of physicians and the income per capita of a particular geographic area of the world [28]. Developing countries lack appropriately recognized or managed acute myocardial infarction care. Ambulance services are often nonexistent; doctors and nurses are lacking; basic thrombolytic therapy is not available; and PPCI is unimaginable. As a result of these drawbacks, mortality from acute myocardial infarction and long-term outcomes are unacceptable [29]. Even in developed countries, despite the availability of a universal healthcare system, socioeconomic status has pronounced effects on access to specialized cardiac services, as well as on mortality 1 year after acute myocardial infarction [30].

Time as a Strong Predictor of Outcomes

Despite efforts to reduce hospital mortality from acute myocardial infarction, globally, 50–75% of mortality will occur in the pre-hospital environment [31]. Total ischemic time is an important predictor of outcomes, 1-year mortality increases by 7% for each 30 minutes of delay in reperfusion [32]. It has been recognized that in-hospital delays have improved such that current reductions in door-to-balloon times no longer impact on mortality. Rather, the challenge lies in the pre-hospital total ischemic time, which is patient and system dependent [33]. Patient awareness is a key factor. Only 23% of STEMI patients activate the emergency medical service during their initial care, but almost 83% of them would use the emergency medical service if they knew that their symptoms were related to a STEMI. Most of these patients are taken to hospital by lay people and 16% drive their own car [34]. System delays and treatment implementation can also be impacted by protocol implementation in a STEMI network [35].

LATIN, A Cloud Computing STEMI Network Supported by Artificial Intelligence

The Lumen Americas Telemedicine Infarct Network is an evolving project that implements tele-EKG machines in low-complexity referral centers that lack cardiologists. These machines record a 12-lead EKG and transmit it via a telemedicine center located in a cloud computing system which provides capillarity to reach the most remote areas in Brazil and Colombia (Figure 25.2). Hosted in the cloud, an integrated telemedicine platform receives the row data from remote referrals and submits them to a knowledge-based clinical support decision system, which then recommends a reperfusion strategy based on the variables and rules collected. During this phase, pre-diagnosis clinical decision support systems are used to help the physician prepare the diagnoses and treatment. The system triggers the processes to the whole network (automatic activation of the ambulance, the catheterization lab team, bypassing the emergency department and the intensive care unit). The during-diagnosis clinical decision

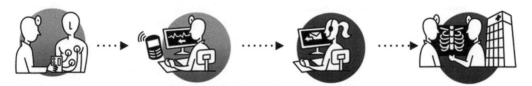

Figure 25.2 An integrated telemedicine platform.

support system helps in filtering the diagnosis and improving it. The post-diagnosis clinical decision support system is used to mine data to derive connections between patients and clinical research to predict future events. One of the post-diagnosis features is the analysis of the area of the ST-elevation behavior as a predictor of reperfusion quality.

Conclusions

Patients at higher risk of suffering a STEMI live in underserved areas. Telemedicine can improve the penetration of diagnosis, increase the universalization of access and decentralization of complexity, and can improve equity and de-hospitalization. Taken together, each of these improvements promotes cost effectiveness. Since the introduction of thrombolysis for STEMI reperfusion, it has been shown that processes, rather than procedures, are the main challenges to be implemented in the care of patients. In addition, data have shown that processes are well developed at the hospital level, and significant reductions in door-to-balloon time are not capable of reducing mortality in STEMI patients, but there is much to implement during the pre-hospital environment.

Patient awareness and patient-related delay is a major challenge. The "internet of things" concept provides a unique opportunity for patient monitoring. Machine-to-machine systems also allow the automatic detection of high-risk ischemic events at the patient's location, in the pre-hospital environment, either at home or at work. Cloud computing technology allows telemedicine centers to be connected to extremely remote areas at low cost, dramatically improving capillarity of these systems. Artificial intelligence, through clinical decision support systems, increase adherence to the most up-to-date guidelines and also improves the sharing of protocols between referral and tertiary hospitals. The final step of brain-technology integration is singularity – a period when there will be no gap between biological neuronal decision and the technological computer intelligence. Mammals have added about 1 cubic inch of brain matter every 100,000 years. Computer power is doubled every 18 months.

References

1 About Telemedicine: The Ultimate Frontier for Superior Healthcare Delivery. American Telemedicine Association. Available at http://www.americantelemed.org/about/about-telemedicine (accessed March 24, 2017).

2 Summary of the HIPAA Privacy Rule. Office for Civil Rights. Available at http://www.hhs.gov/ocr/privacy/hipaa/understanding/summary (accessed March 24, 2017).

3 Molinari G., Reboa G, Frascio M et al. The role of telecardiology in supporting the decision-making process of general practitioners during the management of patients with suspected cardiac events. *J Telemed Telecare*, 2002; 8: 97–101.

4 Bailey JJ, Berson AS, Garson JA, et al. Recommendations for standardization and specifictions in automated electrocardiography: Bandwidth and digital signal processing. A report for health professionals by an ad hoc writing group of the Committee on Electrocardiography and Cardiac Electrophysiology of the Council on clinical Cardiology, American Heart Association. *Circulation*, 1990; 81: 730–739.

5 Kudenchuk PJ, Maynard C, Cobb IA et all. Utility of the pre-hospital electrocardiogram in diagnosing acute coronary syndromes: the myocardial infarction triage and intervention (MITI) project. *J Am Coll Cardiol*, 1998; 32: 17–27.

6 Hasin Y, David D, Rogel S. Diagnostic and therapeutic assessment by telephone electrocardigraphic monitoring of ambulatory patients. *BMJ*, 1976; 2: 612–615.

7 Grim P, Feldman T, Martin M, et al. Cellular telephone transmission of 12-lead electrocardiogram from ambulance to hospital. *Am J Cardiol*, 1987; 60: 715–720.

8 Aufderheide TP, Hendley GE, Woo J, et all. A prospective evaluation of prehospital 12-lead ECG application in chest pain patients. *J Electrocardiol*, 1992; 24: 8–13.

9 Lau J, Loannidis J, Balk E, et al. Diagnosing acute cardiac ischemia in the emergency department: a systematic review of the accuracy and clinical effect of current technologies. *Ann Emerg Med*, 2001; 37: 453–460.

10 Dietrich Meyer-Ebrecht. Picture archiving and communication systems (PACS) for medical applications. *Int J Bio-Med Comput*, 1994; 35(2): 91–124.

11 Michio Kaku. *Physics of the Future: How Science Will Shape Human Destiny and Our Daily Lives by the Year 2100 is a 2011.* Harmondsworth, UK: Penguin; 2011.

12 Eric Topol. *The Creative Destruction of Medicine. How the Digital Revolution will Create Better Health Care.* New York, NY: Basic Books; 2013.

13 Vincent Müller. *Philosophy and Theory of Artificial Intelligence.* New York, NY: Springer; 2012.

14 Miller RA. Medical diagnostic decision support systems- past, present, and future: A threaded bibliography and brief commentary. *J Am Med Informatics Assoc*, 1994; 1: 8–27.

15 Garg AX, Adhikari NKJ, McDonald H, et al. Effects of computerized clinical decision support systems in practitioner performance and patient outcomes A systematic review. *J Am Med Assoc*, 2005; 293: 1223–1238.

16 Olsson SE, Ohlsson M, Öhlin H, et al. Decision support for the initial triage of patients with acute myocardial infarction. *Clin Physiol Funct Imag*, 2006; 26: 151–156.

17 Mell P, Grance T. *The NIST Definition of Cloud Computing* (NIST Special Publication 800-145). Gaithersburg, MD: Computer Security Division Information Technology Laboratory National Institute of Standards and Technology; 2011.

18 Satyanarayanan M. Pervasive Computing: Vision and Challenges. *IEEE Personal Commun*, 2001; 8: 10–17.

19 Chen M, Wan J, Li F. Machine-to-machine communications: architectures, standards and applications. KSII Trans *Internet Inform Syst*, 2012; 6(2): 480–497.

20 Dziubiński M. PocketECG: a new continuous and real-time ambulatory arrhythmia diagnostic method. *Cardiol J*, 2011; 18(4): 454–460.

21 Fletcher GF, Balady GJ, Vogel RA, et al. Preventive Cardiology: How Can We Do Better? Proceedings of the 33rd Bethesda Conference, Bethesda, Maryland, USA. December 18, 2001. *J Am Coll Cardiol*, 2002; 40(4): 579–651.

22 Fiscella K, Tancredi D, Franks P, et al. Adding socioeconomic status to Framingham scoring to reduce disparities in coronary risk assessment. *Am Heart J*, 2009; 157: 988–994.

23 Agency for Healthcare Research and Quality. *2013 National Healthcare Disparities Report* (AHRQ Publication No. 14-0006). Rockville, MD: US Department of Health and Human Services; 2014.

24 Polanczyk CA, Kuntz K, Sacks DB, et al. Cost-effectiveness of triage strategies using CK-MB and troponin I in emergency department patients with acute chest pain. *Ann Intern Med*, 1999; 131: 909–918.

25 Masoudi FA, Magid DJ, Vinson DR, et al. Implications of the failure to identify high-risk electrocardiogram finding for the quality of care of patients with acute myocardial infarction. *Circulation*, 2006; 114: 1565–1571.

26 Office of the National Coordinator for Health Information Technology (ONC). *Federal Health Information Technology Strategic Plan 2011–2015:* Putting the I into Health IT. Washington, DC: ONC. Available at http://www.healthit.gov/sites/default/files/utility/final-federal-health-it-strategic-plan-0911.pdf (accessed March 24, 2017).

27 Alter DA, Naylor D, Phil D, et al. Effects of socioeconomic status on access to invasive cardiac procedures and on mortality after acute myocardial infarction. *N Engl J Med*, 1999; 341: 1359–1367.

28 Physician Shortages to Worsen Without Increases in Residency Training. Association of American Medical Colleges. Available at https://www.aamc.org/download/150584/data (accessed March 24, 2017).

29 Mehta S, Botelho RV, Rodriguez D, et al. A tale of two cities: STEMI interventions in developed and developing countries and the potential of telemedicine to reduce disparities in care. *J Interv Cardiol*, 2014; 27: 155–166.

30 McGovern P, Pankow JS, Shahar E, et al. Recent trends in acute coronary heart disease. mortality, morbidity, medical care, and risk factors. *N Engl J Med*, 1996; 334: 884–890.

31 De Luca G, Suryapranata H, Ottervanger JP, et al. Time delay to treatment and mortality in primary angioplasty for acute myocardial infarction. every minute of delay counts. *Circulation*, 2004; 109: 1223–1225.

32 Bates ER, Jacobs AK. Time to treatment in patients with STEMI. *N Engl J Med*, 2013; 369(10): 889–892.

33 Gibson CM. Time is myocardium and time is outcomes. *Circulation*, 2001; 104: 2632–2634.

34 Task Force on the Management of ST-Segment Elevation Acute Myocardial Infarction of the European Society of Cardiology (ESC). ESC Guidelines for the management of acute myocardial infarction in patients presenting with ST-segment elevation. *Eur Heart J*, 2012; 33(20): 2569–2619.

35 Kurzweil R. *Singularity is Near: When Humans Transcend Biology*. Harmondsworth, UK: Penguin; 2005.

26

Innovative Telemedicine STEMI Protocols

Sameer Mehta MD FACC MBA, Roberto Vieira Botelho MD PhD, Freddy Bojanini MD, Juan Corral MD, Marco Perin MD, María Teresa Bedoya Reina MD, Juliana Giraldo MD, Laura Álvarez MD, Cindy Manotas MD, Sebastián Moreno MD, Sergio Reyes MD, María Botero Urrea MD

Introduction

Charles Dickens' observations in *A Tale of Two Cities* are exemplified in the disparate nature of the management of acute myocardial infarction (AMI) in developed and developing countries. Developed countries have access to sophisticated ambulance networks, pre-hospital management, 24/7 cardiac catheterization suites, a large group of skilled cardiologists, nurses, and technicians, thrombectomy devices, and drug-eluting stents, and a host of financial and infrastructural resources [1,2]. Management of AMI with such an infrastructure results in reliably low mortality and good long-term outcomes. In striking contrast, developing countries lack appropriately recognized or managed AMI care. Ambulances services are often nonexistent; doctors and nurses are lacking; basic thrombolytic therapy is not available; and primary percutaneous coronary intervention (PPCI) is unimaginable [3]. As a result of these drawbacks, mortality and long-term outcomes from AMI are abysmal.

Health economists analyzing such disparities will confidently conclude that it will be decades of sustained growth and development for developing countries to match the economic, scientific, structural, and logistical parity in AMI care in developed countries. As the world awaits these changes, millions of AMI sufferers in developing countries will be denied access to advanced AMI care [4].

Telemedicine offers a novel platform to dramatically narrow the disparities in AMI care in developed and developing countries. Telemedicine can drastically increase access to AMI care, and it may do so cost effectively [5]. Diagnostic interpretation of a STEMI electrocardiogram (EKG) may increase [6]. Even more importantly, telemedicine affords an attractive possibility of comprehensively managing AMI and triaging patients into thrombolytic therapy, pharmacoinvasive, management or PPCI.

To demonstrate the feasibility of telemedicine in evening out inequalities in AMI care in developed and developing countries, the Lumen Americas Telemedicine Infarct Network (LATIN) has been developed and being piloted in 100 LATIN sites in Brazil and Colombia. Table 26.1 [7,8] provides some statistics comparing the United States, Brazil, Colombia, and Mexico in areas relevant to AMI care. Developing countries such as Colombia and Mexico are less urbanized and have a significant proportion of their population living in poverty. Furthermore, while the mortality from heart disease is high, healthcare expenditure in general

Manual of STEMI Interventions, First Edition. Edited by Sameer Mehta.

Table 26.1 Relevant Statistics Comparison between Developed and Developing Countries.

Indicator	Year	United States	Brazil	Colombia	Mexico
Populations (1,000s)	2012	315,791	198,361	47,551	116,147
Urban (%)	2012	82.6	84.9	75.6	78.4
Mortality rate:					
Annual average (1,000s)	2012	2,647	1,270.75	264	557.6
General (per 1,000 population)	2010	125.6[a]	56.1[a]	72.9[a]	60.7[a]
		70.8[b]	79.5[b]	125.9[b]	93.1[b]
Ischemic heart disease (per 100,000 pop.):	2009/2010				
General		125.6[a]	56.1[a]	72.9[a]	60.7[a]
		70.8[b]	62[b]	101.7[b]	74[b]
Male		130.8[a]	65.5[a]	80.1[a]	68.7[a]
		96[b]	79.5[b]	125.9[b]	93.1[b]
Female		113[a]	47[a]	65.9[a]	53[a]
		50.3[b]	47.2[b]	82.3[b]	57.6[b]
Estimated rate:					
– 45–64 years	2009/2010	85.38	102.4	103.01	70.96
– ≥ 65 years		749.55	518.77	1008.3	726.94
Ill-defined and unknown conditions (%)	2009/2010	1.55	6.97	2.16	2.05
Poverty headcount ratio at $1.25 per day (%)	2008–2010	–	6.14	8.16	1.15
Annual national health expenditure as proportion of GDP (%):	2011				
Public		9.9	3.1	3.5	3
Private		5.6	4.1	1.5	3.1
Physician ratio (per 10,000 population)	2009	26	15.1	16.6	22
Hospital bed ratio (per 1,000 population)	2010/2011	3	2.3	1.39	1.7
Outpatient care facilities (*n*)	2001/2010	4,815	67,901	33,029	18,815

[a] Corrected rate
[b] Adjusted rate
[c] Proportion of certified deaths due to ill-defined and unknown conditions

is much lower in those countries. As expected, access to physicians and hospital beds is also considerably lower than in the United States. With most well-equipped medical facilities in the cities, access to quality health care and a reliable ambulance service is problematic for rural residents, which places a large reliance on rural outpatient care facilities.

These differences occur from several factors – financial, infrastructure, logistical and cultural. Several of these elements are interrelated. As an example, the vital factor of ambulance services appears to correlate with economic development of the region [1,2]. This observation is obvious in regions where well-developed ambulance services are entirely absent [3].

Acute Myocardial Infarction and Ambulance Networks

AMI management remains fundamentally dependent upon existing networks of ambulance services, which provide the initial, but critical, first step of managing a patient with AMI [9]. An ambulance provides the following distinct purposes for AMI management, as illustrated in

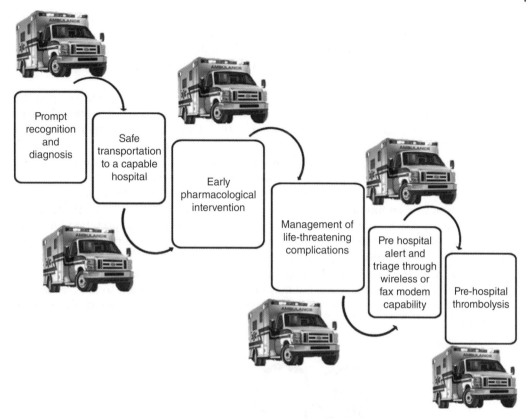

Figure 26.1 Roles of the ambulance in ST-elevation myocardial infarction interventions.

Figure 26.1 [10]. The availability and capability of ambulance resources and networks vary widely, from a complete lack of reliable ambulance to mobile units that provide pre-hospital thrombolysis [9]. Yet despite the vast abilities of the ambulance service, even in developed countries, ambulance care for a patient with AMI merely represents transportation to a hospital [11]. It is tragic that many patients are being transported without a definite diagnosis of AMI [12]. This glaring omission makes it impossible for the ambulance to have an accurate assessment of the patient, let alone the correct management. In some situations, this type of unguided service is dangerous, as poorly equipped ambulances provide a deceptive sense of security for an AMI patient [13].

The major difference between AMI care in Europe and the United States emanates from this specific dissimilarity – in Europe, the vast majority of AMI patients are transported to a hospital in an ambulance, whereas in the United States, the larger percentage of patients are still self-transporting [14]. In various Asian nations, there is a blend of such services; in some poor African countries, ambulance services for AMI are unavailable and/or unreliable.

Telemedicine

What should patients do if there is no reliable ambulance network to transport them to a hospital? In such situations, patients transport themselves to the hospital, which greatly delays the treatment of AMI. Management of AMI, either by thrombolysis or PPCI, is critically time dependent. For thrombolytic therapy, a door-to-needle time of less than 30 minutes, and for PPCI, a door-to-balloon time of less than 90 minute, are the advocated guidelines [5,15,16]. With a qualitative and quantitative absence of ambulances, achieving these mandated treatment times is simply not possible. As a result, both thrombolytic therapy and PPCI will therefore be suboptimal. Unfortunately, this situation is the norm rather than the exception.

Telemedicine effectively reduces these shortcomings [6,17]. It can even improve upon the results of thrombolytic therapy and PPCI through its unique ability to initiate very early management, both within and outside an ambulance [18]. With thoughtful integration into a regional STEMI network [19], telemedicine uses the best of today's technology to advance three pathways of treatment in the comprehensive management of AMI. Figure 26.2 introduces the roles of telemedicine when applied to locations with or without ambulance.

Telemedicine is founded on four distinct attributes. These include increased access, greater accuracy, a comprehensive AMI management strategy, and cost effectiveness. Telemedicine support comprises two components: Accurate EKG interpretation and teleconsultation. Not every EKG interpretation will require a teleconsultation. The role of teleconsultation is to guide triage of patients with a confirmed myocardial infarction. Considering the characteristics of developing countries and their urgent need for improved AMI care, effective use of telemedicine may offer a pragmatic solution to increase access and accuracy of treatment in a cost-effective manner while taking advantage of telemedicine platforms.

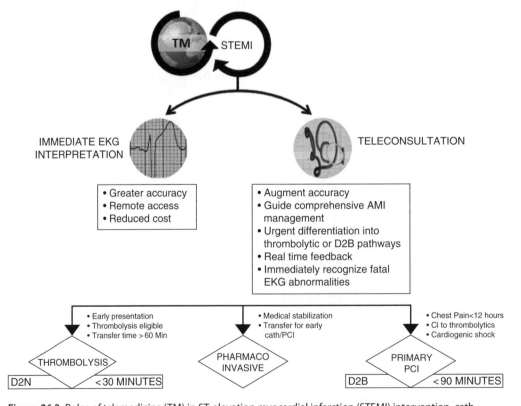

Figure 26.2 Roles of telemedicine (TM) in ST-elevation myocardial infarction (STEMI) intervention. cath, catherization; D2B, door-to-balloon; D2N, door-to-needle; EKG, electrocardiogram; PCI, percutaneous coronary intervention.

Lumen Americas Telemedicine Infarct Network

Integration of telemedicine into the current global infrastructure is paramount to ensuring its success. Telemedicine is used as a foundation pillar to initiate an optimal strategy for world-wide AMI management. As shown in Table 26.1, developing countries rely largely on rural outpatient facilities to provide healthcare. An integrated approach that incorporates these facilities in AMI care is essential.

The Lumen Americas Telemedicine Infarct Network (LATIN) is structured as a hub-and-spoke strategy for comprehensive AMI management. The primary responsibility of the hubs is to deliver and expedite PPCI for STEMI interventions with door-to-balloon times of less than 90 minute. The spokes, up to five sites located 5–250 miles from each hub, may provide thrombolytic therapy or pharmacoinvasive management strategy and expedite transfer for PPCI. Spoke sites lack the ability to provide PPCI. To carry out this strategy, LATIN has three partners with distinct roles. The telemedicine device is provided by ITMS Inc., which is also providing a wireless software platform, Platform Integrated Telemedicine (PIT). Medtronic Inc. provides logistical support for both the pilot and the main phase of LATIN. Lumen provides educational training for LATIN sites.

Telemedicine devices are strategically placed in the ambulance, remote and inaccessible locations, and in places where AMI patients traditionally present (primary clinics, private nursing homes, and the offices of general practitioners) [19]. This strategy eliminates the huge barriers caused by the inadequacies of the ambulance systems to enable the administration of very early, pre-hospital AMI therapy [18].

Methods

Most LATIN methods and protocol are based upon established guidelines; some additionally rely on the vast experience gained with the Single Individual Community Experience Registry (SINCERE), which has accumulated vast experience in performing short door-to-balloon STEMI interventions. LATIN begins when a patient with clinical suspicion and established coronary artery disease risk factors presents to a LATIN site. Great clinical prudence is required at this critical juncture. Good clinical decision making optimally and cost-effectively employs telemedicine and eliminates false positive responses.

Step 1: The Electrocardiogram and Pre-hospital Management

Patients presenting with chest pain will be given a 12-lead EKG on the telemedicine device within 10 minutes of presentation, as per clinical guidelines. Neither a clear STEMI presentation nor a case with atypical history and normal EKG would require assistance from the telemedicine strategy, and would not be sent for telemedicine consultation. Uncertainty arises when the EKG includes early repolarization pattern, pericarditis, left anterior hemiblock and left bundle branch block, left ventricular hypertrophy with strain, and left ventricular aneurysm. A clinical AMI presentation and suspicious EKG immediately involves use of the telemedicine protocol.

While seeking an accurate EKG diagnosis, numerous critical tasks are performed in an ambulance, as described in Figure 26.1. Early pharmacology is initiated in the ambulance and includes aspirin (325 mg), clopidogrel (300 mg, prasugrel and ticagrelor are even better options), sublingual nitroglycerine, supplemental oxygen, statins, beta-blockers, and an anticoagulant. The latter may include a bolus of unfractionated heparin (60 µg/kg) or a bolus of bivalirudin. Low molecular weight heparin may also be used, but would be less ideal.

Step 2: Teleconsultation-Based LATIN Triage

Two documents are required to initiate teleconsultation. These include the presenting EKG and the LATIN clinical short form. Remotely located (in-hospital, at telemedicine centers or at home), expert cardiologists access these documents from the PIT platform and provide immediate EKG diagnosis based upon a true vector analysis. Pre-notification of STEMI to hub sites is performed after accurate EKG diagnosis (as described above) primarily by telemedicine transmission and if needed by verbal communication or fax/modem. Telemedicine simultaneously delivers the STEMI EKG and the LATIN clinical short form to all three LATIN locations: Hub, spoke, and in the ambulance. The teleconsultation cardiologist will communicate with the spoke site or ambulance to provide pre-hospital AMI management. Once the patient arrives at a hub site, EMS will have a record of the pre-hospital intervention and contact information of the teleconsultation cardiologist who diagnosed the STEMI and facilitated pre-hospital STEMI care.

Step 3: Pre-Hospital Early Thrombolysis

The hubs initiate the STEMI protocol immediately upon confirmation of a STEMI diagnosis. Each LATIN site has advanced directives for either PPCI or thrombolytic strategies based upon their location. As a general strategy, thrombolytic therapy is recommended for very early presentation (less than 2 hours from onset of pain), while PPCI is recommended when transfer to a hub is readily available and for patients with cardiogenic shock.

The choice of lytic agents is left to the discretion of the physician seeking telemedicine consultation. These agents include streptokinase, alteplase or tenecteplase; adjunctive treatment includes antiplatelet and anticoagulants. Analgesia, narcotics, supplemental oxygen, and intravenous access are mandatory. Beta-blockers are often used. Spoke sites are encouraged to develop their individual thrombolytic protocols. Successful lysis is marked by relief of chest pain and ST-segment resolution (greater than 60% ST-segment lowering). Failed lysis provides an absolute indication for transfer to a PCI institution for salvage rescue PCI. All patients with successful thrombolysis are transferred to a PCI institution within a reasonable period of time (4–24 hours).

Figure 26.2 is a more detailed description of the thrombolytic pathway where specific roles of telemedicine are highlighted. Two specific roles for telemedicine can be appreciated. First, an EKG is accurately interpreted by an accredited cardiologist [21], who uses a vector tracing for quick and comprehensive diagnosis and reports it in a secure, format compatible with the US Health Insurance Portability and Accountability Act of 1996 (HIPAA). With the EKG automatically converted to a standardized format, it is directly incorporated into the electronic medical record and serves as a historical template to be used for clinical management and research. The second specific role of telemedicine during thrombolytic therapy is the immediate availability to obtain a consultation for expert guidance during triage and treatment.

Step 4: Pharmacoinvasive Pathway

A pharmacoinvasive pathway mandates early transfer of thrombolytic therapy patients for a PCI strategy. As a result, every patient who receives thrombolytic therapy is expedited for adjunctive PCI. The cardiovascular laboratory at the PCI institution is immediately notified and catheterization laboratory/STEMI activation expedited. Again, choice of thrombolytic therapy is left to the discretion of the operator. Adjunctive therapy is as described for thrombolytic therapy. Figure 26.3 demonstrates a pharmacoinvasive strategy as compared with the thrombolysis pathway with the use of telemedicine. The role of teleconsultation is foremost in this pathway for the remote expert to guide the consulting physicians regarding the timing of

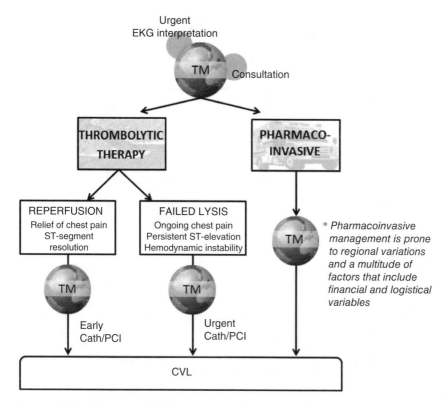

Figure 26.3 Enhancement of thrombolysis and pharmacoinvasive management with telemedicine. Cath, catherization; CVL, central venous line; PCI, percutaneous coronary intervention; TM, telemedicine.

transfer for PCI and the interim clinical management of the patient. Guideline recommendations are followed during this process and decisions such as use of anti-platelets, antithrombotics, glycoprotein IIb/IIIa therapy are discussed.

Step 5: STEMI Intervention Pathway: Door-to-Balloon Interventions

The essence of the STEMI Intervention pathway is the mandated door-to-balloon time of less than 90 minutes. Accurate STEMI diagnosis, intelligent ambulance transport, pre-hospital activation, and emergency department bypass are the four tenets of this strategy. False activation is considerably minimized through an accurate LATIN short form and remote EKG interpretation by expert cardiologists of the telemedicine network. Telemedicine further accomplishes intelligent EMS transport and pre-hospital activation. Advanced directives between LATIN hubs and spokes determine a unidirectional or bidirectional ambulance strategy. Certain LATIN sites have a centralized ambulance network, in addition. An accurate diagnosis triggers prompt ambulance transfer if the patient presents at a spoke site that has rapid PCI access. For patients presenting at the hub sites, remote EKG diagnosis automatically triggers a STEMI alert. Optimal response time for cardiac catheterization laboratory personnel is less than 30 minutes. With early pre-hospital activation, the desirable strategy is either complete or partial bypass of the emergency department. In a complete emergency department bypass, the patient is wheeled from the ambulance to the cardiac catheterization laboratory without stopping at the emergency room. In a partial strategy, an emergency physician rapidly assesses the patient and confirms availability of the cardiac catheterization laboratory.

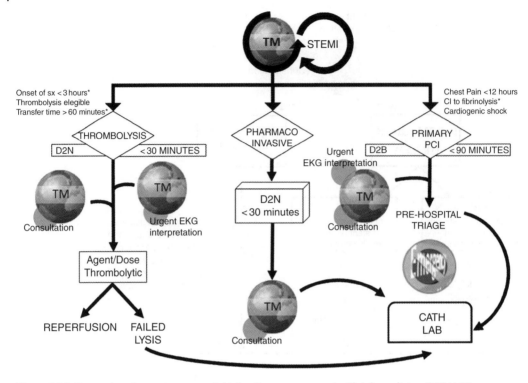

Figure 26.4 Comprehensive acute myocardial infarction management with telemedicine. CATH LAB, catheterization laboratory; CI, contraindication; D2B, door-to-balloon; D2N, door-to-needle; EKG, electrocardiogram; PCI, percutaneous coronary intervention; Sx, symptoms; TH, thrombolysis; TM, telemedicine; * [15,32].

There is scientific evidence that emergency department bypass in suitable cases with accurate and early pre-hospital triage greatly contributes to reducing door-to-balloon times. Figure 26.4 combines the three previous LATIN figures in a master blueprint, demonstrating the novel and comprehensive algorithm that uses a telemedicine platform to facilitate any of the three AMI management pathways – thrombolytic therapy, pharmacoinvasive management and PPCI.

Results

Creation of LATIN Hubs and Spokes

During the pilot phase of LATIN, conducted between April 1, 2014 to June 15, 2015, 84 active LATIN centers have been created (Figure 26.5). These include 54 in Colombia and 32 in Brazil. Maximum spokes per hub was nine in Colombia and seven in Brazil. Mean hub-to-spoke distance was 26 miles in Colombia and 38 miles in Brazil. Maximum population coverage for the hub and spoke was in São Paulo, Brazil, and in Barranquilla, Colombia. Gradual activation of the hubs and spokes was progressed during the pilot phase with the following essential requirements:

- hub: PPCI capability with 24/7 on-call team, ability to bypass the emergency department, feedback mechanisms, single-call activation, and on-site cardiac surgery;
- spoke: transfer protocols, telemedicine setup and training, ambulance network, and STEMI coordinator.

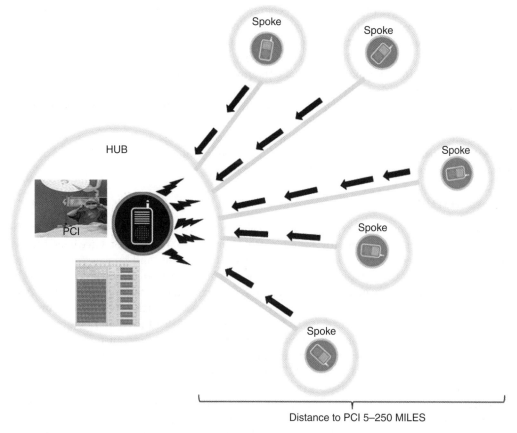

Figure 26.5 The Lumen Americas Telemedicine Infarct Network hub and spokes model. PCI, percutaneous coronary intervention.

Site activation was meticulous and included telemedicine hardware and software platform installation; incorporation of LATIN telemedicine protocols; standardization of transmission methodology; establishing three-way communication channels between telemedicine center, hub, and spoke; feedback pathways; creating reliable ambulance network; Lumen STEMI training; verification of emergency department bypass capabilities; and mandated trial runs. Different challenges were encountered in establishing LATIN centers in Brazil and Colombia. In Brazil, the largest constraint arose from bureaucratic delays although adoption of telemedicine protocol was smooth and gratifying. In addition, establishing telemedicine technology was seamless in Brazil where we encountered early adopters of the technology. LATIN centers in Colombia have been challenged by insurance hurdles, technology gaps, lack of intensive care beds, and an overall slow adoption of technology. A total of six LATIN centers were discontinued as they had inadequate telecommunication capabilities, lacked reliable ambulance transfer, and had low enrollment. Additional requests for approximately 30 new centers are being evaluated. Plans are also underway for expansion of LATIN in Mexico.

LATIN Protocol

Although the LATIN protocol has only required minor revisions, there has been an overall change in strategy. This revision has sought more PPCI than thrombolytic therapy or pharmacoinvasive management, which was proposed after recognizing massive delays to thrombolytic adminis-tration, use of first-generation thrombolytics, and delayed presentation. As opposed to the very narrow window of opportunity for treating patients with thrombolytic therapy, the longer treatment time of 12 hours for PPCI was particularly advantageous. This latter observation was more pronounced in Colombia. Individual personnel were trained at each hub and spoke, and the essential components of the LATIN protocol were incorporated into a standardized AMI management strategy. Standardization was exceptionally challenging, as it required adminis-trative changes at most hubs and spokes. In several cases, this required structural realignment of emergency rooms, ambulance notification, allocation of triage nurses, and the creation of STEMI coordinators. In addition to the scientific incorporation of the LATIN STEMI protocols, a gradual adoption of a 24/7 STEMI culture was affected.

Telemedicine Platform

Standardized equipment and software, web-based protocols, backup trans-telephonic meth-odology, continuous quality initiatives, and text-message (SMS) notification have been the five essential LATIN technology components installed at each hub and spoke. An innovative STEMI parameter of transmission to telemedicine diagnosis has been established, and it is the single, best parameter to measure the efficiency and accuracy of telemedicine-based AMI management. Telemedicine diagnosis is scrupulously followed at each LATIN site. It involves three critical components: Immediate transmission of the 12-lead EKG and clinical history form from the spoke; processing, filtration, and standardization of the transmission EKG into a telemedicine STEMI vector; and simultaneous, dual SMS notification of the EKG diagnosis to the hub and spoke. The 84 active LATIN centers have been connected to 3 telemedicine hubs from where expert cardiologists perform 24/7 LATIN telemedicine diagnoses and tele-consultation. These LATIN telemedicine hubs are located in Bogota, Colombia, São Paulo, Brazil, and Santiago, Chile. Each LATIN EKG is assigned a red alert priority, and the remote cardiologist is immediately notified. Training of telemedicine cardiologists is an ongoing initiative that incorporates all aspects of the Lumen process and procedure protocols. This particular educational activity has been performed on a monthly basis. Each LATIN expert cardiologist undergoes rigorous quality assurance.

Ambulance Networks

Creation of reliable ambulance networks has been the single most daunting task during the pilot phase of LATIN. It has required local, state, and even federal changes of healthcare delivery to individual hospitals. Often, this task was further complicated by cumbersome insurance directives. In terms of LATIN time and resource allocation, this task has required the greatest commitment. These challenges were present equally in Brazil and Colombia. In both countries, there was a complete absence of intelligent, organized ambulance networks, including a lack of ambulances, lack of paramedics, and lack of ambulance notification path-ways. An entirely new STEMI process was created by LATIN. This included the following six-step process:

1) immediate triage of a patient with chest pain;
2) urgent 12-lead EKG;
3) transmission of EKG and clinical history form to telemedicine center;
4) receipt of expert-guided accurate EKG diagnosis for immediate ambulance notification;
5) LATIN hub alert;
6) medical stabilization and transfer of patients.

Not only have ambulance availability and delays been a constraint during the LATIN pilot phase, but we also anticipate these to be ongoing future challenges in both countries. It is a deep appreciation of this particular constraint that has raised the goals of LATIN. Creating efficient ambulance networks within the LATIN population has now emerged as a top goal for this program. Several protocol, strategy, and logistic improvements are now being considered, which will further streamline ambulance operations. These include LATIN training for paramedics and incorporation of LATIN hardware and platforms in individual ambulances.

STEMI Procedure

The following components of the LATIN procedure have been individually taught to all LATIN interventional cardiologists: early dual antiplatelet therapy; preference for transradial access; 6 Fr arterial access sheaths; obtaining complete angiographic studies including angiography of non-culprit vessel; selection of appropriate guiding catheter and guide wires; compulsive selective thrombectomy techniques based on thrombus grade; bare-metal or drug-eluting stents; intracoronary vasodilators; quick assessment of left ventricular function; early sheath removal and ambulation.

Using the above five steps of LATIN, 601 patients have been treated during the pilot phase of LATIN; 374 patients in Brazil and 227 patients in Colombia; 91% of the patients were treated with PPCI. Hospital Santa Marcelina in São Paulo, Brazil, and the CAMINO Universitario Distrital Adelita de Char in Barranquilla, Colombia, have been the largest enrollers. Mean time to telemedicine diagnosis of 5.8 minutes was achieved. The extremely difficult and meticulous process of collecting data across 84 centers in 19 cities and 2 countries is in progress.

Discussion

Current methods for ambulance pre-hospital triage and transfer of PPCI with a mandated door-to-balloon time of less than 90 minutes are hampered by several drawbacks [23]. Pre-hospital triage with in-ambulance personnel either, advanced paramedics (Ottawa, Canada) or physicians (France) is clearly an inefficient and expensive method that has not gained greater acceptance globally. The current wireless transmission models use a software-only diagnosis of AMI, heavily hampered by both false positive and false negative results [24]. The telemedicine model, in contrast, obtains a 12-lead EKG for real-time interpretation by a cardiologist, thus avoiding delays and ensuring accuracy [25]. The carefully designed platforms and network of dedicated cardiologists at the other end of the transmission make telemedicine an attractive option [26]. Figure 26.6 compares the three pathways of triage.

Telemedicine (ITMS, Inc.) has developed an EKG device with multi-port transmission capabilities, a patented telemedicine-integrated platform with its own network and server support. Each EKG received is vectored into a standard format with correct dimensions, crucial for accurately reading QT interval. The standardization of an EKG makes it ready for the electronic medical record (EMR) and coding compatible with the billing system and with the International Statistical Classification of Diseases and Related Health Problems, 10th edition. This vectoring, if performed on mobile phones with third party software, is much more time consuming. The telemedicine platform also takes painstaking measures to be HIPPA compliant, while ensuring security of transmission and including time stamps and confirmation of receipt for record keeping. A massive staff of accredited cardiologists is scheduled on shifts to maintain 24/7 availability for immediate EKG interpretation. Trained personnel perform a preliminary filter based on urgency of the received EKG's to further streamline the process.

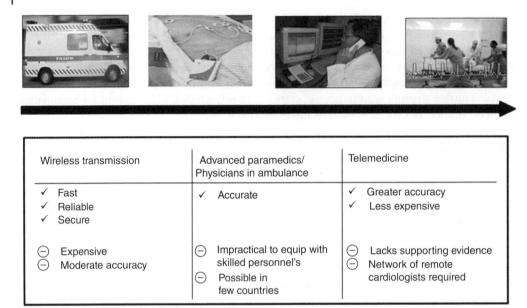

Wireless transmission	Advanced paramedics/ Physicians in ambulance	Telemedicine
✓ Fast ✓ Reliable ✓ Secure	✓ Accurate	✓ Greater accuracy ✓ Less expensive
⊖ Expensive ⊖ Moderate accuracy	⊖ Impractical to equip with skilled personnel's ⊖ Possible in few countries	⊖ Lacks supporting evidence ⊖ Network of remote cardiologists required

Figure 26.6 Comparison of three methods of pre-hospital diagnosis and triage.

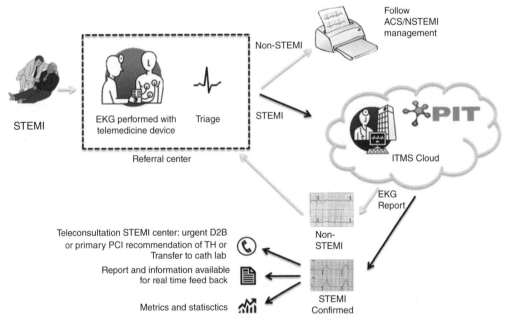

Figure 26.7 ITMS Telemedicine ST-elevation myocardial infarction (STEMI) diagnosis and triage. ACS, acute coronary syndrome; Cath Lab, catheterization laboratory; EKG, electrocardiogram; PCI, percutaneous coronary intervention; PIT, Platform Integrated Telemedicine; TH, thrombolysis.

Figure 26.7 highlights the advantages of the ITMS telemedicine platform, where each EKG is interpreted with maximum accuracy, stored in a robust database, and immediately compatible with other healthcare facilities' medical records. Finally, the cost of telemedicine devices (ITMS, Inc.) is considerably less than the cost of standard wireless transmission devices.

Understanding the prevalent modes of telecommunication as they pertain to AMI management is imperative to evaluate telemedicine as an effective strategy for global AMI management.
Present modes of inter-physician and inter-facility transportation include telephone conversation, FAX, wireless communication and telemedicine. Telemedicine ensures rapid and clear
communication on the status of AMI patient, who may require careful management of his or her
life-threatening complications or critical condition during the lengthy transport from emergency
rooms to catheterization laboratories. From our present understanding of the various modalities,
telemedicine affords distinct advantages as a comprehensive strategy for facilitating AMI
communications for seamless navigating through a STEMI process and the STEMI procedure.

Telemedicine provides comprehensive management of AMI by facilitating thrombolytic
therapy, pharmacoinvasive management and PPCI with mandated door-to-balloon times. In
the thrombolytic pathway, the critical function of teleconsultation provides the less appreciated and cost-effective benefits of remote consultation [28]. The reviewer or remote consultant
obtains a clearer history from the recipient physician and guides the latter through an urgent
triage into a thrombolytic or a PPCI pathway [29], the current bottleneck in STEMI care. As
timeliness is of critical importance in STEMI intervention, it is immensely valuable to triage
the patient scientifically, cost effectively and rapidly through either a mandated door-to-needle
time or a door-to-balloon time with this remote but prompt discussion [30,31]. The consultation
primarily uses the following criteria:

- Thrombolysis is indicated by a very early presentation (less than 3 hours from symptom
  onset), long transfer times (less than 90 minutes to reach PCI facility) for PPCI, unavailability
  of PPCI and no contraindications for thrombolytic therapy.
- P PCI is guided by presentation within 12 hours from the onset of chest pain, contraindication to thrombolytic therapy, presentation with cardiogenic shock and transfer times of less
  than 90 minutes.

Limitations

The potential of teleconsultation for advancing the pharmacoinvasive management is not as
prominent, as local cardiologists are often involved with the management of the case by this
stage under less time constraint. Yet, discussions are likely to contribute to better clinical management and more efficient transfer. Often repeat EKGs are also compared during this process,
where having consultative options may aid the decision process.

While the proposed LATIN study will test the practicality and effectiveness of a STEMI
network with deep integration of telemedicine and will make observations on its most useful
features, applying such a controlled system to the Latin American region at large will be
challenging. In areas with a severely lacking ambulance service, the transfer of patients for PCI
still requires fundamental improvements in infrastructure. Public health mandates will be
essential to ensure that scientifically proven guidelines being followed uniformly. Finally, financial inadequacy will still preclude patients from accessing proper treatment without increased
insurance coverage and public healthcare expenditure.

Conclusions

Major inequalities exist in the care of AMI in developed and developing countries. Telemedicine
provides a strong rationale for reducing these differences. LATIN provides the world's first and
comprehensive population-based AMI strategy that uses telemedicine to provide global AMI care.
LATIN may be the revolutionary start to bridging the gap between the disparate levels of AMI care.

References

1 Henry TD, Atkins JM, Cunningham MS, et al. ST elevation myocardial infarction: recommendations on triage of patients to cardiovascular centers of excellence. *J Am Coll Cardiol*, 2006; 47: 1339–1345.

2 Ting HH, Rihal CS, Gersh BJ, et al. Regional systems of care to optimize timeliness of reperfusion therapy for ST-elevation myocardial infarction: the Mayo Clinic STEMI protocol. *Circulation*, 2007; 116: 729–736.

3 Ayrik C, Ergene U, Kinay O, et al. Factors influencing emergency department arrival time and in-hospital management of patients with acute myocardial infarction. *Adv Ther*, 2006; 23: c244–c255.

4 Morrison LJ, Verbeek PR, McDonald AC, et al. Mortality and pre-hospital thrombolysis for acute myocardial infarction: a meta-analysis. *JAMA*, 2000; 283: 2686–2692.

5 Brunetti ND, De Gennaro L, Dellegrottaglie G, et al. A regional prehospital electrocardiogram network with a single telecardiology "Hhb" for public emergency medical service: technical requirements, logistics, manpower, and preliminary results. *Telemed e-Health*, 2011; 17: 727–733.

6 Sejersten M, Sillesen M, Hansen PR, et al. Effect on treatment delay of prehospital teletransmission of 12-lead electrocardiogram to a cardiologist for immediate triage and direct referral of patients with ST- segment elevation acute myocardial infarction to primary percutaneous coronary intervention. *Am J Cardiol*, 2008; 101: 941–946.

7 Pan American Health Organization, *Health in the Americas*. Washington, DC: Pan American Health Organization; 2012.

8 Pan American Health Organization. Health Indicators Database. Basic indicator browser: Indicators by countries and years. http://ais.paho.org/phip/viz/indicatorsbycountryandyears.asp. (accessed March 27, 2017).

9 Ingarfield SL, Jacobs IG, Jelinek GA, et al. Patient delay and use of ambulance by patients with chest pain. *Emerg Med Austr*, 2005; 17: 218–223.

10 Mehta S, Kostela JC, Oliveros E, et al. Global acute myocardial infarction perspectives: Beyond door-to-balloon interventions. *Interv Cardiology Clin*, 2012; 1: 479–484.

11 Solla, DJF, de Mattos Paiva Filho I, Delisle JE, et al. Integrated regional networks for ST-Segment Elevation Myocardial Infarction care in developing countries the experience of Salvador, Bahia, Brazil. *Circulation*, 2013; 6(1): 9–17.

12 McCabe, JM, Armstrong, EJ, Kulkarni, A, et al. Prevalence and factors associated with false-positive ST-Segment Elevation Myocardial Infarction diagnoses at Primary Percutaneous Coronary intervention-capable centers, a report from the Activate-SF Registry. *Arch Intern Med*, 2012; 172(11): 864–871.

13 Thuresson M, Berglin Jarlöv M, Lindahl B, et al. Factors that influence the use of ambulance in acute coronary syndrome. *Am Heart J*, 2008; 156: 170–176.

14 Herlitz J, Thuresson M, Svensson L, et al. Factors of importance for patients' decision time in acute coronary syndrome. *Int J Cardiol*, 2010; 141: 236–242.

15 Antman EM, Anbe DT, Armstrong PW, et al. ACC/AHA guidelines for the management of patients with ST-elevation myocardial infarction: executive summary. A report of the American College of Cardiology/American Heart Association Task Force on Practice Guidelines (Writing Committee to Revise the 1999 Guidelines for the Management of Patients With Acute Myocardial Infarction). *Circulation*, 2004; 110: 588–636.

16 Antman EM, Hand M, Armstrong PW, et al. Focused update of the ACC/AHA 2004 guidelines for the management of patients with ST-elevation myocardial infarction: a report of the American College of Cardiology/American Heart Association Task Force on Practice Guidelines. *Circulation*, 2008; 117: 296–329.

17 Terkelsen CJ, Lassen JF, Nørgaard BL, et al. Reduction of treatment delay in patients with ST-elevation myocardial infarction: impact of pre-.hospital diagnosis and direct referral to primary percutanous coronary intervention. *Eur Heart J*, 2005; 26: 770–777.

18 Brunetti, ND, De Gennaro, L, Amodio, et al. Telecardiology improves quality of diagnosis and reduces delay to treatment in elderly patients with acute myocardial infarction and atypical presentation. *Eur J Cardiovasc Prev Rehab*, 2010; 17(6): 615–620.

19 Rokos, IC, Larson, DM, Henry, TD, et al. Rationale for establishing regional ST-elevation myocardial infarction receiving center (SRC) networks. *Am Heart J*, 2006; 152(4): 661–667.

20 Ting HH, Krumholz HM, Bradley EH, et al. Implementation and integration of prehospital ECGs into systems of care for acute coronary syndrome: a Scientific Statement from the American Heart Association Interdisciplinary Council on Quality of Care and Outcomes Research, Emergency Cardiovascular Care Committee, Council on Cardiovascular Nursing, and Council on Clinical Cardiology. *Circulation*, 2008; 118: 1066–1079.

21 Brown JP, Mahmud E, Dunford JV, et al. Effect of prehospital 12-lead electrocardiogram on activation of the cardiac catheterization laboratory and door-to-balloon time in ST-segment elevation acute myocardial infarction. *Am J Cardiol*, 2008; 101: 158–161.

22 Gershlick AH, Stephens-Lloyd A, Hughes S, et al. for the REACT Trial Investigators Rescue angioplasty after failed thrombolytic therapy for acute myocardial infarction. *N Engl J Med*, 2005; 353: 2758–2768.

23 Amit G, Cafri C, Gilutz H, et al. Benefit of direct ambulance to coronary care unit admission of acute myocardial infarction patients undergoing primary percutaneous intervention. *Int J Cardiol*, 2007; 119: 355–358.

24 Schoos MM, Sejersten M, Hvelplund A, et al. Reperfusion delay in patients treated with primary percutaneous coronary intervention: insight from a real world Danish ST-segment elevation myocardial infarction population in the era of telemedicine. *Eur Heart J*, 2012; 1(3): 200–209.

25 Le May MR, Davies RF, Labinaz M. Hospitalization costs of primary stenting versus thrombolysis in acute myocardial infarction: cost analysis of the Canadian STAT Study. *Circulation*, 2003; 108: 2624–2630.

26 Ilczak T, Mikulska M. Telematic systems in emergency medical services, applied in treatment of acute coronary syndrome of STEMI type. In Mikulski J. (ed.) *Telematics in the Transport Environment 2012* (Communications in Computer and Information Science, vol. 329), pp. 87–93. Heidelburg: Springer; 2012.

27 Steg PG, Cambou JP, Goldstein P, et al. Bypassing the emergency room reduces delays and mortality in ST elevation myocardial infarction: the USIC 2000 registry. *Heart*, 2006; 92: 1378–1383.

28 Hailey D, Ohinmaa A, Roine R. Published evidence on the success of telecardiology: A mixed record. *J Telemed Telecare*, 2004; 10: 36–38.

29 Clemmensen, P, Loumann-Nielsen, S, Sejersten, M. Telemedicine fighting acute coronary syndromes. *J Electrocardiol*, 2010; 43(6): 615–618.

30 Welsh RC, Westerhout CM, Buller CE, et al. Anticoagulation after subcutaneous enoxaparin is time sensitive in STEMI patients treated with tenecteplase. *J Thromb Thrombol*, 2012; 34(1): 126–131.

31 Bhatt D. Timely PCI for STEMI – Still the treatment of Choice. *N Engl J Med*, 2013; 368: 1446–1447.

32 Wu AH, Parsons L, Every NR, et al; Second National Registry of Myocardial Infarction. Hospital outcomes in patients presenting with congestive heart failure complicating acute myocardial infarction: A report from the Second National Registry of Myocardial Infarction (NRMI-2). *J Am Coll Cardiol*, 2002; 40(8): 1389–1394.

Part V

Future Perspectives

27

STEMI Interventions, Beyond the Culprit Lesion

Neil Ruparelia PhD MRCP, Antonio Colombo MD, Azeem Latib MD

Introduction

Primary percutaneous coronary intervention (PPCI) of the culprit infarct-related artery (IRA) in a timely manner is the reperfusion therapy of choice for patients presenting with ST-elevation myocardial infarction (STEMI) [1,2]. While the decision to treat the culprit lesion in the acute setting is usually uncomplicated, the best treatment strategy for significant 'bystander' coronary lesions has yet to be established.

The Clinical Conundrum

The treatment of the culprit artery with PPCI in the acute setting for STEMI has been unequivocally demonstrated to be the reperfusion therapy of choice [1]. However, 40–70% of patients present with significant coronary disease which extends beyond the culprit vessel [3], as illustrated by the case example in Figure 27.1. The debate over the optimal management of non-culprit lesions in the emergency setting of STEMI has arisen due to observations that a conservative approach may be advantageous for the management of stable lesions [4]. However, the presence of significant non-culprit coronary lesions is associated with higher mortality rates, a higher incidence of recurrent myocardial infarction and worse prognosis [5,6] following STEMI. These patients may therefore represent a different clinical group to stable patients with no prior history of plaque rupture and acute vessel occlusion. The reasons for this are multifactorial and include plaque instability at sites beyond that in the culprit vessel [7], greater ischemic burden and impaired contractility of remote zones in the presence of significant untreated coronary disease [6].

By performing multivessel percutaneous coronary intervention (MV-PCI) in the acute setting, any concerns with regards to bystander lesion instability are immediately addressed, and at the same time obviate the requirement for further procedures resulting in reduced hospital stay and associated cost. On the other hand, these advantages are offset by the risks associated with longer procedure times, increased contrast doses and increased procedural complexity in patients that may be hemodynamically unstable in the setting of a biologically milieu of proinflammatory and prothrombotic mediators that may predispose the patients to subsequent stent thrombosis [8,9]. Additionally, in the acute setting of STEMI, the severity of non-culprit lesions is often overestimated, with up to 40% of these lesions not being hemodynamically significant when assessed by fractional flow reserve at follow-up [10] and may result in patients being treated unnecessarily without the benefit.

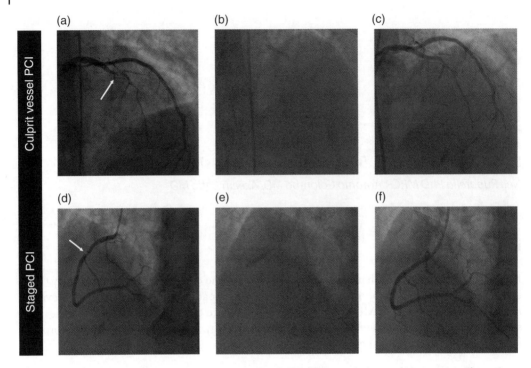

(a) (b) (c)

(d) (e) (f)

Culprit vessel PCI

Staged PCI

Figure 27.1 Staged percutaneous coronary intervention (PCI) following culprit vessel intervention. The patient presented with posterior ST-elevation myocardial infarction. The patient proceeded to primary percutaneous coronary intervention and the culprit vessel was identified as the left anterior descending artery (arrow, a). This was treated successfully with the implantation of a 3.0 × 18 mm drug-eluting stent (b), with an excellent final result (c). The patient was hemodynamically stable and the critical bystander lesion in the right coronary artery (d) was successfully treated as a staged procedure 6 weeks after the index procedure with the implantation of a 3.0 × 23 mm drug-eluting stent (e), with an excellent final angiographic result (f). By current evidence, the lesions in the right coronary artery could have been treated during the index procedure or admission.

In summary, there are a number of possible management strategies following culprit vessel PCI for the treatment of non-culprit 'bystander' coronary lesions, and these include:

- MV-PCI in the acute setting;
- staged PCI to the non-culprit lesion(s) during the same hospital admission;
- staged PCI to the non-culprit lesion(s) in the weeks or months after the acute event;
- medical therapy only, with revascularization of non-culprit lesions if clinically indicated.

Current Evidence

The current guidelines from the European Society of Cardiology (ESC) [11], and the American College of Cardiology (ACC)/American Heart Association (AHA) are summarized in Table 27.1. Both these guidelines strongly support the treatment of the culprit artery only in patients who are hemodynamically stable, with a staged approach for the management of non-culprit lesions and are predominantly based upon results from retrospective registry data with few data coming from randomized controlled trials.

Table 27.1 Current guidelines for the management of non-culprit bystander coronary lesions.

Guideline	Recommendation	Class	Level
European Society of Cardiology [11]	PPCI should be limited to the culprit vessel with the exception of cardiogenic shock and persistent ischemia after PCI of the supposed culprit lesion.	IIa	B
	Staged revascularization of non-culprit lesions should be considered in STEMI with multivessel disease in case of symptoms or ischemia within days to weeks after PPCI.	IIa	B
	Immediate revascularization of significant non-culprit lesions during the same procedure as PPCI of the culprit vessel may be considered in selected patients.	IIb	B
American College of Cardiology/American Heart Association	PCI should not be performed in a non-infarct artery at the time of PPCI in patients with STEMI who are hemodynamically stable.	III	B
	PCI is reasonable in a non-infarct artery at a time separate from PPCI in patients who have spontaneous symptoms of myocardial ischemia.	I	C
	PCI is reasonable in a non-infarct artery at a time separate from PPCI in patients with intermediate or high-risk findings on noninvasive testing.	IIa	B

PCI, percutaneous coronary intervention; PPCI, primary PCI; STEMI: ST-elevation myocardial infarction.

Retrospective Studies

Retrospective studies have reported contradictory findings with regards to the best management strategy of non-culprit lesions. In the HORIZONS-AMI (Harmonizing Outcomes with RevasculariZatiON and Stents in Acute Myocardial Infarction) trial [12], PCI of the non-culprit vessel at the time of PPCI was associated with a higher 1-year mortality (9.2% vs. 2.3%, $P < 0.0001$), cardiac mortality (6.2% vs. 2.0%, $P = 0.005$) and stent thrombosis rate (5.7% vs. 2.3%, $P = 0.02$) when compared with a staged approach, which supported findings from other retrospective clinical studies [13,14]. However, other smaller studies have suggested MV-PCI may be safely performed and be associated with some benefit [15,16].

Prospective Studies

A number of prospective randomized studies have been carried out to further clarify the optimal strategy in this patient group and are summarized in Table 27.2. The PRAMI (Preventative Angioplasty in Acute Myocardial Infarction) study [17] was a multicenter prospective randomized trial that enrolled 465 patients with STEMI who underwent culprit vessel PCI and then were subsequently randomized to MV-PCI ($n = 234$) of any additional angiographically significant lesion (> 50% angiographic stenosis) or no additional intervention ($n = 231$). Patients with cardiogenic shock, previous coronary artery bypass grafting, and non-infarct chronic total occlusions were excluded. Over the 23-month follow-up period, the combined incidence of cardiac death, nonfatal myocardial infraction and refractory angina occurred in 21 MV-PCI patients and 53 patients treated with a strategy of culprit vessel only PCI (CO-PCI), which translated to a significant 65% relative reduction in this combined endpoint. These results were predominantly driven by a 65% reduction in refractory angina and a 68% reduction in non-fatal myocardial infarction. However, this study was underpowered and the event rate in the control arm was very high (possibly as a result of the open-label nature of the study), while the "intermediate" option of

Table 27.2 Prospective clinical trials of the management of non-culprit bystander coronary lesions.

Study	Design	Patients (n)	Groups	In-hospital mortality	Long-term mortality	Other outcomes
Di Mario et al. [31]	Multicenter RCT	69	CO-PCI, MV-PCI	CO-PCI: 0% vs. MV-PCI: 1.9%, $P = 0.754$	1 year CO-PCI: 0% vs. MV-PCI: 1.9%, $P = 0.754$	MACE (1 year): CO-PCI: 35.3% vs. MV-PCI: 21.1% ($p = 0.33$). Repeat revascularization or CABG: CO-PCI: 35.3% vs. MV-PCI: 17.3%; $P = 0.174$.
Politi et al. [32]	Single-center RCT	214	CO-PCI, staged PCI, MV-PCI, CO-PCI	8.3% vs. staged PCI: 0% vs. MV-PCI: 3.1%, $P = 0.037$	2.5 years CO-PCI: 15.5% vs. staged PCI: 6.2% vs. MV-PCI: 9.2%, $P = 0.17$	MACE (2.5 years): CO-PCI: 50.0% vs. staged-PCI: 20.0% vs. MV-PCI: 23.1%; $P < 0.001$). Repeat revascularization: CO-PCI: 33.3% vs. staged PCI: 12.3% vs. MV-PCI: 9.2%; $P < 0.001$.
PRAMI [17]	Multicenter RCT	465	CO-PCI, MV-PCI	Not reported	23 months: MV-PCI: 1.7% vs. CO-PCI: 2.6%, $P = 0.86$	Non-cardiac mortality (3 years): MV-PCI: 3.4% vs. CO-PCI: 2.6%; $P = 0.86$. Repeat revascularization: MV-PCI: 16% vs. CO-PCI: 19.9% (HR: 0.30, 95% CI 0.17–0.56; $P < 0.001$).
CVLPRIT [18]	Multicenter RCT	296	CO-PCI, MV-PCI (in hospital)	Not reported	1 year: MV-PCI: 2.7% vs. CO-PCI: 6.9%, $P = 0.09$	Time to first MACE (1 year): MV-PCI: 10% vs. CO-PCI: 21.2% (HR:0.45, 95% CI 0.24–0.84; $P = 0.009$). Repeat revascularization: MV-PCI: 5.3% vs. CO-PCI: 11.0% (HR 0.46, 95% CI 0.20–1.08; $P = 0.07$).

CABG, coronary artery bypass grafts; CI, confidence interval; CO-PCI, culprit-only percutaneous coronary intervention; HR, hazard ratio; MACE, major adverse cardiovascular events; MV-PCI, multivessel percutaneous coronary intervention; RCT: randomized controlled trial.

a staged-PCI approach was not tested. Importantly, in patients who underwent MV-PCI in the acute setting, there was no increase in stent thrombosis.

The more recent CVLPRIT (the Complete Versus Lesion-only PRImary PCI Trial) [18] study did have a staged 'PCI' arm; 296 patients were randomized to either in-hospital revascularization (n = 150), which mandated MV-PCI during hospital admission (either at the time of STEMI or "staged" but during the same admission), or to CO-PCI revascularization (n = 146). The primary endpoint was a composite of all-cause death, recurrent myocardial infarction, heart failure and ischemic-driven revascularization within 12 months. The primary endpoint occurred in 10.0% of the MV-PCI group compared with 21.2% in the CO-PCI group (hazard ratio, HR 0.45, 0.24–0.84; P = 0.009). However, while there was a trend toward an improvement in each of the primary endpoints, there was no statistically significant difference between groups with regards to death or myocardial infarction.

Both of these well-conducted trials indicate that MV-PCI is not harmful and may even be associated with benefit, although due to their modest size it is still unclear if this approach is associated with improved survival and larger adequately powered trials are required to answer these remaining concerns.

Meta-Analyses

A number of meta-analyses have also been performed in a bid to resolve some of the uncertainties from these retrospective and prospective studies but again have reported conflicting results. A recent large meta-analysis conducted by Bainey et al. compared outcomes following MV-PCI in 7886 patients and CO-PCI in 38,438 patients [19]. They found that there was no significant difference in hospital mortality with MV-PCI compared with CO-PCI (odds ratio, OR, 1.11, 1.00–1.27; P = 0.6. However, MV-PCI at the index procedure was associated with a significant increase in hospital mortality (OR 1.35, 1.19–1.54; P < 0.001). When MV-PCI was performed as a staged procedure this was associated with lower hospital mortality (OR 0.35, 0.21–0.59; P < 0.001), reduced long-term mortality (OR 0.74, 0.65–0.85; P < 0.001) and repeat PCI (OR 0.65, 0.46–0.90, P = 0.01) suggesting that a staged PCI strategy may be beneficial in this patient group over MV-PCI in the acute setting.

On the other hand, a meta-analysis conducted by El-Hayek et al. looking at data obtained only from randomized controlled trials (RCT) and including both the PRAMI and CVLPRIT studies, compared 566 patients that underwent MV-PCI compared with 478 that underwent CO-PCI. MV-PCI was associated with a significant reduction in all-cause mortality (relative risk, RR, 0.57, 0.36–0.92; P = 0.02) and in cardiac death (RR 0.38, 0.20–0.73; P = 0.004) [20]. In addition, there was a significantly lower risk of recurrent myocardial infarction (RR 0.41, 0.23–0.75; P = 0.004) and future revascularization (RR 0.37, 0.27–0.52; P < 0.00001) supporting MV-PCI in the acute setting. These findings were supported by another meta-analysis of RCT that studies 628 patients treated with MV-PCI and 562 patients with CO-PCI only. MV-PCI resulted in a significant reduction in major adverse cardiac events (RR 0.57, 0.42–0.78; P < 0.001), which was driven by a lower risk of urgent revascularization in the MV-PCI group (RR 0.55, 0.35–0.86; P = 0.01) [21]. Owing to the uncertainties about the general applicability of the results of these studies to routine clinical practice, there are a number of larger prospective randomized studies in progress. These are summarized in Table 27.3 and discussed in further detail below.

Special Circumstances

Data from randomized trials and meta-analyses have included "uncomplicated" patients presenting with STEMI, where a number of different management strategies could be employed. However, there are certain clinical scenarios that deserve special attention.

Table 27.3 Current prospective clinical trials of the management of non-culprit bystander coronary lesions.

Study	Design	Patients	Groups	Primary endpoint	Follow-up duration (years)
DANAMI-3 [25]	Multi-center RCT	627	CO-PCI MV-PCI	All cause mortality, hospitalization for heart failure	2
PRAGUE-13 [26]	Multi-center RCT	400	CO-PCI and staged PCI CO-PCI	Death, non fatal MI, stroke	2
COMPLETE [27]	Multi-center RCT	3,900	CO-PCI and staged PCI CO-PCI	Cardiovascular death, myocardial infarction	4
COCUA [28]	Multi-center RCT	646	MV-PCI CO-PCI and staged PCI	Cardiac mortality, STEMI, target lesion revascularization	3
CROSS-AMI [30]	Multi-center RCT	400	CO-PCI and staged PCI during index admission COR and stress echo guided revascularization	Cardiovascular death, recurrent MI, any revascularization, hospitalization for heart failure	1
COMPARE-ACUTE [29]	Multi-center RCT	885	MV-PCI (FFR-guided) CO-PCI and FFR-guided staged PCI	All-cause mortality, nonfatal MI, any revascularization, stroke	3

CO-PCI, culprit only percutaneous coronary intervention; FFR: fractional flow reserve; MI, myocardial infarction; MV-PCI, multivessel percutaneous coronary intervention; PCI: percutaneous coronary intervention, RCT: randomized controlled trial; STEMI: ST-elevation myocardial infarction.

Cardiogenic Shock

A significant minority of patients present with STEMI in cardiogenic shock (as in the case example in Figure 27.2) and in these individuals a MV-PCI approach appears to be associated with improved outcomes. Data from the SHOCK (Should We Emergently Revascularize Occluded Coronaries for Cardiogenic Shock) trial provided a basis for complete revascularization where MV-PCI at the index event was associated with a significant reduction in mortality at 6-months (50.3% vs. 63.1%, $P = 0.027$) [22]. This approach was further supported by a 2015 meta-analysis that identified 386 patients treated with CO-PCI and 124 patients with MV-PCI who presented with STEMI in cardiogenic shock [23]. The MV-PCI approach resulted in a significantly lower adjusted risk of in-hospital mortality (9.3% vs. 2.4%, HR 0.263, 0.149–0.462; $P < 0.001$) and death from all causes (13.1% vs. 4.8%, HR 0.4, 0.264–0.606; $P < 0.001$). Additionally MV-PCI significantly decreased the adjusted risk of the composite endpoint of death from all causes, recurrent myocardial infarction and any revascularization (20.3% vs. 18.1%, HR 0.728, 0.55–0.965; $P = 0.026$).

The Presence of Ongoing Ischemia

As supported by the guidelines [11,24], after the treatment of the presumptive culprit lesion, treatment of 'bystander' lesions is indicated in the presence of ongoing ischemia (e.g. electro-cardiographic changes, patient symptoms).

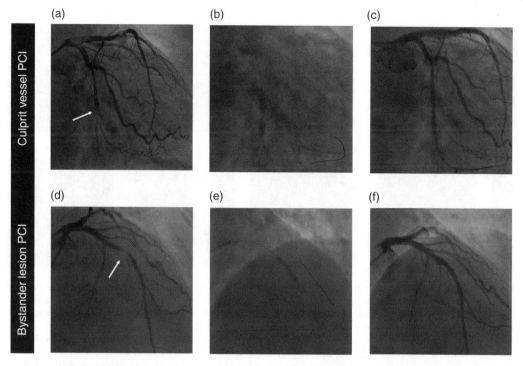

Figure 27.2 Multivessel percutaneous coronary intervention (PCI) in the setting of acute myocardial infarction with cardiogenic shock. The patient presented with an inferoposterior ST-elevation myocardial infarction and proceeded to emergency primary percutaneous coronary intervention. The culprit circumflex artery (arrow, a) was successfully treated with implantation of a 2.75 × 28 mm drug-eluting stent (b), with a good final angiographic result (c). In view of the hazy appearance of the critical mid left anterior descending artery lesion (arrow, d), this was treated at the index procedure with implantation of a 3.5 × 28 mm drug-eluting stent (e), with an excellent final angiographic result (f).

Unstable Lesions

Following treatment of the culprit vessel, because of the angiographic appearance of an unstable lesion (ulcerated plaque, hazy appearance, presence of thrombus) in a non-culprit lesion (Figure 27.3), it may also be appropriate to treat this lesion in an attempt to reduce the risk of a further acute plaque event.

Areas of Uncertainty

There are a number of areas of remaining uncertainty with regard to the optimal treatment of non-culprit lesions. While emergency MV-PCI might be necessary in some patients (e.g. cardiogenic shock), a staged approach may be beneficial in others. It is however, currently unclear when this second procedure should be performed and whether it should be deferred for a few days or longer. It is also unclear how best to identify patients (and lesions) in non-culprit arteries that would most benefit from treatment. Perhaps hemodynamic assessment with fractional flow reserve or the use of intravascular imaging with optical coherence tomography, intravascular ultrasound or even newer techniques, such as near infrared spectroscopy, may enable more accurate identification of vulnerable lesions and therefore may offer an advantage over angiography-only guided intervention.

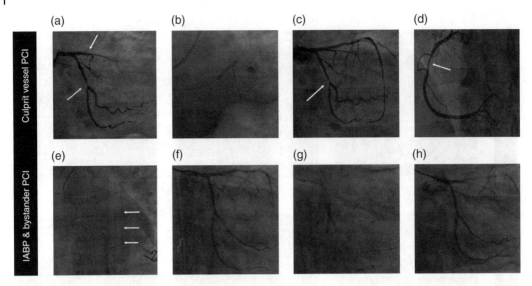

Figure 27.3 Multivessel percutaneous coronary intervention (PCI) following culprit vessel intervention due to unstable features of bystander disease. The patient presented as an emergency with anterior ST-elevation myocardial infarction with cardiogenic shock. Angiography revealed the left anterior descending artery to the culprit vessel (arrow, a), with a critical circumflex lesion (arrow, a). The patient proceeded to primary percutaneous coronary intervention of the left anterior descending artery with successful implantation of a 3.5 × 23 mm drug-eluting stent (DES, b) with an excellent result (c). The right coronary artery was noted to have mild atheroma only (d). In view of continuing hemodynamic instability, an intra-aortic balloon pump (IABP) was inserted (arrows, e), and the critical bystander disease (arrow, c) was treated (f) with implantation of a 3.0 × 38 mm DES with final kissing balloon post-dilatation (g) with an excellent final angiographic result (h).

In an attempt to answer some of these questions, a number of trials are currently being conducted and are summarized in Table 27.3. Studies including the DANAMI-3 (DANish study of optimal acute treatment of patients with ST-elevation Myocardial Infarction 3) trial [25], PRAGUE-13 [26] and COMPLETE [27] trials are testing whether or not to treat non-culprit lesions following successful PPCI of the culprit vessel, while the COCUA trial is investigating outcomes following acute MV-PCI versus staged PCI of the non-culprit vessel [28]. To investigate the role of coronary physiology in the revascularization of the non-culprit vessels, the COMPARE-ACUTE study is comparing fractional flow reserve (FFR)-guided revascularization versus angiographically guided intervention [29], and the CROSS-AMI study is investigating the role of non-invasive imaging (stress echocardiography) in guiding staged non-culprit vessel PCI [30].

Conclusions

Following successful treatment of the culprit lesion, it is clear that, in some patients, MV-PCI is associated with benefit. However this is not performed without risk, and there are no currently available tools that can help clinicians in selecting patients (and lesions) who would have most to benefit from this strategy. In view of the heterogeneity of patients presenting with STEMI, the final revascularization strategy should be decided upon on an individual basis, taking into account both the potential benefits and associated risks.

Based on the currently available evidence, a reasonable approach would be to treat the culprit lesion and to proceed immediately to MV-PCI in the presence of ongoing ischemia or cardiogenic shock. In patients who are hemodynamically stable, it would be acceptable to stop following treatment of the culprit vessel and defer treatment of bystander lesions. The timing of this staged procedure should be decided on an individual basis taking into account lesion severity, vascular access, left ventricular ejection fraction, renal function, bleeding risks and patient wishes.

Larger randomized studies are needed to further define the impact of MV-PCI on long-term clinical outcomes (specifically mortality), to determine the optimal timing of non-culprit vessel intervention and to identify patients who would have most to benefit from treatment of bystander coronary lesions.

References

1 Keeley EC, Boura JA, Grines CL. Primary angioplasty versus intravenous thrombolytic therapy for acute myocardial infarction: a quantitative review of 23 randomised trials. *Lancet*, 2003; 361(9351): 13–20.

2 De Luca G, Suryapranata H, Ottervanger JP, et al. Time delay to treatment and mortality in primary angioplasty for acute myocardial infarction: every minute of delay counts. *Circulation*, 2004; 109(10): 1223–1225.

3 Kahn JK, Rutherford BD, McConahay DR, et al. Results of primary angioplasty for acute myocardial infarction in patients with multivessel coronary artery disease. *J Am Coll Cardiol*, 1990; 16(5): 1089–1096.

4 Boden WE, O'Rourke RA, Teo KK, et al. Optimal medical therapy with or without PCI for stable coronary disease. *N Engl J Med*, 2007; 356(15): 1503–1516.

5 Sorajja P, Gersh BJ, Cox DA, et al. Impact of multivessel disease on reperfusion success and clinical outcomes in patients undergoing primary percutaneous coronary intervention for acute myocardial infarction. *Eur Heart J*, 2007; 28(14): 1709–1716.

6 Goldstein JA, Demetriou D, Grines CL, et al. Multiple complex coronary plaques in patients with acute myocardial infarction. *N Engl J Med*, 2000; 343(13): 915–322.

7 Stone GW, Maehara A, Lansky AJ, et al. A prospective natural-history study of coronary atherosclerosis. *N Engl J Med*, 2011; 364(3): 226–235.

8 Frangogiannis NG, Smith CW, Entman ML. The inflammatory response in myocardial infarction. *Cardiovasc Res*, 2002; 53(1): 31–47.

9 Katayama T, Nakashima H, Takagi C, et al. Predictors of sub-acute stent thrombosis in acute myocardial infarction patients following primary coronary stenting with bare metal stent. *Circ J*, 2006; 70(2): 151–155.

10 Dambrink JH, Debrauwere JP, van't Hof AW, et al. Non-culprit lesions detected during primary PCI: treat invasively or follow the guidelines? *EuroIntervention*, 2010; 5(8): 968–975.

11 Windecker S, Kolh P, Alfonso F, et al. 2014 ESC/EACTS guidelines on myocardial revascularization. *Eur Heart J*, 2014; 35(37): 2541–2619.

12 Kornowski R, Mehran R, Dangas G, et al. Prognostic impact of staged versus "one-time" multivessel percutaneous intervention in acute myocardial infarction: analysis from the HORIZONS-AMI (harmonizing outcomes with revascularization and stents in acute myocardial infarction) trial. *J Am Coll Cardiol*, 2011; 58(7): 704–11.

13 Toma M, Buller CE, Westerhout CM, et al. Non-culprit coronary artery percutaneous coronary intervention during acute ST-segment elevation myocardial infarction: insights from the APEX-AMI trial. *Eur Heart J*, 2010; 31(14): 1701–1707.

14 Hannan EL, Samadashvili Z, Walford G, et al. Culprit vessel percutaneous coronary intervention versus multivessel and staged percutaneous coronary intervention for ST-segment elevation myocardial infarction patients with multivessel disease. *JACC Cardiovasc Interv*, 2010; 3(1): 22–31.

15 Qarawani D, Nahir M, Abboud M, et al. Culprit only versus complete coronary revascularization during primary PCI. *Int J Cardiol*, 2008; B(3): 288–292.

16 Khattab AA, Abdel-Wahab M, Rother C, et al. Multi-vessel stenting during primary percutaneous coronary intervention for acute myocardial infarction. A single-center experience. *Clin Res Cardiol*, 2008; 97(1): 32–38.

17 Wald DS, Morris JK, Wald NJ, et al. Randomized trial of preventive angioplasty in myocardial infarction. *N Engl J Med*, 2013; 369(12): 1115–1123.

18 Gershlick AH, Khan JN, Kelly DJ, et al. Randomized Trial of Complete Versus Lesion-Only Revascularization in Patients Undergoing Primary Percutaneous Coronary Intervention for STEMI and Multivessel Disease: The CvLPRIT Trial. *J Am Coll Cardiol*, 2015; 65(10): 963–972.

19 Bainey KR, Mehta SR, Lai T, et al. Complete vs culprit-only revascularization for patients with multivessel disease undergoing primary percutaneous coronary intervention for ST-segment elevation myocardial infarction: a systematic review and meta-analysis. *Am Heart J*, 2014; 167(1): 1–14 e2.

20 El-Hayek GE, Gershlick AH, Hong MK, et al. Meta-Analysis of Randomized Controlled Trials Comparing Multivessel Versus Culprit-Only Revascularization for Patients With ST-Segment Elevation Myocardial Infarction and Multivessel Disease Undergoing Primary Percutaneous Coronary Intervention. *Am J Cardiol*, 2015; 115(11): 1481–1486.

21 Elgendy IY, Huo T, Mahmoud A, et al. Complete versus culprit-only revascularization in patients with multi-vessel disease undergoing primary percutaneous coronary intervention: A meta-analysis of randomized trials. *Int J Cardiol*, 2015; 186: 98–103.

22 Hochman JS, Sleeper LA, Webb JG, et al. Early revascularization in acute myocardial infarction complicated by cardiogenic shock. SHOCK Investigators. Should We Emergently Revascularize Occluded Coronaries for Cardiogenic Shock. *N Engl J Med*, 1999; 341(9): 625–634.

23 Park JS, Cha KS, Lee DS, et al. Culprit or multivessel revascularisation in ST-elevation myocardial infarction with cardiogenic shock. *Heart*, 2015; 101(15): 1225–1232.

24 O'Gara PT, Kushner FG, Ascheim DD, et al. 2013 ACCF/AHA guideline for the management of ST-elevation myocardial infarction: executive summary: a report of the American College of Cardiology Foundation/American Heart Association Task Force on Practice Guidelines. *J Am Coll Cardiol*, 2013; 61(4): 485–510.

25 Hofsten DE, Kelbaek H, Helqvist S, et al. The Third DANish Study of Optimal Acute Treatment of Patients with ST-segment Elevation Myocardial Infarction: Ischemic postconditioning or deferred stent implantation versus conventional primary angioplasty and complete revascularization versus treatment of culprit lesion only: Rationale and design of the DANAMI 3 trial program. *Am Heart J*, 2015; 169(5): 613–621.

26 Multivessel coronary disease diagnosed at the time of primary PCI for STEMI: complete revascularization versus conservative strategy (PRAGUE 13). ClinicalTrials.gov. Available at https://clinicaltrials.gov/ct2/show/NCT01332591 (accessed March 26, 2017).

27 Complete versus culprit-only revascularization to treat multivessel disease after primary PCI for STEMI (COMPLETE). ClinicalTrials.gov. Available at https://clinicaltrials.gov/ct2/show/NCT01740479 (accessed March 26, 2017).

28 Complete lesion versus culprit lesion revascularization (COCUA). ClinicalTrials.gov. Available at https://clinicaltrials.gov/ct2/show/NCT01180218 (accessed March 26, 2017).

29 Comparison between FFR guided revascularization versus conventional strategy in acute STEMI patients with MVD. (COMPARE-ACUTE). ClinicalTrials.gov. Available at https://clinicaltrials.gov/ct2/show/NCT01399736 (accessed March 26, 2017).

30 Strategies of revascularization in patients with ST-segment elevation myocardial infarction (STEMI) and multivessel disease (CROSS-AMI). ClinicalTrials.gov. Available at https://clinicaltrials.gov/ct2/show/NCT01179126/(accessed March 26, 2017).

31 Di Mario C, Mara S, Flavio A, et al. Single vs multivessel treatment during primary angioplasty: results of the multicentre randomised HEpacoat for cuLPrit or multivessel stenting for Acute Myocardial Infarction (HELP AMI) Study. *Int J Cardiovasc Interv*, 2004; 6(3–4): 128–133.

32 Politi L, Sgura F, Rossi R, et al. A randomised trial of target-vessel versus multi-vessel revascularisation in ST-elevation myocardial infarction: major adverse cardiac events during long-term follow-up. *Heart*, 2010; 96(9): 662–667.

28

Promising Technologies for STEMI Interventions
Joshua PY Loh MD, HC Tan

Introduction

Stenting is recommended over balloon angioplasty for patients undergoing primary percutaneous coronary intervention (PPCI) and new-generation drug-eluting stents (DES) are recommended over bare-metal stents (BMS) under the latest 2014 European guidelines on myocardial revascularization [1]. Evidence has suggested that the new-generation everolimus -eluting stent (EES) is superior to first generation sirolimus-eluting stents (SES) in reducing major acute vascular events in patients with ST-elevation myocardial infarction (STEMI) [2]. However, new technologies emerging in the stent industry, such as the pro-healing endothelial progenitor capture stent and bioresorbable scaffold, may provide new treatment options in the choice of stent during primary PCI.

Endothelial Progenitor Cell Capture Stent

The endothelial progenitor cell (EPC) capture stent (Genous™ stent) is a stainless steel bioactive stent coated with covalently bound murine monoclonal anti-human CD34 antibodies (Figure 28.1). The target of these antibodies is the CD34 antigen, which is a hematopoietic stem/progenitor cell marker expressed on the surface of EPCs. The EPC capture stent is designed to attract CD34-positive cells, which include EPCs, from the coronary circulation. The captured EPCs have the ability to differentiate and establish a functioning endothelial cell layer over the stent. Preclinical studies demonstrate complete coverage of the EPC capture stent by a functioning layer of endothelium after seven to 14 days [3]. The first EPC capture stent was implanted in Rotterdam during EuroPCR in 2003, and was subsequently awarded the Conformité Européenne (CE) mark in 2005. Since then, it has been commercially available in many countries in Europe and Asia, but not in the United States. Since 2010, the dual-helix stent platform of the EPC capture stent has been changed from stainless steel to cobalt chromium, with a reduced stent strut thickness of 0.0040 inches to 0.0032 inches [4].

Potential Advantages of the EPC Capture Stent in STEMI

There are several potential advantages in using the EPC capture stent in STEMI. First, stenting in PPCI occurs in a highly thrombotic milieu, and this poses the risk of delayed endothelial healing, especially with the use of DES [5]. The delay in endothelial healing leads to uncovered stent struts,

Manual of STEMI Interventions, First Edition. Edited by Sameer Mehta.
© 2017 John Wiley & Sons Ltd. Published 2017 by John Wiley & Sons Ltd.

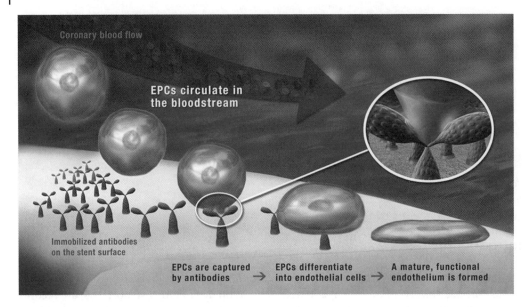

Figure 28.1 Genous™ endothelial progenitor cell capture (EPC) stent (reproduced with permission from OrbusNeich Wanchai, Hong Kong).

and these exposed struts serve as a nidus for stent thrombosis [6]. Several large, real-world registries have demonstrated that patients presenting with STEMI and undergoing PCI have an increased risk of both early and late stent thrombosis [7–10]. EPCs have been shown to contribute to endothelial cell regeneration and restoring the endothelium [11]. Consequently, the rapid restoration of a functional endothelium is proposed to minimize the risk of stent thrombosis and excessive neointimal proliferation [12]. The pro-healing property of the EPC capture stent restores vascular function, prevents platelet aggregation, and decreases thrombogenicity. In addition, it inhibits of smooth muscle cell migration and proliferation, thus preventing neointimal hyperplasia [13,14].These properties make the EPC capture stent an attractive choice in STEMI.

Second, EPCs are mobilized in large numbers from the bone marrow acutely during STEMI, and their numbers continue to increase and peak at day seven [15]. Other factors shown to increase circulating EPC count are PCI and administration of statins [16,17]. Implanting the EPC capture stent during primary PCI will optimally harness the increased levels of circulating EPC count and will improve endothelial healing.

Third, the rapid endothelialization properties of the EPC capture stent may be highly advantageous in the event of early discontinuation of dual antiplatelet therapy (DAPT). The operator is often especially challenged at the time of PPCI to fully ascertain the patient's suitability for prolonged DAPT [18]. Acquiring a detailed history of bleeding risks, assessment of drug compliance, and the need for urgent noncardiac surgery is usually not feasible during PPCI. Hence, EPC capture stents may prove to be safer in the event of short DAPT duration or early DAPT discontinuation [19].

EPC Capture Stent in STEMI

Table 28.1 shows a summary of published clinical studies evaluating the EPC capture stent in STEMI. The majority of the data come from small single-center registries with intermediate to long-term clinical follow-up.

Table 28.1 Published studies on endothelial progenitor cell capture stent in STEMI.

Study	Design	Patients (n)	Intended DAPT duration (months)	Primary outcome (%)	Follow-up (months)	Stent thrombosis (%)	TLR (%)	Late luminal loss (mm)	Binary re-stenosis (%)
Co et al. [20]	Single-center registry	120	1	MACE 5.8	6	1.7	2.5	–	–
Lee et al. [21]	Single-center registry	321	1	MACE 12.2	12	0.9	4.1	–	–
Chong et al. [22]	Single-center registry	95	1	MACE 13.7	24	1.1	4.2	–	–
Low et al. [27]	Single-center registry	95	1	MACE 16	34	0	10.5	0.87 ± 0.67	28
Kaul et al. [28]	Single-center case series	11	–	Angiography	8	0	10	0.97 ± 0.94	50
Santas-Alvarez et al. [23]	Single-center registry	139	12	Death 3.6	12	1.4	3.8	–	–
Scacciatella et al. [25]	Single-center registry	50	1	MACE 18	6	0	10	–	–
Pereira-da-Silva et al. [24]	Single-center registry	109	12	MACE 6.4	12	2.8	3.7	–	–
Bystron et al. [26]	Single-center RCT of Genous vs. CoCr stent	100[a]	1	MACE 24	6	6 (vs. 0)	14 (vs. 4)	0.98 ± 0.70 (vs.0.79 ± 0.47)	18 (vs. 12)

[a] 50 patients in each arm.
CoCr, chromium/cobalt; DAPT, dual antiplatelet therapy; MACE, major adverse cardiac events; RCT, randomized controlled trial.

Clinical Data

The National University Heart Centre, Singapore, was one of the first centers to evaluate EPC capture stent in PPCI. In the initial report by Co et al. [20], 120 STEMI patients without cardiogenic shock received 129 EPC capture stents with high procedural success (95%). Major adverse cardiac event (MACE) rates were 1.6% inpatient, and 5.8% at 6 months. Stent thrombosis rates were 1.7% at 6 months (1 acute, and 1 subacute). An extended cohort study by Lee et al. [21] of 321 patients followed up for 1 year demonstrated MACE rates of 12.2%, and low rates of stent thrombosis of 0.9%. Of note, there were no incidences of late stent thrombosis. This confirmed the feasibility of EPC capture stent implantation in PPCI. A 2-year follow up of 95 patients receiving EPC capture stents (compared with 53 patients receiving bioabsorbable polymer SES and 218 patients receiving BMS) demonstrated long-term safety with MACE rates of 13.7% and stent thrombosis rates of 1.1% [22]. Target lesion revascularization rates were 2.5% at 6 months, 4.1% at 1 year and 4.2% at 2 years across these three studies. These results were generally consistent with other registries [23–25]. Stent thrombosis rates were 0–2.8% up to 1 year follow-up, with the majority of thromboses occurring early. Target lesion revascularization (TLR) rates were generally less than 5% at 1 year across the registries, with the exception of that reported by Scacciatella et al. (10% at 6 months).

Dual Antiplatelet Therapy

The intended DAPT duration in our institution was 1 month. Despite this short duration, stent thrombosis rates were low with no late thromboses [20–22]. In contrast, in two other registries, DAPT was administered for up to 1 year [23,24]. From these registries with extended DAPT duration, only one patient suffered a late stent thrombosis at 7 months due to discontinuation of DAPT, with the few other patients experiencing early stent thrombosis either on DAPT or having discontinued DAPT. The only randomized controlled trial evaluated 100 patients from a single-center randomized to EPC capture stent or cobalt chromium stent during primary PCI [26]. DAPT was given for 1 month in both groups. At 6-month clinical follow-up, MACE and TLR rates were 24% compared with 10% ($P=0.06$), and 14% compared with 4% ($P=0.08$). In contrast to the safety data shown in the above registries, the rates of stent thrombosis were not insignificant at 6% (three cases: one early and two late) in the EPC capture stent group versus none in the cobalt chromium stent group.

Angiographic Follow-Up

Routine angiographic follow-up was limited to even fewer studies. In general, the EPC capture stent suffered from high late lumen loss comparable with BMS, and inferior to DES. Angiographic follow-up was performed on the first 95 consenting patients implanted with EPC capture stents during PPCI in our center at a mean follow-up of 245 days [27]. Quantitative coronary angiography analysis was performed by an independent core laboratory (Cardiovascular Research Foundation, NY). The angiographic in-stent late lumen loss was 0.87 ± 0.67 mm, with a binary restenosis rate of 28%; 50% of the patients with binary restenosis were symptomatic. The most common pattern of in-stent re-stenosis was diffuse re-stenosis (62%). MACE at 34 months was 16%, and TLR was 10.5%, likely driven by routine angiographic follow-up. In another small series of 10 patients (28), late lumen loss was 0.97 ± 0.94 mm at 8 months, and binary restenosis was 50%, leading to a clinical TLR of 10%. In the single randomized controlled trial evaluating EPC capture stent versus cobalt chromium stent [26], late lumen loss was 0.98 ± 0.70 mm, compared with 0.79 ± 0.47 mm at 6 months. These findings are consistent with other published data on the use of EPC capture stents in a variety of settings with late lumen loss of 0.63–1.14 mm [29–32], which are far inferior to the new-generation DES [33–35].

In summary, the EPC capture stent appeared to live up to its promise of low rates of stent thrombosis despite a short DAPT duration. However, initial hope that the rapid endothelialization may favor late lumen loss has not materialized in the clinical studies. In terms of clinical efficacy, the EPC capture stent does not offer any added advantage over BMS, even in the setting of PPCI.

The Combo Stent: A Combined DES and EPC Capture Stent

To capitalize on the theoretical benefit of promoting endothelialization with EPC capture technology, a combined approach using an antiproliferative drug to address the late lumen loss has been developed. The Combo™ Bioengineered SES (OrbusNeich) combines sirolimus elution from an abluminal biodegradable polymer matrix with covalently bound CD34 antibody layer designed for control of neointimal proliferation and promote accelerated stent endothelialization (Figure 28.2). The first randomized controlled trial in humans has been published, demonstrating non-inferiority of the Combo stent to the paclitaxel-eluting stent in a 9-month angiographic follow-up (late lumen loss of 0.39 ± 0.45 mm vs. 0.44 ± 0.56 mm) [36], no difference in MACE at 12 months, and no stent thrombosis in either group. The National University Heart Centre currently has a program evaluating Combo stent use in PPCI. The preliminary data have been presented at the EuroPCR 2015 conference. In the first 61 STEMI patients receiving Combo stent, the procedural success was 100%. There was one acute stent thrombosis (2.1%), with none up to 6 months. MACE at 6 months was 4.3%.

The REDUCE study [37] is a multicenter randomized controlled trial in 1500 patients with acute coronary syndrome receiving a Combo stent, randomized one to one to either short-term

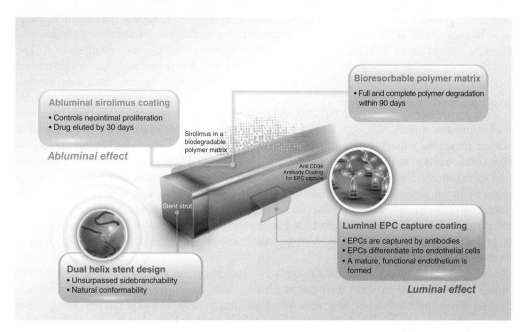

Figure 28.2 Combo™ bioengineered sirolimus-eluting stent (reproduced with permission from OrbusNeich, Wanchai, Hong Kong).

(3 months) or standard (12 months) DAPT. The HARMONEE study [38] is a joint Japan and United States multicenter stent study which aims to randomize close to 600 patients undergoing elective or urgent PCI to Combo stent versus EES, including an optical coherence tomography substudy. It is hoped that these studies will address the efficacy and safety of this novel combination stent.

Bioresorbable Vascular Scaffold

The use of the bioresorbable vascular scaffold (BVS) has gained increasing popularity among interventionists, with the technology being continually pushed beyond its current recommended indications. The BVS is designed to resorb naturally into the body, leaving no permanent scaffold. This method can overcome the general limitations of the metallic stents, such as permanent caging of the vessel with permanent impairment of coronary vasomotion, side-branch jailing, the impossibility of late lumen enlargement (positive remodeling), obscuring of non-invasive computed tomographic (CT) or magnetic resonance images, and preclusion of future surgical revascularization.

BVS works in three phases (revascularization, restoration and resorption) to deliver vascular reparative therapy and it may have the potential to treat patients with acute coronary syndrome. There are several reasons why BVS may be advantages in patients with STEMI. STEMI patients are frequently younger, have less extensive coronary atherosclerotic burden and may live many years after successful PPCI. They will thus derive the benefit of not having a permanent rigid metallic structure in their coronary arteries and will retain the option of future surgical revascularization. The second reason is that incomplete stent apposition, early or late, occurs commonly in the setting of PPCI. This is because operators may frequently undersize the stent because the vessels may appear "smaller" than they actually are. The vessel may "grow" when there is dissolution of jailed thrombus or plaque debris, or when vasoconstriction in the acute phase resolves. Incomplete stent apposition may not be recognized at the time of implantation but may be detected at follow-up, and could be a possible cause of late stent thrombosis [39]. The resorption of BVS after 2 years obviates the issue of late stent malapposition. The third reason is that, as BVS carries a larger stent strut width, it is postulated that less thrombus embolization may result from a different pattern of thrombus dislodgement and compression to the arterial wall. The percentage of vessel wall area covered by the BVS polymer (scaffold/vessel ratio) has been evaluated to be 26%, which is considerably higher than what was observed for conventional metallic DES (about 12%) [40]. This characteristic of BVS might be associated with an increased capacity of capturing debris and thrombotic material behind the struts before embolization to distal microcirculation. This so-called "snow-racket" concept (entrapment of thrombotic material between the stent and the vessel) is currently the basis for the design of novel devices, such as MGuard [41]. Finally, the physiological advantages of late lumen enlargement and vasomotion appear appealing to STEMI patients.

At present, there are two lactic acid-based devices which have received CE mark approval for use in Europe: the EES ABSORB (Abbott Vascular) and the novolimus-eluting DESolve stent (Elixir Medical Corporation).

There have been many institutional registry reports of the use of BVS ABSORB stent (Figure 28.3) in STEMI patients, the most prothrombotic condition among all forms of atherosclerosis. The culprit lesions in these patients almost universally have angiographic evidence of thrombus before and after PPCI. The consistent experience has been that the use of the biodegradable stent is feasible, safe and with high rate of final thrombolysis in myocardial infarction III flow and good scaffold apposition. One of the earliest series of feasibility report was from

Figure 28.3 ABSORB bioresorbable vascular scaffold (reproduced with permission from Abbot Vascular, Santa Clara, CA).

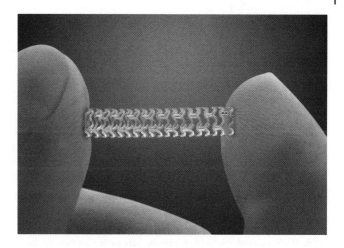

the National University Heart Centre, where we reported 11 patients who had BVS stents successfully implanted during PPCI with no major complications [42]. Wiebe et al. also reported low incidence of MACE at median follow up duration of 137 days for their series of 25 patients [43].

Kocka et al. reported a retrospective series of 41 STEMI patients who were treated with BVS and found that the device success rate was 98%, with a very low rate of strut malapposition seen on optical coherence tomography. Edge dissection was present in 38% of patients, but this was mostly small and clinically silent. In addition, the investigators showed that a strategy of significant scaffold oversizing in that setting results in excellent acute procedural results [44]. Diletti et al. also showed that strut malapposition (defined as greater than 5%) was observed in 22.6% of scaffolds compared with reported metallic balloon expandable stent malapposition rate of 37.1% in STEMI patients [45].

Randomized direct head-to-head comparison in establishing the true efficacy of BVS stent vis-à-vis metallic DES is still lacking, however. The ABSORB II trial comparing the ABSORB scaffold with metallic EES suggested that there is inferior acute luminal gain, post-procedural minimal lumen area on angiography and intravascular ultrasound with the BVS [46]. This was, however, in the context that the protocol did not recommend post-dilatation of the bioresorbable scaffold device. The conformability of the coronary anatomy is better for a bioresorbable scaffold than for a metallic stent. Onuma et al. further showed that there was no difference in acute recoil between bioresorbable scaffold and metallic EES on quantitative coronary angiography measurement [47]. A retrospective propensity-matching study of 290 patients who received BVS implantation during STEMI in six institutions was compared with the patient dataset from the EXAMINATION trial (which compared EES and BMS), and found no difference in device-oriented endpoints including cardiac death, target vessel myocardial infarction and target lesion revascularization between the BVS and EES or BMS at 30 days (3.1% vs. 2.4%, $P = 0.593$; vs. 2.8%, $P = 0.776$, respectively) and 1 year (4.1% vs. 4.1%, $P = 0.994$; vs. 5.9%, $P = 0.301$). Definite or probable scaffold BVS thrombosis rate was numerically higher at either 30 days (2.1% vs. 0.3%, $P = 0.059$; vs. 1.0%, $P = 0.324$, respectively) or at 1 year (2.4% vs. 1.4%, $P = 0.948$; vs. 1.7%, p=0.825, respectively), as compared with EES or BMS.

The observation of higher incidence of scaffold thrombosis is of concern, as it has been reported in registry and randomized controlled studies. Jaguszewski et al. reported a case of acute scaffold thrombosis from poor scaffold expansion in patient with ACS treated with ABSORB [48]. The GHOST-EU registry reported acceptable "real-world" outcomes of 1189 patients who received BVS with target lesion failure of only 4.4% at 6 months, but the rates of early and midterm scaffold thrombosis, mostly clustered within 30 days, were not negligible [49].The cumulative incidence of definite or probable scaffold thrombosis was 1.5% at 30 days and 2.1% at six months, with 16 of 23 cases occurring within 30 days. Even the ABSORB II trial had reported numerically higher number of scaffold thrombosis, albeit statistically insignificant. A new entity of very late scaffold thrombosis is also increasingly being recognized, for which the mechanism is not clearly known [50]. Incomplete tissue coverage, in-scaffold neoatherosclerosis, and scaffold disruption have all been purported to be the cause of such rare but clinically important occurrences. It seems prudent that long-term safety data may be needed prior to widespread clinical use of BVS.

The present iteration of ABSORB, with its thick strut of 150 μm and larger crossing profile requires special consideration to achieve optimal short- and long-term results. The need for a standardized approach for BVS use and optimal implantation techniques to blunt the rates of early and late scaffold failure was clearly spelt out in a consensus document by a group of high BVS operators [51]. Careful attention needs to be paid to patient and lesion selection, vessel sizing, scaffold selection, lesion preparation, scaffold implantation and optimization, and use of intravascular imaging. Treatment of a long lesion with overlapping stenting is of particular concern because of the relatively thick struts which may prolong the healing process [52]. Careful application of overlapping techniques to ensure less than 1 mm of overlap is recommended.

Conclusions

The benefit of BVS is quite intuitive. To have a stent that disappears after its useful function has been served, with the additional benefits of restoring normal vasomotor tone and increasing lumen caliber with positive vessel remodeling is attractive. While the short-term results are encouraging, most of the reported series of BVS in STEMI patients are small in sample size, with no head-to head comparison with the current standard of care. A longer-term study with a larger patient population will certainly be needed.

References

1 Windecker S, Kolh P, Alfonso F, et al. 2014 ESC/EACTS Guidelines on myocardial revascularization. *Eur Heart J*, 2014; 35: 2541–2619.

2 Hofma SH, Brouwer J, Velders MA, et al. Second-generation everolimus-eluting stents versus first-generation sirolimus-eluting stents in acute myocardial infarction. 1-year results of the randomized XAMI (XienceV Stent vs. Cypher Stent in Primary PCI for Acute Myocardial Infarction) trial. *J Am Coll Cardiol*, 2012; 60(5): 381–387.

3 Kutryk MJ, Kuliszewski MA. In vivo endothelial progenitor cell seeding for the accelerated endothelialization of endovascular devices. *Am J Cardiol*, 2003; 92: 94L–95L.

4 Sethi R, Lee CH. Endothelial progenitor cell capture stent: safety and effectiveness. *J Interv Cardiol*, 2012; 25: 493–500.

5 Nakazawa G, Finn AV, Joner M, et al. Delayed arterial healing and increased late stent thrombosis at culprit sites after drug-eluting stent placement for acute myocardial infarction patients: an autopsy study. *Circulation*, 2008; 118: 1138–1145.

6 Finn AV, Joner M, Nakazawa G, et al. Pathological correlates of late drug-eluting stent thrombosis: strut coverage as a marker of endothelialization. *Circulation*, 2007; 115: 2435–2441.

7 Loh JP, Pendyala LK, Kitabata H, et al. Comparison of outcomes after percutaneous coronary intervention among different coronary subsets (stable and unstable angina pectoris and ST-segment and non-ST-segment myocardial infarction). *Am J Cardiol*, 2014; 113:1794–1801.

8 de la Torre-Hernández JM, Alfonso F, Hernández F, et al. Drug-eluting stent thrombosis: Results from the multicenter Spanish registry ESTROFA (Estudio ESpañol sobre TROmbosis de stents FArmacoactivos). *J Am Coll Cardiol*, 2008; 51:986–990.

9 Iqbal J, Sumaya W, Tatman V, et al. Incidence and predictors of stent thrombosis: a single-centre study of 5,833 consecutive patients undergoing coronary artery stenting. *EuroIntervention*, 2013; 9: 62–69.

10 van Werkum JW, Heestermans AA, Zomer AC, et al. Predictors of coronary stent thrombosis: the Dutch Stent Thrombosis Registry. *J Am Coll Cardiol*, 2009; 53:1399–1409.

11 Asahara T, Murohara T, Sullivan A, et al. Isolation of putative progenitor endothelial cells for angiogenesis. *Science*, 1997; 275: 964–967.

12 Kipshidze N, Dangas G, Tsapenko M, et al. Role of the endothelium in modulating neointimal formation: vasculoprotective approaches to attenuate restenosis after percutaneous coronary interventions. *J Am Coll Cardiol*, 2004; 44: 733–739.

13 Roy-Chaudhury P. Endothelial progenitor cells, neointimal hyperplasia, and hemodialysis vascular access dysfunction: novel therapies for a recalcitrant clinical problem. *Circulation*, 2005; 112: 3–5.

14 Duckers HJ, Soullié T, den Heijer P, et al. Accelerated vascular repair following percutaneous coronary intervention by capture of endothelial progenitor cells promotes regression of neointimal growth at long term follow-up: final results of the Healing II trial using an endothelial progenitor cell capturing stent (Genous R stent). *EuroIntervention*, 2007; 3: 350–358.

15 Shintani S, Murohara T, Ikeda H, et al. Mobilization of endothelial progenitor cells in patients with acute myocardial infarction. *Circulation*, 2001; 103: 2776–2779.

16 Banerjee S, Brilakis E, Zhang S, et al. Endothelial progenitor cell mobilization after percutaneous coronary intervention. *Atherosclerosis*, 2006; 189: 70–75.

17 Ii M, Losordo DW. Statins and the endothelium. *Vascul Pharmacol*, 2007; 46: 1–9.

18 Latry P, Martin-Latry K, Lafitte M, et al. Dual antiplatelet therapy after myocardial infarction and percutaneous coronary intervention: analysis of patient adherence using a French health insurance reimbursement database. *EuroIntervention*, 2012; 7: 1413–1419.

19 Sangiorgi GM, Morice MC, Bramucci E, et al. Evaluating the safety of very short-term (10 days) dual antiplatelet therapy after Genous™ bio-engineered R stent™ implantation: the multicentre pilot Genous trial. *EuroIntervention* 2011; 7: 813–819.

20 Co M, Tay E, Lee CH, et al. Use of endothelial progenitor cell capture stent (Genous Bio-Engineered R Stent) during primary percutaneous coronary intervention in acute myocardial infarction: intermediate- to long-term clinical follow-up. *Am Heart J*, 2008; 155: 128–132.

21 Lee YP, Tay E, Lee CH, et al. Endothelial progenitor cell capture stent implantation in patients with ST-segment elevation acute myocardial infarction: one year follow-up. *EuroIntervention*, 2010; 5: 698–702.

22 Chong E, Poh KK, Liang S, et al. Two-year clinical registry follow-up of endothelial progenitor cell capture stent versus sirolimus-eluting bioabsorbable polymer-coated stent versus bare metal stents in patients undergoing primary percutaneous coronary intervention for ST elevation myocardial infarction. *J Interv Cardiol*, 2010; 23: 101–108.

23 Santas-Alvarez M, Lopez-Otero D, Cid-Alvarez AB, et al. Safety and efficacy of endothelial progenitor cell capture stent in ST-elevation acute myocardial infarction. GENIA Study. *Rev Esp Cardiol*, 2012; 65: 670–671.

24 Pereira-da-Silva T, Bernardes L, Cacela D, et al. Safety and effectiveness of the Genous™ endothelial progenitor cell-capture stent in the first year following ST-elevation acute myocardial infarction: A single center experience and review of the literature. *Cardiovasc Revasc Med*, 2013; 14: 338–342.

25 Scacciatella P, D'Amico M, Pennone M, et al. Effects of EPC capture stent and CD34+ mobilization in acute myocardial infarction. *Minerva Cardioangiol*, 2013; 61: 211–219.

26 Bystroň M, Cervinka P, Spaček R, et al. Randomized comparison of endothelial progenitor cells capture stent versus cobalt-chromium stent for treatment of ST-elevation myocardial infarction. Six-month clinical, angiographic, and IVUS follow-up. *Catheter Cardiovasc Interv*, 2010; 76: 627–631.

27 Low AF, Lee CH, Teo SG, et al. Effectiveness and safety of the genous endothelial progenitor cell-capture stent in acute ST-elevation myocardial infarction. *Am J Cardiol*, 2011; 108: 202–205.

28 Kaul U, Bhatia V, Ghose T, et al. Angiographic follow-up of genous bioengineered stent in acute myocardial infarction (GENAMI)-a pilot study. *Indian Heart J*, 2008; 60: 532–535.

29 Miglionico M, Patti G, D'Ambrosio A, et al. Percutaneous coronary intervention utilizing a new endothelial progenitor cells antibody-coated stent: a prospective single-center registry in high-risk patients. *Catheter Cardiovasc Interv*, 2008; 71: 600–604.

30 Aoki J, Serruys PW, van Beusekom H, et al. Endothelial progenitor cell capture by stents coated with antibody against CD34: the HEALING-FIM (Healthy Endothelial Accelerated Lining Inhibits Neointimal Growth-First In Man) Registry. *J Am Coll Cardiol*, 2005; 45: 1574–1579.

31 den Dekker WK, Houtgraaf JH, Onuma Y, et al. Final results of the HEALING IIB trial to evaluate a bio-engineered CD34 antibody coated stent (Genous™ Stent) designed to promote vascular healing by capture of circulating endothelial progenitor cells in CAD patients. *Atherosclerosis*, 2011; 219: 245–252.

32 Beijk MA, Klomp M, Verouden NJ, et al. Genous endothelial progenitor cell capturing stent vs. the Taxus Liberte stent in patients with de novo coronary lesions with a high-risk of coronary restenosis: a randomized, single-centre, pilot study. *Eur Heart J*, 2010; 31: 1055–1064.

33 Stone GW, Midei M, Newman W, et al. Comparison of an everolimus-eluting stent and a paclitaxel-eluting stent in patients with coronary artery disease. *JAMA*, 2008; 299: 1903–1913.

34 Windecker S, Serruys PW, Wandel S, et al. Biolimus-eluting stent with biodegradable polymer versus sirolimus-eluting stent with durable polymer for coronary revascularisation (LEADERS): a randomised non-inferiority trial. *Lancet*, 2008; 372: 1163–1173.

35 Meredith IT, Worthley S, Whitbourn R, et al. RESOLUTE Investigators. Clinical and angiographic results with the next-generation resolute stent system: a prospective, multicenter, first-in-human trial. *JACC Cardiovasc Interv*, 2009; 2: 977–985.

36 Haude M, Lee SW, Worthley SG, et al. The REMEDEE trial: a randomized comparison of a combination sirolimus-eluting endothelial progenitor cell capture stent with a paclitaxel-eluting stent. *JACC Cardiovasc Interv*, 2013; 6: 334–343.

37 Short-term Dual Anti Platelet Therapy in Patients With ACS Treated With the COMBO Dual-therapy Stent (REDUCE): NCT02118870. Available at https://clinicaltrials.gov/ct2/show/NCT02118870 (accessed March 26, 2017).

38 Japan–USA Harmonized Assessment by Randomized, Multi-Center Study of OrbusNEich's Combo StEnt (HARMONEE): NCT02073565. Available at https://clinicaltrials.gov/ct2/show/NCT02073565?term=NCT02073565&rank=1 (accessed March 26, 2017).

39 Hong MK, Mintz GS, Lee CW, et al. Impact of late drug-eluting stent malapposition on 3-year clinical events. *J Am Coll Cardiol*, 2007; 50: 1515–1516.

40 Muramatsu T, Onuma Y, Garcia-Garcia HM, et al. Incidence and short-term clinical outcomes of small side branch occlusion after implantation of an everolimus-eluting bioresorbable vascular scaffold: an interim report of 435 patients in the ABSORB-EXTEND single-arm trial in comparison with an everolimus-eluting metallic stent in the SPIRIT first and II trials. *JACC Cardiovasc Interv*, 2013; 6: 247–257.

41 Stone GW, Abizaid A, Silber S, et al. Prospective, randomized, multicenter evaluation of a polyethylene terephthalate micronet mesh-covered stent (MGuard) in ST-segment elevation myocardial infarction: the MASTER trial. *J Am Coll Cardiol*, 2012; 60: 1975–1984.

42 Kajiya T, Linag M, Sharma RK, et al. Everolimus-eluting bioresorbable vascular scaffold (BVS) implantation in patients with ST segment elevation myocardial infarction (STEMI). *EuroIntervention*, 2013; 9: 501–504.

43 Wiebe J, Möllmann H, Most A, et al. Short-term outcome of patients with ST-segment elevation myocardial infarction (STEMI) treated with an everolimus-eluting bioresorbable vascular scaffold. *Clin Res Cardiol*, 2014; 103: 141–148.

44 Kočka V, Malý M, Toušek P, et al. Bioresorbable vascular scaffolds in acute ST-segment elevation myocardial infarction: a prospective multicentre study 'Prague 19'. *Eur Heart J*, 2014; 35: 787–794.

45 Diletti R, Karanasos A, Muramatsu T, et al. Everolimus-eluting bioresorbable vascular scaffolds for treatment of patients presenting with ST-segment elevation myocardial infarction: BVS STEMI first study. *Eur Heart J*, 2014; 35: 777–786.

46 Serruys PW, Chevalier B, Dudek D, et al. A bioresorbable everolimus-eluting scaffold versus a metallic everolimus-eluting stent for ischaemic heart disease caused by de-novo native coronary artery lesions (ABSORB II): an interim 1-year analysis of clinical and procedural secondary outcomes from a randomised controlled trial. *Lancet*, 2015; 385: 43–54.

47 Onuma Y, Serruys PW, Gomez J, et al. Comparison of in vivo acute stent recoil between the bioresorbable everolimus-eluting coronary scaffolds (revision 1.0 and 1.1) and the metallic everolimus-eluting stent. *Catheter Cardiovasc Interv*, 2011; 78: 3–12.

48 Jaguszewski M, Wyss C, Alibegovic J, et al. Acute thrombosis of bioabsorbable scaffold in a patient with acute coronary syndrome. *Eur Heart J*, 2013; 34: 2046.

49 Capodanno D, Gori T, Nef H, et al. Percutaneous coronary intervention with everolimus-eluting bioresorbable vascular scaffolds in routine clinical practice: early and midterm outcomes from the European multicentre GHOST-EU registry. *EuroIntervention*, 2015; 10: 1144–1153.

50 Azzalini L, Al-Hawwas M, L'Allier PL. Very late bioresorbable vascular scaffold thrombosis: A new clinical entity. *EuroIntervention*, 2015; 11: e1–2.

51 Tamburino C, Latib A, van Geuns RJ, et al. Contemporary practice and technical aspects in coronary intervention with bioresorbable scaffolds: a European perspective. *EuroIntervention*, 2015; 11: 45–52.

52 Farooq V, Serruys PW, Heo JH, et al. Intracoronary optical coherence tomography and histology of overlapping everolimus-eluting bioresorbable vascular scaffolds in a porcine coronary artery model: the potential implications for clinical practice. *JACC Cardiovasc Interv*, 2013; 6: 523–532.

Index

Manual of STEMI Interventions, First Edition. Edited by Sameer Mehta.
© 2017 John Wiley & Sons Ltd. Published 2017 by John Wiley & Sons Ltd.